Breast Cancer: Advances in Molecular Imaging

Editors

GARY A. ULANER
AMY M. FOWLER

PET CLINICS

www.pet.theclinics.com

Consulting Editor
ABASS ALAVI

October 2023 • Volume 18 • Number 4

ELSEVIER

1600 John F. Kennedy Boulevard • Suite 1800 • Philadelphia, Pennsylvania, 19103-2899

http://www.pet.theclinics.com

PET CLINICS Volume 18, Number 4
October 2023 ISSN 1556-8598, ISBN-13: 978-0-443-18203-7

Editor: John Vassallo (j.vassallo@elsevier.com)
Developmental Editor: Varun Gopal

PET Clinics (ISSN 1556-8598) is published quarterly by Elsevier Inc., 360 Park Avenue South, New York, NY 10010-1710. Months of issue are January, April, July, and October. Periodicals postage paid at New York, NY, and additional mailing offices. Subscription prices per year are $275.00 (US individuals), $500.00 (US institutions), $100.00 (US students), $304.00 (Canadian individuals), $563.00 (Canadian institutions), $100.00 (Canadian students), $297.00 (foreign individuals), $563.00 (foreign institutions), and $140.00 (foreign students). To receive student and resident rate, orders must be accompanied by name of affiliated institution, date of term, and the signature of program/residency coordinator on institution letterhead. Orders will be billed at individual rate until proof of status is received. Foreign air speed delivery is included in all Clinics subscription prices. All prices are subject to change without notice. POSTMASTER: Send address changes to PET Clinics, Elsevier Health Sciences Division, Subscription Customer Service, 3251 Riverport Lane, Maryland Heights, MO 63043. **Customer Service: 1-800-654-2452 (U.S. and Canada); 314-447-8871 (outside U.S. and Canada). Fax: 314-447-8029. E-mail: journalscustomerservice-usa@elsevier.com (for print support); journalsonlinesupport-usa@elsevier.com (for online support).**

Reprints. For copies of 100 or more of articles in this publication, please contact the Commercial Reprints Department, Elsevier Inc., 360 Park Avenue South, New York, NY 10010-1710. Tel.: 212-633-3874; Fax: 212-633-3820; E-mail: reprints@elsevier.com.

PET Clinics is covered in MEDLINE/PubMed (Index Medicus).

Contributors

CONSULTING EDITOR

ABASS ALAVI, MD, MD (Hon), PhD (Hon), DSc (Hon)
Professor of Radiology and Neurology, Director of Research Education, Division of Nuclear Medicine, Department of Radiology, Hospital of the University of Pennsylvania, Perelman School of Medicine, University of Pennsylvania, Philadelphia, Pennsylvania, USA

EDITORS

GARY A. ULANER, MD, PhD, FACNM
James and Pamela Muzzy Endowed Chair in Molecular Imaging and Therapy, Hoag Family Cancer Institute, Irvine, California, USA; Molecular Imaging and Therapy, Hoag Family Cancer Institute, Newport Beach, California, USA; Department of Radiology, Department of Translational Genomics, University of Southern California, Los Angeles, California, USA

AMY M. FOWLER, MD, PhD, FSBI
Associate Professor, Section of Breast Imaging and Intervention, Department of Radiology, University of Wisconsin-Madison School of Medicine and Public Health, University of Wisconsin Carbone Cancer Center, Department of Medical Physics, University of Wisconsin-Madison, Madison, Wisconsin, USA

AUTHORS

BEATRIZ ELENA ADRADA, MD, FSBI
Professor, Department of Breast Imaging, The University of Texas MD Anderson Cancer Center, Houston, Texas, USA

SINA BAGHERI, MD
Postdoctoral Researcher, Department of Radiology, Breast Cancer Translational Research Group, Philadelphia, Pennsylvania, USA

KATHERINE CECIL, MD
Department of Radiology and Biomedical Imaging, University of California, San Francisco, San Francisco, California, USA

ASHRIT CHALLA
Undergraduate Researcher, Department of Radiology, Breast Cancer Translational Research Group, Hospital of the University of Pennsylvania, Philadelphia, Pennsylvania, USA

AMY S. CLARK, MD
Assistant Professor, Division of Hematology/Oncology, University of Pennsylvania, Philadelphia, Pennsylvania, USA

ELIZABETH H. DIBBLE, MD
Assistant professor, Department of Diagnostic Imaging, The Warren Alpert Medical School of Brown University/Rhode Island Hospital, Providence, Rhode Island, USA

MAXWELL DUCHARME, BS
Department of Radiology, The University of Alabama at Birmingham, Birmingham, Alabama, USA

AMY M. FOWLER, MD, PhD, FSBI
Associate Professor, Section of Breast Imaging and Intervention, Department of Radiology, University of Wisconsin-Madison School of Medicine and Public Health, University of

Wisconsin Carbone Cancer Center,
Department of Medical Physics, University of
Wisconsin-Madison, Madison, Wisconsin,
USA

ALISON R. GEGIOS, MD
Assistant Professor, Section of Breast Imaging
and Intervention, Department of Radiology,
University of Wisconsin-Madison School of
Medicine and Public Health, Madison,
Wisconsin, USA

DAVID GROHEUX, MD, PhD
Department of Nuclear Medicine, Saint-Louis
Hospital, University Paris-Diderot, INSERM
U976, HIPI, Paris, France; Centre d'Imagerie
Radio-isotopique, La Rochelle, France

LAURA HUPPERT, MD
Assistant Professor, Department of Medicine,
Helen Diller Family Comprehensive Cancer
Center, University of California, San Francisco,
San Francisco, California, USA

MAHSA KIANI, MD
Postdoctoral Researcher, Department of
Radiology, Breast Cancer Translational
Research Group, Hospital of the University of
Pennsylvania, Philadelphia, Pennsylvania, USA

SUZANNE E. LAPI, PhD
Departments of Radiology and Chemistry, The
University of Alabama at Birmingham,
Birmingham, Alabama, USA

COURTNEY LAWHN-HEATH, MD
Assistant Professor, Department of Radiology
and Biomedical Imaging, Helen Diller Family
Comprehensive Cancer Center, University of
California, San Francisco, San Francisco,
California, USA

HANNAH LINDEN, MD
Medical Oncology, University of Washington,
Seattle, Washington, USA

APARNA MAHAJAN, MD
Associate Professor, Department of Pathology
and Laboratory Medicine, University of
Wisconsin-Madison, Madison, Wisconsin,
USA

AMEER MANSUR, BS
Departments of Radiology and Biomedical
Engineering, The University of Alabama at
Birmingham, Birmingham, Alabama, USA

ELIZABETH S. McDONALD, MD, PhD, FSBI
Associate Professor of Radiology, Breast
Imaging Divisions, Department of Radiology,
Breast Cancer Translational Research Group,
Hospital of the University of Pennsylvania,
Philadelphia, Pennsylvania, USA

LINDA MOY, MD
Professor, Department of Radiology, NYU
Grossman School of Medicine, New York, New
York, USA

RITA MUKHTAR, MD
Helen Diller Family Comprehensive Cancer
Center, Department of Surgery, University of
California, San Francisco, San Francisco,
California, USA

SAIMA MUZAHIR, MD, FCPS, FRCPE
Assistant Professor of Radiology, Enterprise
Theranostic Lead, Division of Nuclear Medicine
and Molecular Imaging, Department of `
Radiology and Imaging Sciences, Emory
University Hospital, Atlanta, Georgia, USA

SOPHIA R. O'BRIEN, MD
Assistant Professor, Divisions of Molecular
Imaging and Therapy Breast Imaging,
Department of Radiology, Hospital of the
University of Pennsylvania, Philadelphia,
Pennsylvania, USA

AUSTIN R. PANTEL, MD, MSTR
Assistant Professor of Radiology, Division of
Nuclear Medicine Imaging and Therapy,
Department of Radiology, Hospital of the
University of Pennsylvania, Philadelphia,
Pennsylvania, USA

MIRAL M. PATEL, MD
Assistant Professor, Department of Breast
Imaging, The University of Texas MD
Anderson Cancer Center, Houston, Texas,
USA

MOLLY S. PETERSON, MD
Clinical Fellow, Section of Breast Imaging and
Intervention, Department of Radiology,
University of Wisconsin-Madison School of

Medicine and Public Health, Madison, Wisconsin, USA

KATJA PINKER, MD, PhD
Department of Radiology, Director of Breast MRI and Breast Imaging Service, Memorial Sloan Kettering Cancer Center, New York, New York, USA

GAIANE M. RAUCH, MD, PhD, FSBI, FSABI
Professor, Departments of Abdominal Imaging and Breast Imaging, The University of Texas MD Anderson Cancer Center, Houston, Texas, USA

VALERIA ROMEO, MD, PhD
Department of Advanced Biomedical Sciences, University of Naples Federico Naples, Italy

MADHUCHHANDA ROY, MBBS, PhD
Clinical Assistant Professor, Department of Pathology and Laboratory Medicine, University of Wisconsin-Madison, Madison, Wisconsin, USA

DAVID M. SCHUSTER, MD, FACR
Professor of Radiology and Imaging Sciences and Urology, GRA Distinguished Cancer Scientist, Director, Division of Nuclear Medicine and Molecular Imaging, Department of Radiology and Imaging Sciences, Emory University Hospital, Atlanta, Georgia, USA

LUKE SLIGH, BS
Department of Radiology, The University of Alabama at Birmingham, Birmingham, Alabama, USA

ANNA G. SORACE, PhD
Associate Professor, Departments of Radiology and Biomedical Engineering, The University of Alabama at Birmingham, Birmingham, Alabama, USA

GARY A. ULANER, MD, PhD, FACNM
James and Pamela Muzzy Endowed Chair in Molecular Imaging and Therapy, Hoag Family Cancer Institute, Irvine, California, USA; Molecular Imaging and Therapy, Hoag Family Cancer Institute, Newport Beach, California, USA; Department of Radiology, Department of Translational Genomics, University of Southern California, Los Angeles, California, USA

REBECCA WARD, MD
Diagnostic Radiology Resident, Department of Radiology, Hospital of the University of Pennsylvania, Philadelphia, Pennsylvania, USA

GRACE G. WU, BA
Medical Student Researcher, Department of Radiology, Breast Cancer Translational Research Group, Hospital of the University of Pennsylvania, Philadelphia, Pennsylvania, USA

Medicine and Public Health, Madison, Wisconsin, USA

KATJA PINKER, MD, PhD
Department of Radiology, Director of Breast MRI and Breast Imaging Service, Memorial Sloan Kettering Cancer Center, New York, New York, USA

GAIANE M. RAUCH, MD, PhD, FSBI, FSABI
Professor, Departments of Abdominal Imaging and Breast Imaging, The University of Texas MD Anderson Cancer Center, Houston, Texas, USA

VALERIA ROMEO, MD, PhD
Department of Advanced Biomedical Sciences, University of Naples Federico II, Naples, Italy

MADHUCHHANDA ROY, MBBS, PhD
Clinical Assistant Professor, Department of Pathology and Laboratory Medicine, University of Wisconsin-Madison, Madison, Wisconsin, USA

DAVID M. SCHUSTER, MD, FACR
Professor of Radiology and Imaging Sciences and Urology, GRA Distinguished Cancer Scientist, Director, Division of Nuclear Medicine and Molecular Imaging, Department of Radiology and Imaging Sciences, Emory University Hospital, Atlanta, Georgia, USA

LUKE SUGH, BS
Department of Radiology, The University of Alabama at Birmingham, Birmingham, Alabama, USA

ANNA G. SORACE, PhD
Associate Professor, Departments of Radiology and Biomedical Engineering, The University of Alabama at Birmingham, Birmingham, Alabama, USA

GARY A. ULANER, MD, PhD, FACNM
James and Pamela Muzzy Endowed Chair in Molecular Imaging and Therapy, Hoag Family Cancer Institute, Irvine, California, USA; Molecular Imaging and Therapy, Hoag Family Cancer Institute, Newport Beach, California, USA; Department of Radiology, Department of Translational Genomics, University of Southern California, Los Angeles, California, USA

REBECCA WARD, MD
Diagnostic Radiology Resident, Department of Radiology, Hospital of the University of Pennsylvania, Philadelphia, Pennsylvania, USA

GRACE G. WU, BA
Medical Student Researcher, Department of Radiology, Breast Cancer Translational Research Group, Hospital of the University of Pennsylvania, Philadelphia, Pennsylvania, USA

Contents

Human Epidermal Growth Factor Receptor 2/Human Epidermal Growth Factor Receptor 3 PET Imaging: Challenges and Opportunities

Maxwell Ducharme, Ameer Mansur, Luke Sligh, Gary A. Ulaner, Suzanne E. Lapi, and Anna G. Sorace

Human epidermal growth factor receptor 2 (HER2) and HER3 provide actionable targets for both therapy and imaging in breast cancer. Further, clinical trials have shown the prognostic impact of receptor status discordance in breast cancer. Intra- and intertumoral heterogeneity of both HER and hormone receptor expression contributes to inherent errors in tissue sampling, and single biopsies are incapable of identifying discordance in biomarker expression. Numerous PET radiopharmaceuticals have been developed to evaluate (or target for therapy) HER2 and HER3 expression. This review seeks to inform on challenges and opportunities in HER2 and HER3 PET imaging in both clinical and preclinical settings.

Other Novel PET Radiotracers for Breast Cancer

Sophia R. O'Brien, Rebecca Ward, Grace G. Wu, Sina Bagheri, Mahsa Kiani, Ashrit Challa, Gary A. Ulaner, Austin R. Pantel, and Elizabeth S. McDonald

Many novel PET radiotracers have demonstrated potential use in breast cancer. Although not currently approved for clinical use in the breast cancer population, these innovative imaging agents may one day play a role in the diagnosis, staging, management, and even treatment of breast cancer.

AI-Enhanced PET and MR Imaging for Patients with Breast Cancer

Valeria Romeo, Linda Moy, and Katja Pinker

New challenges are currently faced by clinical and surgical oncologists in the management of patients with breast cancer, mainly related to the need for molecular and prognostic data. Recent technological advances in diagnostic imaging and informatics have led to the introduction of functional imaging modalities, such as hybrid PET/MR imaging, and artificial intelligence (AI) software, aimed at the extraction of quantitative radiomics data, which may reflect tumor biology and behavior. In this article, the most recent applications of radiomics and AI to PET/MR imaging are described to address the new needs of clinical and surgical oncology.

PET CLINICS

PROGRAM OBJECTIVE

The goal of the *PET Clinics* is to keep practicing radiologists and radiology residents up to date with current clinical practice in positron emission tomography by providing timely articles reviewing the state of the art in patient care.

TARGET AUDIENCE

Practicing radiologists, radiology residents, and other health care professionals who provide patient care utilizing radiologic findings.

LEARNING OBJECTIVES

Upon completion of this activity, participants will be able to:
1. Review breast cancer screening, staging, treatment response evaluation, and problem-solving.
2. Discuss the various breast imagining modalities used to screen for breast cancer.
3. Recognize challenges and opportunities faced by clinical and surgical oncologists in the management of breast cancer patients.

ACCREDITATION

The Elsevier Office of Continuing Medical Education (EOCME) is accredited by the Accreditation Council for Continuing Medical Education (ACCME) to provide continuing medical education for physicians.

The EOCME designates this journal-based CME activity for a maximum of 10 *AMA PRA Category 1 Credit*(s)™. Physicians should claim only the credit commensurate with the extent of their participation in the activity.

All other health care professionals requesting continuing education credit for this enduring material will be issued a certificate of participation.

DISCLOSURE OF CONFLICTS OF INTEREST

The EOCME assesses conflict of interest with its instructors, faculty, planners, and other individuals who are in a position to control the content of CME activities. All relevant conflicts of interest that are identified are thoroughly vetted by EOCME for fair balance, scientific objectivity, and patient care recommendations. EOCME is committed to providing its learners with CME activities that promote improvements or quality in healthcare and not a specific proprietary business or a commercial interest.

The planning committee, staff, authors, and editors listed below have identified no financial relationships or relationships to products or devices they or their spouse/life partner have with commercial interest related to the content of this CME activity:

Beatriz Elena Adrada, MD, FSBI; Sina Bagheri, MD; Katherine Cecil, MD; Ashrit Challa; Amy S. Clark, MD; Elizabeth H. Dibble, MD; Maxwell Ducharme, PhD; Alison R. Gegios, MD; David Groheux, MD, PhD; Laura Huppert, MD; Mahsa Kiani, MD; Kothainayaki Kulanthaivelu, BCA, MBA; Suzanne E. Lapi, PhD; Courtney Lawhn-Heath, MD; Hannah Linden, MD; Michelle Littlejohn; Aparna Mahajan, MD; Ameer Mansur, BS; Elizabeth S. McDonald, MD, PhD, FSBI; Linda Moy, MD; Rita Mukhtar, MD; Saima Muzahir, MD, FCPS, FRCPE; Sophia R. O'Brien, MD; Austin R. Pantel, MD, MSTR; Miral M. Patel, MD; Molly S. Peterson, MD; Katja Pinker, MD, PhD; Valeria Romeo, MD, PhD; Madhuchhanda Roy, MBBS, PhD; David M. Schuster, MD, FACR; Luke Sligh, BS; Anna Sorace, PhD; Rebecca Ward, MD; Grace G. Wu, BA

The planning committee, staff, authors, and editors listed below have identified financial relationships or relationships to products or devices they or their spouse/life partner have with commercial interest related to the content of this CME activity:

Amy M. Fowler, MD, PhD: Advisor, Researcher: GE Healthcare

Gaiane M. Rauch, MD, PhD, FSBI, FSABI: Researcher: GE Healthcare

Gary A. Ulaner, MD, PhD, FACNM: Researcher, Consultant, and/or Speaker: Lantheus, GE Heathcare, Curium, POINT Biopharma, RayzeBio, BriaCell, and ImaginAb

UNAPPROVED/OFF-LABEL USE DISCLOSURE

The EOCME requires CME faculty to disclose to the participants:
1. When products or procedures being discussed are off-label, unlabelled, experimental, and/or investigational (not US Food and Drug Administration [FDA] approved); and
2. Any limitations on the information presented, such as data that are preliminary or that represent ongoing research, interim analyses, and/or unsupported opinions. Faculty may discuss information about pharmaceutical agents that is outside of FDA-approved labelling. This information is intended solely for CME and is not intended to promote off-label use of these medications. If you have any questions, contact the medical affairs department of the manufacturer for the most recent prescribing information.

TO ENROLL

To enroll in the *PET Clinics* Continuing Medical Education program, call customer service at 1-800-654-2452 or sign up online at http://www.theclinics.com/home/cme. The CME program is available to subscribers for an additional annual fee of USD 254.00

METHOD OF PARTICIPATION

In order to claim credit, participants must complete the following:
1. Complete enrolment as indicated above.
2. Read the activity.
3. Complete the CME Test and Evaluation. Participants must achieve a score of 70% on the test. All CME Tests and Evaluations must be completed online.

CME INQUIRIES/SPECIAL NEEDS

For all CME inquiries or special needs, please contact elsevierCME@elsevier.com.

Preface

Breast Cancer: Advances in Molecular Imaging

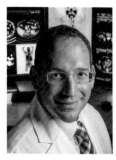 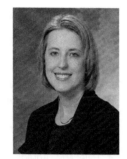

Gary A. Ulaner, MD, PhD   Amy M. Fowler, MD, PhD

Editors

Molecular imaging plays an essential clinical role for staging and for informing treatment decisions for patients with breast cancer. Since the previous *PET Clinics* issue published in 2018 on the uses and opportunities for molecular imaging in patients with breast cancer,[1] several advances have been achieved. We are excited to share these updates from the past 5 years in this new *PET Clinics* issue.

The articles in this issue are presented in a progressive manner from established approaches that are routinely used in clinic, toward newly approved radiopharmaceuticals and other novel tracers undergoing evaluation in clinical trials, and conclude with artificial intelligence methods to enhance imaging. The opening article by Roy and colleagues provides an important framework from the pathologist's perspective on how the various molecular and histologic subtypes of breast cancer may affect the appearance on various imaging modalities.[2] Next, the review by Gegios and colleagues highlights the recent advances in conventional, dedicated breast imaging techniques for screening and diagnosis of breast cancer and discusses the current limitations of these anatomic-based modalities.[3] The article by Patel and colleagues discusses dedicated breast imaging modalities based on functional imaging that can detect mammographically occult malignancy and may be a helpful alternative for patients who cannot obtain breast MR imaging.[4]

The next group of articles focuses on whole-body imaging for systemic staging and treatment response assessment. The article by Cecil and colleagues reviews the literature regarding the appropriate use of metabolic imaging with FDG-PET/computed tomography (CT) for patients with breast cancer and when it may outperform conventional imaging.[5] Next, the review by Groheux summarizes the utility of contrast-enhanced CT, bone scintigraphy, and FDG-PET/CT for systemic staging of breast cancer and discusses the advantages and limitations of these modalities.[6] This section concludes with an article by Muzahir and colleagues, which focuses on the diagnostic accuracy and clinical utility of molecular imaging compared with conventional imaging for the assessment of tumor response to therapy.[7]

The next thematic group of articles reviews radiopharmaceuticals beyond FDG for targeted molecular imaging of receptor-based and other biomarkers that play key roles in breast cancer tumor biology. The article by Ulaner and colleagues focuses on PET tracers targeting estrogen receptor and progesterone receptor, which are important determinants for endocrine therapy response.[8] The clinical applications for the recently approved agent for estrogen receptor PET imaging, ^{18}F-fluoroestradiol, are discussed. Human epidermal growth factor receptor (HER) is another key biomarker that is used for targeted

PET Clin 18 (2023) xiii–xiv
https://doi.org/10.1016/j.cpet.2023.05.003
1556-8598/23/© 2023 Published by Elsevier Inc.

therapy in HER2-amplified breast cancer. The review by Ducharme and colleagues focuses on the challenges and opportunities in HER2 and HER3 PET imaging in both clinical and preclinical settings.[9] There are many novel radiopharmaceuticals that are actively being investigated with potential clinical use in breast cancer. The article by O'Brien and colleagues highlights several of these agents that target amino acid metabolism, DNA damage repair proteins, tumor proliferation and hypoxia, cancer-associated fibroblasts, and the immune microenvironment.[10]

The exploration into how artificial intelligence and radiomics can enhance current molecular imaging techniques continues to progress. The final article in this issue by Romeo and colleagues delves into the most recent applications of artificial intelligence and radiomics to hybrid molecular imaging with PET/MR imaging for patients with breast cancer.[11]

We have greatly enjoyed editing this issue of *PET Clinics*. This issue provides a historical account of the role of molecular imaging for patients with breast cancer, the current standards of care in our field, and frames many of the unanswered questions that clinicians and researchers will be addressing for the future.

Gary A. Ulaner, MD, PhD
Molecular Imaging and Therapy
Hoag Family Cancer Institute
16105 Sand Canyon
Irvine, CA 92618, USA

Departments of Radiology and Translational Genomics
University of Southern California
Los Angeles, CA 90033, USA

Amy M. Fowler, MD, PhD
University of Wisconsin School of Medicine and Public Health
600 Highland Avenue
Madison, WI 53792-3252, USA

E-mail addresses:
gary.ulaner@hoag.org (G.A. Ulaner)
afowler@uwhealth.org (A.M. Fowler)

REFERENCES

1. McDonald ES, Ulaner GA. Uses and opportunities for molecular imaging in patients with breast cancer. PET Clin 2018;13(3):xi–xii.
2. Roy M, Fowler AM, Ulaner GA, Mahajan A. Molecular classification of breast cancer. PET Clin 2023; 18(4). [Epub ahead of print].
3. Gegios AR, Peterson MS, Fowler AM. Breast cancer screening and diagnosis: recent advances in imaging and current limitations. PET Clin 2023;18(4). [Epub ahead of print].
4. Patel MM, Adrada BE, Fowler AM, Rauch GM. Molecular breast imaging and positron emission mammography. PET Clin 2023;18(4). [Epub ahead of print].
5. Cecil K, Huppert L, Mukhtar R, et al. Metabolic positron emission tomography (PET) in breast cancer. PET Clin 2023;18(4). [Epub ahead of print].
6. Groheux D. Breast cancer systemic staging (comparison of CT, bone scan and FDG PET/CT). PET Clin 2023;18(4). [Epub ahead of print].
7. Muzahir S, Ulaner G, Schuster DM. Evaluation of treatment response in patients with breast cancer. PET Clin 2023;18(4). [Epub ahead of print].
8. Ulaner GA, Fowler AM, Clark AS, Linden H. Estrogen receptor (ER)- and progesterone receptor (PR)-targeted PET for patients with breast cancer. PET Clin 2023;18(4). [Epub ahead of print].
9. Ducharme M, Mansur A, Sligh L, Ulaner GA, Lapi SE, Sorace AG. HER2/HER3 PET imaging: challenges and opportunities. PET Clin 2023;18(4). [Epub ahead of print].
10. O'Brien SR, Ward R, Wu GG, et al. Other novel PET radiotracers for breast cancer. PET Clin 2023;18(4). [Epub ahead of print].
11. Romeo V, Moy L, Pinker K. AI-enhanced PET and MRI for patients with breast cancer. PET Clin 2023; 18(4). [Epub ahead of print].

Molecular Classification of Breast Cancer

Madhuchhanda Roy, MBBS, PhD[a],*, Amy M. Fowler, MD, PhD[b,c], Gary A. Ulaner, MD, PhD[d,e], Aparna Mahajan, MD[f]

KEYWORDS

- Breast cancer • Luminal breast carcinoma • HER2-positive breast carcinoma
- Triple-negative breast carcinoma • Basal-like breast carcinoma

KEY POINTS

- Breast carcinomas are a heterogenous group of tumors that have traditionally been classified based on tumor morphology, that is, histological type and grade.
- Recent advances in molecular pathology have facilitated the classification of breast carcinoma into four distinct types based on intrinsic gene expression profile: luminal A, luminal B, ERBB2/human epidermal growth factor receptor 2-enriched, and basal-like.
- The unique molecular pathology of breast cancers influences their appearance on imaging, including FDG and FES PET.
- Improved understanding of molecular pathogenesis of cancer has helped in identifying unique molecular targets for specific morphologic types of breast cancer.
- Although predicting outcome and response to therapy continues to be a challenge for individual patients with breast cancer, combining the traditional morphologic evaluation with the molecular profile have paved the path for expanding treatment outcomes and improved management.

INTRODUCTION

Breast cancer is the most common carcinoma in women worldwide. It encompasses a large and heterogeneous group of tumors. Based on morphologic appearance, most (80%–85%) invasive breast carcinomas (IBC) are traditionally classified as invasive ductal carcinoma of no special type (invasive ductal carcinoma [IDC]), followed by invasive lobular carcinoma (ILC, 5%–15%), and a very small percentage of tumors are classified as other special subtype carcinomas. Although all carcinomas arise within the terminal duct lobular unit, that is, share the same site of origin, the classification of IDC or ILC is based on the ability to form tubules or ducts and cellular cohesiveness. IBC are graded on their morphology by applying the Nottingham grading system with grade I tumors having an excellent prognosis when compared with survival rates for grade II and III tumors.[1–4] In addition to histologic classification and Nottingham grading, other important parameters include patient age, tumor size, hormone receptor, and human epidermal growth factor receptor 2 (HER2) status, Ki-67 proliferation index, presence of lymphovascular invasion, and lymph node status. These clinicopathologic parameters in conjunction with algorithms such as Nottingham Prognostic Index,

[a] Department of Pathology and Laboratory Medicine, University of Wisconsin - Madison, B1761 WIMR, 1111 Highland Avenue, Madison, WI 53705, USA; [b] Department of Radiology, Section of Breast Imaging and Intervention, University of Wisconsin – Madison, 600 Highland Avenue, Madison, WI 53792-3252, USA; [c] Department of Medical Physics, University of Wisconsin Carbone Cancer Center, University of Wisconsin-Madison, 600 Highland Avenue, Madison, WI 53792-3252, USA; [d] Hoag Family Cancer Institute, 16105 Sand Canyon Avenue, Ste 215, Irvine, CA 92618, USA; [e] Department of Radiology, Department of Translational Genomics, University of Southern California, Los Angeles, CA 90007, USA; [f] Department of Pathology and Laboratory Medicine, University of Wisconsin – Madison, B1781 WIMR, 1111 Highland Avenue, Madison, WI 53705, USA
* Corresponding author.
E-mail address: miroy@wisc.edu

PET Clin 18 (2023) 441–458
https://doi.org/10.1016/j.cpet.2023.04.002

Predict, or Adjuvant! Online are taken into consideration to discuss prognosis and adjuvant treatment decisions for individual patients.

Owing to the heterogeneous nature of IBC, grade-matched tumors may vary considerably with respect to their hormone and HER2 receptor status. In addition, despite significant differences based on morphology, the disease free and the overall survival between stage-matched IDC and ILC are comparable[5–7]; however, long-term follow-up studies provide data to support a worse prognosis in patients with lobular histology in the metastatic setting.[8,9] All these challenges along with the need to identify new prognostic and predictive factors and the revolution of molecular pathology over the last two decades have facilitated the development of molecular classification of IBC, and multigene assays to predict tumor behavior and guide therapeutic decisions with the goal of achieving more personalized treatment options. Here, the authors discuss the utility of molecular classification in expanding our knowledge of breast cancer and optimizing their clinical management.

Molecular Classification of Breast Cancer

Perou and colleagues[10] initially described the breast cancer "molecular portraits" in 2000. In this seminal study, the authors demonstrated that despite their phenotypic diversity, human breast cancers could be grouped into distinct categories based on intrinsic gene expression patterns, and subsequent extended analyses revealed five distinct subtypes of breast carcinoma: luminal A, luminal B, erythroblastic oncogene B (ERBB2), basal-like, and normal-breast-like.[11,12] In 2012, The Cancer Genome Atlas Network (TCGA) study analyzed a diverse set of breast tumors using six different technology platforms and further established that the diverse group of breast cancers phenotypically converge into four main breast cancer subtypes: luminal A, luminal B, ERBB2/HER2-enriched (HER2E), and basal-like.[13]

Tumor subtypes based on this classification system portray distinct clinicopathologic features and response to neoadjuvant chemotherapy (Table 1).[13,14] Luminal tumors are the most numerous and diverse with several multigene assays clinically approved to assist in predicting outcomes for patients receiving endocrine therapy and chemotherapy in high-risk patients (Figs. 1–4; Table 2).[15–25] The HER2E/amplified group (Fig. 5) is a great clinical success due to effective therapeutic targeting of HER2, and these continue to evolve to include HER2-low tumors.[25–27] Triple-negative/basal-like breast carcinomas (Fig. 6) are treated

with chemotherapy, and most recently have shown great response to immunotherapy.[28–32] Although molecular tests offer the potential to revolutionize patient management, their interpretation and application are complex and require significant expertise, which is still evolving. The practical and standardized approach is to classify IBC based on combined morphologic evaluation and immunohistochemical studies, which serve as a surrogate for molecular subtyping in routine practice, and is discussed below.

Luminal Subtype

The luminal tumors were named as such because of the high expression of genes normally expressed by luminal epithelium of the breast with a characteristic signature containing keratins 8 and 18. Luminal IBC is the most common subtype with the most diverse array of gene expression, mutation spectrum, copy number changes, and clinical outcomes.[15,18] These tumors demonstrate high mRNA and protein expression of the luminal expression signature ESR1, GATA3, FOXA1, XBP1, and MYB and high frequency of PIK3CA mutation.[33,34] In addition, TP53 mutation frequency is low in luminal A compared with luminal B cancers, and several other pathway-inactivating events, including ATM loss, MDM2 amplification, and cyclin D1 amplification, occur more frequently within luminal B cancers.[13]

Because of the high cost associated with commercially available multigene assays (see Table 2), surrogate markers by immunohistochemistry (IHC) are used to classify the luminal A and B subtypes. Initially, the surrogate IHC definition of luminal A tumors was estrogen receptor (ER)-positive and HER2-negative with a Ki-67 index of less than 14%, and the definition of luminal B tumors was ER-positive and HER2-negative with a Ki-67 index of greater than 14% or HER2-positive.[35] This was subsequently modified to classify luminal A tumors as ER-positive, HER2-negative with a Ki-67 index less than 14%, and progesterone receptor (PR) more than 20%.[36] Of note, not all luminal tumors can be accurately classified by these criteria in routine practice, and although Ki-67 index is used in the assessment of prognosis, the American Society of Clinical Oncology currently does not accept this as a routine prognostic marker in breast cancer due to lack of a standardized scoring method.[37–39]

Tubular carcinoma (TC), cribriform carcinoma, mucinous carcinoma (MC), grade 1 and 2 IDC, and grade 1 and 2 ILC usually fall under the luminal A subtype, whereas grade 2 or 3 IDC, grade 2 and 3 ILC, and invasive micropapillary carcinoma

Table 1
Clinicopathologic features based on molecular classification of breast cancer

	Luminal A (55%)	Luminal B (15%)	HER2-Enriched (15%–20%)	Basal-Like (10%)
Demographics	Marked increase in incidence with age	Younger patients, *BRCA2* mutation carriers	Younger patients	Younger patients, *BRCA1* mutation carriers
FDG-avidity	Low	Low-medium	High	High
Morphologic grade	Grade 1 and 2	Grade 2 and 3	Grade 3	Grade 3
Common IBC types	Tubular carcinoma, grade 1 and 2 ILC and IDC, mucinous carcinoma	Grade 2 and 3 ILC and IDC, micropapillary carcinoma	IDC grade 3	IDC grade 3, metaplastic carcinoma
Receptor expression	High ER+, High PR+, HER2–	Low ER+, low PR+, HER2+/–	ER–, PR–, HER2+	ER–, PR–, HER2–
Ki-67 index	Low	Intermediate	High	High
Prognosis	Good	Intermediate	Poor	Poor
Distant relapse	Low rate of recurrence after long-disease free interval	5 years for HER2– tumors; 5–7 years for HER2+ tumors	Peak recurrence 2 y	Peak recurrence 3–5 y
Most common site of relapse	Bone	Bone	Visceral organs	Visceral organs
Response to endocrine therapy	Good	Poor; may respond better to aromatase inhibitors than tamoxifen	No	No
Response to chemotherapy	pCR in 8%–10%	pCR in 20%	pCR in 30%–60%, superior with HER2-directed therapy	pCR in 30%–40%; superior with use of immunotherapy
Genetic alteration	*PIK3CA* mutation common, rare *TP53*	*TP53* mutation more common; *PIK3CA* mutation less common compared with luminal A	*TP53* and *PIK3CA* mutation	*TP53* mutation frequent, *PIK3CA* mutation less common
Oncotype DX/MammaPrint	Low risk	High risk	High risk	High risk

Abbreviations: EP, endoPredict; pCR, pathological complete response; qRT-PCR, quantitative reverse transcription polymerase chain reaction.

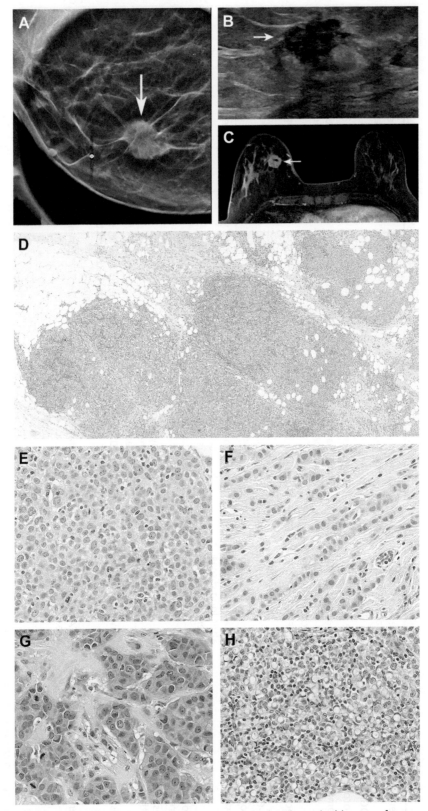

Fig. 1. Invasive lobular carcinoma. A 45-year-old woman presented with a palpable area of concern in the right breast. (*A*) Spot mediolateral oblique view from diagnostic mammogram demonstrates an irregular mass with

(IMPC) fall under the luminal B subtype. Luminal B is the most common subtype associated with *BRCA2* mutation.

HER2-Enriched Subtype

These tumors are characterized by expression of genes in the *ERBB2* or *HER2* amplicon at 17q12. DNA amplification of *HER2* was readily evident in these tumors in the TCGA study and the HER2E-mRNA-subtype also typically demonstrated high aneuploidy, the highest somatic mutation rate, and DNA amplification of other potential therapeutic targets including *FGFRs*, *EGFR*, *CDK4*, and *CCND1*.[13] Of note, HER2E subtype tumors defined by gene expression profile did not entirely overlap with HER2E tumors clinically defined by IHC and FISH assays. Only 50% of clinically defined HER2+ tumors fell into this HER2E-mRNA-subtype, and the remaining clinically HER2+ tumors were observed predominantly in the luminal mRNA subtypes.[13]

Basal-Like Subtype

The basal-like tumors were so named because they express genes expressed by the basal myoepithelial cells of the breast. Expression features of basal-like tumors include a characteristic signature containing keratins 5, 6, and 17 and high expression of genes associated with cellular proliferation. The basal-like subtype tumors are also often referred to as triple-negative breast cancers (TNBC) because most are typically negative for ER, PR, and HER2. However, only 75% of TNBC are basal-like with the remaining 25% composed of all other mRNA subtypes.[40] Basal-like tumors demonstrate a high frequency of *TP53* mutation, loss of *RB1*, *BRCA1* inactivation, *PIK3CA* mutation, *ATM* mutation, high *MYC* activation, and *cyclin E1* amplification.[13,41,42] These tumors are seen with an increased incidence in patients with germline *BRCA1* mutations[12,43] and in patients of African ancestry.[42,44]

Although most basal-type carcinomas are aggressive and triple negative, they have a wide morphologic spectrum, and it is the grade of the tumor that determines prognosis in this subtype. Of note, TNBCs that express androgen receptor (AR), are not considered basal-type carcinoma, and are best classified as luminal AR subtype.[45] TNBCs have a gene expression profile similar to basal-like breast cancers and also express high levels of epithelial-to-mesenchymal transition markers and low levels of the epithelial tight junction proteins claudin-3, -4, and -7[46–49]; hence their designation as claudin-low tumors. These tumors also express cancer stem cell markers and immune response genes and show low to absent expression of E-cadherin protein but are nevertheless morphologically distinct from lobular carcinomas.[48,49] Finally, salivary gland type tumors are another type of TNBC; however, these are rare and have a favorable prognosis except in higher grade examples.[50–53]

There are noticeable effects of molecular subtypes on PET imaging of breast cancer. Luminal subtype breast carcinomas tend to have lower 18F-Fluorodeoxyglucose (FDG)-avidity than HER2E and basal-like subtypes,[54,55] although there are no standardized uptake value (SUV) cut-offs that reliably distinguish them. Propensity for sites of distant metastases also varies by subtype, with luminal subtypes demonstrating a greater propensity for osseous metastases, whereas basal-like subtypes are more likely to metastasize to visceral organs. There are specific PET radiotracers which target ER[56,57] and HER2,[58,59] which are also reviewed in separate articles in this issue (see *Estrogen Receptor (ER)- and Progesterone Receptor (PR)-targeted PET for Patients with Breast Cancer* and *HER2/HER3 PET Imaging: Challenges and Opportunities*).

Special Histologic Subtypes

Several special histologic subtypes of breast cancer are associated with a distinct histologic appearance and clinical behavior. A few of these special-type tumors have been associated with characteristic genetic changes; however, there is also considerable genetic heterogeneity within many special-type cancers despite their distinct morphology. Some of these special histologic subtypes are discussed below.

Invasive lobular carcinoma

ILC is composed of dyshesive cells that are most often individually dispersed or arranged in a single-

---

spiculated margins at 4 o'clock (*arrow*). (*B*) Ultrasound demonstrates a corresponding irregular heterogeneous mass with angular margins (*arrow*). Core needle biopsy demonstrated invasive lobular carcinoma, grade 3 (positive for ER, positive for PR, negative for HER2 overexpression by IHC, Ki-67 index of 60%). (*C*) Preoperative breast MR imaging demonstrated an irregular mass with irregular margins and heterogeneous internal enhancement. (*D–G*) Surgical specimen demonstrated non-cohesive tumor cells predominantly growing in solid pattern (*D*: H&E, original magnification × 4 and *E*: H&E, original magnification × 20), and cells arranged in linear cords invading the stroma (*F*: H&E, original magnification × 20). Note pleomorphic (*G*: H&E, original magnification × 20) and signet ring cell morphology (*H*: H&E, original magnification × 20).

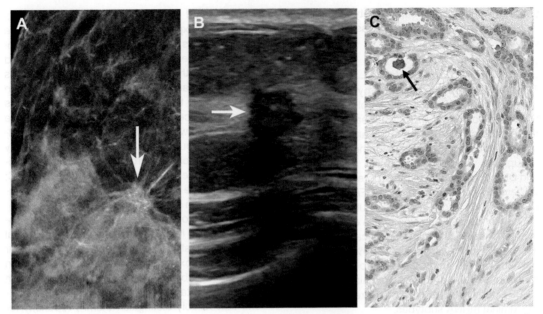

Fig. 2. Tubular carcinoma. A 50-year-old woman presented for routine screening mammography. (*A*) Spot medio-lateral oblique view from subsequent diagnostic mammogram demonstrates an irregular mass with spiculated margins and associated calcifications (*arrow*) in the right breast at 12 o'clock posterior depth. (*B*) Ultrasound demonstrates a corresponding irregular hypoechoic mass with spiculated margins and posterior acoustic shadowing (*arrow*). Core needle biopsy demonstrated invasive ductal carcinoma, grade 1 (positive for ER, positive for PR, negative for HER2 overexpression by IHC, Ki-67 index of 5%). The mass was localized under ultrasound guidance. (*C*) Surgical specimen demonstrated tubular carcinoma, characterized by a haphazard distribution of rounded and angulated tubules with open lumina, lined by a single layer of epithelial cells separated by abundant reactive, fibroblastic stroma and microcalcifications (*arrow*, H&E, original magnification × 20).

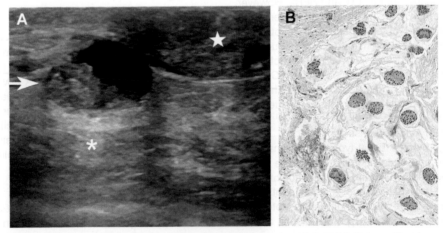

Fig. 3. Mucinous carcinoma. A 88-year-old woman presenting for short-interval follow-up imaging recommended from an outside institution for a probably benign complicated cyst. (*A*) Ultrasound demonstrates a 12 mm complex cystic and solid mass (*arrow*) with circumscribed margins and posterior acoustic enhancement (*) in the right breast 7 o'clock adjacent to the nipple (*star*). The mass did not contain internal vascularity on color flow Doppler images (not shown). Diagnostic mammography (not shown) showed heterogeneously dense breast tissue without a mammographic correlate for the mass on ultrasound. Ultrasound-guided core needle biopsy demonstrated invasive carcinoma with mucinous features, grade 2 (positive for ER, positive for PR, negative for HER2 overexpression by IHC, Ki-67 index of 5%) and focal intermediate grade ductal carcinoma in situ. (*B*) Surgical specimen demonstrated mucinous carcinoma characterized by hypocellular and sparse clusters of tumor cells in large pools of extracellular mucin (H&E, original magnification × 10).

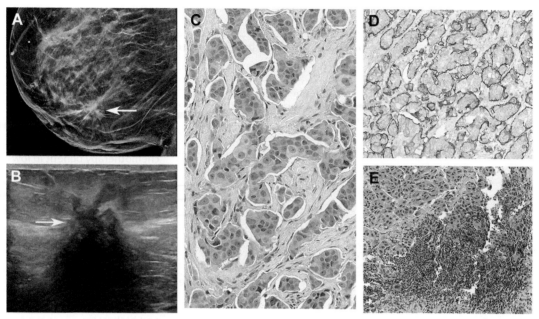

Fig. 4. Invasive micropapillary carcinoma. A 63-year-old woman presented with a palpable area of concern in the right breast. (*A*) Mediolateral view from the diagnostic mammogram demonstrates an irregular mass with spiculated margins (*arrow*) in the right breast at 4 o'clock middle depth with associated nipple retraction. (*B*) Ultrasound demonstrates a corresponding irregular hypoechoic mass with indistinct margins and marked posterior acoustic shadowing (*arrow*). (*C–E*) Ultrasound-guided core needle biopsy demonstrated invasive mammary carcinoma with micropapillary features, grade 2 (positive for ER, positive for PR, equivocal for HER2 overexpression by IHC [score 2+], and negative for *HER2 gene* amplification by in situ hybridization, Ki-67 index of 20%). (*C, D*) Note clusters of tumor cells within empty spaces with inside-out polarity (H&E, original magnification × 20), accentuated by epithelial membrane antigen (EMA) IHC along the periphery facing the stroma (IHC, original magnification × 10), and (*E*) lymph node metastasis (H&E, original magnification × 10). Surgical specimen demonstrated invasive micropapillary carcinoma with extensive axillary lymph node metastasis.

file linear pattern often with minimal to no stromal reaction. Other patterns seen are trabecular, alveolar, and solid (see **Fig. 1**). Classic ILC demonstrates low-to intermediate nuclear grade morphology and a low mitotic count (Nottingham grade 1 or 2, majority being grade 2). Pleomorphic ILC demonstrates intermediate-high or high nuclear grade and marked pleomorphism (Nottingham grade 2 or 3). Signet ring cell features may be present intermixed with these other morphologic patterns. Nottingham grade is an independent predictor of patient outcome in ILC, and of the three components of tumor grading, a high mitotic count is associated with a worse prognosis.[3] Most patients present with a poorly defined palpable breast mass. ILC demonstrates propensity for metastases to the bone, skin, gastrointestinal tract, gynecologic tract, meninges, and serosa.[8,60,61]

Radiologically, the most common mammographic findings are a spiculated mass or an architectural distortion; some cases being clinically and radiologically occult (attributed to the lack of a stromal reaction and therefore, a lack of disruption to the background breast architecture), presenting

with metastases.[62–64] Mammography has a lower sensitivity for the detection of ILC when compared with IDC. Although the addition of ultrasonography improves sensitivity, MR imaging is superior for the detection of multifocal disease and extent of disease.[65–70] Contrast-enhanced spectral mammography is a promising emerging imaging modality for detection of ILC, although data are limited.[70]

The most notable deleterious germline mutations seen in ILC involve *CDH1*, the gene encoding the E-cadherin protein.[71] ILC also displays somatic genetic alterations including gains of 1q and 16p and losses of 16q, which includes the *CDH1* gene locus on 16q22.1 as well as mutations of PIK3CA[72]. The loss of function of E-cadherin results in the characteristic lack of cohesiveness and the invasive pattern of ILC, and in a minority of cases lacking *CDH1* mutations, alterations affecting α-catenin, and other components of the cadherin-catenin family have been reported.[73] Most of classic ILC is classified as luminal A subtype and expresses ER and PR and lacks *HER2* gene amplification/HER2 overexpression.[72] Pleomorphic ILC may lack hormone receptors and

Table 2
Commercially available multigene assays for prognostic/predictive assessment of early-stage ER-positive invasive breast carcinoma on formalin-fixed paraffin-embedded tissue sections

Assay/Company	Assay Type	Indication	Prognostic/Predictive Value
Oncotype DX, Genomic Health	qRT-PCR, 21 gene recurrence score (RS)	ER +, HER2– 0–3 node positive	Prognostic for distant recurrence in 10 years treated with adjuvant tamoxifen Predictive for chemotherapy in high-RS group; no chemotherapy benefit in low-RS group Determination of chemotherapy benefit depends on patients age ($\leq$50 or >50 y, and the RS continuous variable (0–100)
PAM 50/Prosigna, NanoString Technologies[a]	qRT-PCR, 50 gene signature	ER + , HER2– Tumor size 0–3 node positive	Prognostic for distant recurrence based on four intrinsic molecular subtypes Node negative: three risk categories, low, intermediate, and high Node positive: two risk categories, low and high Patients with low-risk scores may not benefit from chemotherapy
Mammaprint, Agendia Inc[a]	Microarray, 70 gene signature	ER + , HER2– 0–3 node positive	Prognostic for early distant recurrence within 5 years of diagnosis Good and poor prognosis group; predictive of chemotherapy benefit in poor prognosis group
EndoPredict (EP) and EndoPredict Clinical (EPclin) Risk Score Myriad Genetics, Inc	qRT-PCR, 12 gene score	ER+, HER2– Tumor size 0–3 node positive	Prognostic for distant recurrence in 5–10 years treated with endocrine therapy
Breast Cancer Index Biotheranostics, Inc	qRT-PCR, 2 gene HOXB13:IL17BR and 5 gene molecular grade index	ER+, HER2– Node-negative	Prognostic in ER + tumors Predictive for tamoxifen response in low-risk groups

[a] Assay was developed to also include ER-negative tumors; however, there are insufficient evidence to recommend use in this patient population per the 2022 ASCO guidelines.
Abbreviations: EP, endoPredict; pCR, pathological complete response; qRT-PCR, quantitative reverse transcription polymerase chain reaction.

overexpress HER2 or be of luminal AR subtype.[74,75] Following neoadjuvant chemotherapy, rates of pathological complete response are typically lower than for IDC, which may be attributed to the molecular characteristics and lower proliferation index of ILC rather than the histological pattern itself.[76,77]

The unique pathology of ILC results in important imaging characteristics. Primary ILC is more difficult to detect than IDC by mammography, breast ultrasound, breast MRI, and FDG PET.[68,78] Metastases from ILC likewise demonstrate lower FDG-avidity.[79,80] The molecular phenotype of ILC may make this histologic subtype of breast cancer amenable to imaging with PET radiotracers for other metabolic pathways or targets. PET agents targeting amino acid metabolism may better visualize ILC compared with FDG PET.[81,82] As nearly all ILCs are ER-positive, ER-targeted imaging agents have been used with success.[83] Fibroblast-activating protein

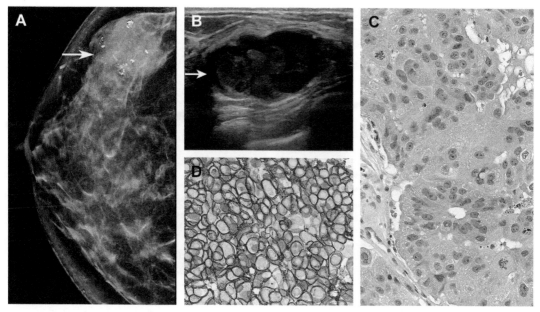

Fig. 5. Invasive ductal carcinoma, Nottingham grade 3, HER2-enriched. A 51-year-old woman presented for routine screening mammography. (*A*) Spot craniocaudal view from subsequent diagnostic mammogram demonstrates an irregular mass with obscured margins and associated calcifications (*arrow*) in the right breast at 10 o'clock posterior depth. (*B*) Ultrasound demonstrates a corresponding complex cystic and solid mass with posterior acoustic enhancement (*arrow*). (*C*) Core needle biopsy demonstrated invasive ductal carcinoma, grade 3, with apocrine features (H&E, original magnification × 20), negative for ER, negative for PR, and (*D*) positive for HER2 overexpression by IHC (score 3+), Ki67 index of 40%. The patient is undergoing neoadjuvant HER2-directed therapy.

agents have been used in a pilot trial.[84] Given the difficulty imaging ILC with most current imaging methods, trials of novel PET radiotracers are likely to continue (**Fig. 7**).

Tubular carcinoma
TC is a low-grade IBC composed of well-formed tubules with open lumina lined by a single layer of neoplastic cells in greater than 90% of the tumor (see **Fig. 2**). These account for about 1.6% of all IBC and are more likely to occur in older patients and tend to be small in size.[85] Most TCs are detected incidentally by mammographic screening as a small spiculated mass, architectural distortion, or focal asymmetry, with calcifications variably present.[85–87] On ultrasonography, TC usually appears as a hypoechoic mass with poorly defined margins and posterior acoustic shadowing.[87]

Based on gene expression profiling studies, TC belongs to the luminal A subtype and is diffusely and strongly ER-positive and PR-positive and HER2-negative with a low Ki-67 index (typically less than 10%).[88] The most frequent alterations detected in TC include concurrent loss of 16q and gain of 1q.[89] The prognosis of TC is better than that of grade I IDC, and long-term outcome is similar to that of age-matched women without

IBC.[85,90,91] Despite small size, clinically occult axillary lymph node metastasis can occur, rarely involving more than one lymph node.[92] Based on available clinical data, adjuvant systemic therapy or axillary dissection may not be indicated in patients with TC given its excellent prognosis.[90]

Mucinous carcinoma
MC is an IBC characterized by clusters of epithelial tumor cells suspended in pools of abundant extracellular mucin (see **Fig. 3**). Pure MC is characterized by a greater than 90% component of mucin with tumor cells of low to intermediate nuclear grade. MC accounts for approximately 2% of all breast carcinomas with a median patient age of 71 years.[93,94] Mixed MCs are classified with a mucin component of 10% to 90%, and tumors with a mucinous component of less than 10% or tumors with high nuclear grade are best classified as IBC with focal mucin production. On mammography, MC may mimic a benign process.[95] On ultrasound, most tumors are hypoechoic, and MR imaging reveals a persistent enhancement pattern and hyperintensity on T2-weighted images.[96]

Pure MC belongs to the luminal A subtype and is positive for ER and PR and lacks HER2 overexpression. MC is transcriptionally different from

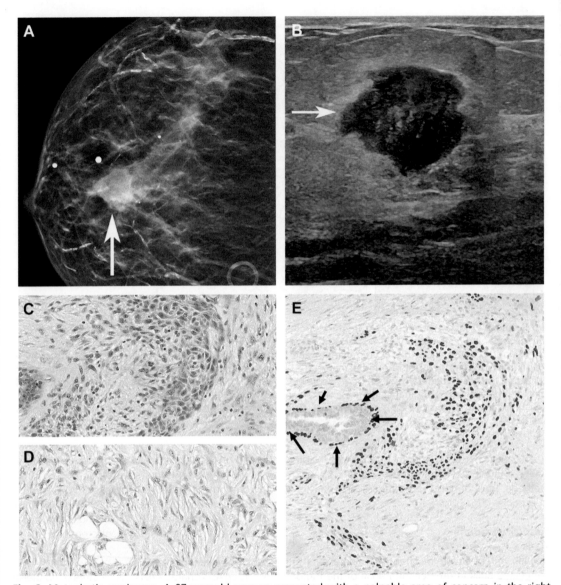

Fig. 6. Metaplastic carcinoma. A 97-year-old woman presented with a palpable area of concern in the right breast. (*A*) Craniocaudal mammographic view of the right breast demonstrates an irregular mass with indistinct margins (*arrow*) at 12 o'clock which corresponds with the palpable area of concern. (*B*) Ultrasound demonstrates a corresponding irregular hypoechoic mass with microlobulated margins (*arrow*). Core needle biopsy demonstrated metaplastic carcinoma (TNBC, Ki67 index of 10%). (*C–E*) Surgical specimen demonstrated a biphasic metaplastic carcinoma of squamous (*C*) and spindle cell (*D*) components (H&E, original magnification × 20), both components are immunoreactive for p63 as are basal myoepithelial cells of entrapped normal breast epithelium (*arrows*).

grade- and molecular subtype-matched IDC and demonstrates lower genetic instability, lower frequency of concurrent 1p gains and 16q losses, lower frequency of somatic mutations of *PIK3CA* and *AKT1* and exhibits aberrant DNA methylation of *MUC2*.[97–100] Of note, mammary MC lacks microsatellite instability, which is a common feature of colorectal, endometrial, and ovarian MC.[101] In mixed MC, the different morphological components are clonal with genomic profiles similar to those of pure MC.[97,99] Pure MC is generally associated with low rates of local and distant recurrence and has excellent 5-year disease-free survival.[93]

Invasive micropapillary carcinoma

Pure IMPCs are rare, accounting for less than 2% of all IBC; however, a micropapillary component intermixed with IBC in mixed forms are more

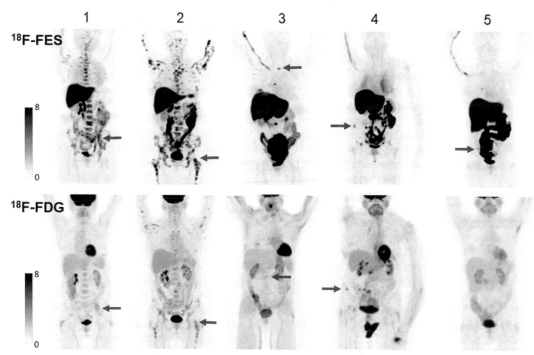

Fig. 7. Comparison of FES PET and FDG PET. Comparison of FES PET and FDG PET in five patients with metastatic ILC. Maximum intensity projection (MIP) images from 18F FES PET scans (top row) and 18F FDG PET scans (bottom row) from five patients are shown. FES PET detected more metastatic lesions (*arrows*) and greater avidity than FDG PET in these patients. In patient 5, active disease was only seen on FES PET, no active disease was seen on FDG PET. (This research was originally published in JNM. Ulaner GA, Jhaveri K, Chandarlapaty S, et al. Head-to-Head Evaluation of 18F-FES and 18F-FDG PET/CT in Metastatic Invasive Lobular Breast Cancer. J Nucl Med. 2021;62(3):326-331. © SNMMI.)

frequent.[102–104] IMPCs have a high propensity for extensive peritumoral lymphovascular invasion and axillary lymph node metastases, the latter of which is present in more than two-thirds of patients at diagnosis (see **Fig. 4**).[103,104] Of note, similar morphology may also be seen in the carcinomas of the lung, bladder, and ovary, and it is important to keep the possibilities of metastases from these sites in mind in the appropriate clinical context.

IMPC usually presents as a palpable mass with imaging features highly suggestive of malignancy.[105] On mammography, the tumor appears as a dense, irregular mass with indistinct margins with or without calcifications; on ultrasound, IMPC appears as a hypoechoic mass, and on MR imaging, the tumor usually appears as an irregular spiculated mass with washout patterns and may be multifocal.[105–107] FDG PET-CT exhibits a high maximum SUV.[106]

IMPC belongs to luminal A or B subtype.[88] Array comparative genomic hybridization analysis has demonstrated recurrent gains of 8q, 17q, and 20q; copy-number alterations different from grade- and ER-matched IBC; *MYC, CCND1,* and

FGFR1 amplifications may also be present.[108,109] The non-micropapillary component of mixed micropapillary IBC harbors genetic alterations similar to those found in the micropapillary areas.[110] In addition, the spectrum of mutations observed in IMPC is similar to those found in other luminal B subtype IBC with recurrent mutations in *PIK3CA, TP53, GATA3,* and *MAP2K4.*[111,112] In keeping with its luminal subtype, most IMPCs are ER-positive and PR-positive; HER2 overexpression and amplification are reported in a variable proportion of cases.[109,110] Although IMPC is associated with advanced locoregional disease, the micropapillary histological type is not an independent variable for disease recurrence or overall survival when compared with age and stage-matched IBC.[102,113,114] Patients with ER-negative disease or those with four or more positive lymph nodes have a worse prognosis.[104]

Metaplastic carcinoma
Metaplastic carcinoma (MBC) is a heterogeneous group of IBC characterized by differentiation of the neoplastic epithelium toward squamous cells and/or mesenchymal elements. MBC may be

monophasic with only one metaplastic component, biphasic with two or more metaplastic components, or mixed with a component of IBC. MBC accounts for 0.2% to 1% of all IBC.[115,116] The clinical features of MBC are similar to those of ER-negative IBC; however, these are more likely to present at an advanced stage.[116] Most patients present with a palpable mass. A mass lesion is detected on ultrasonography, mammography, and MR imaging; calcifications are uncommon.[117]

Although MBC is a heterogeneous group of tumors with marked intertumoral and intratumoral heterogeneity, molecular studies support a monoclonal origin.[118–120] Some authors postulate a late-step tumor dedifferentiation rather than origin from basal-like stem cells.[121] The most frequent mutations in MBC include TP53 and PIK3CA, PTEN, and overexpression and mutations of EGFR.[122,123]

MBC is classified as basal-like or claudin-low subtype using the intrinsic gene classification.[13,46,47,124] The vast majority are TNBC and express high-molecular-weight cytokeratins (CK5/6 and CK14), p63, and EGFR.[122,125]

Specific subtypes of MBC are associated with distinct outcomes; fibromatosis-like MBC and low-grade adenosquamous carcinoma are indolent variants, whereas high-grade spindle cell, squamous cell, and high-grade adenosquamous carcinomas are associated with the worst prognosis, matrix-producing carcinomas have an intermediate prognosis.[126–132] Overall, MBC has lower response rates to conventional chemotherapy and a worse clinical outcome after traditional chemotherapy than other forms of TNBC. Recent trials with immunotherapy have shown promising results.[28–32]

Rare salivary gland-type tumors

Normal breast and salivary glands share similar histologic architecture consisting of luminal epithelial cells and outer myoepithelial cells. They also share a similar immunoprofile including expression of low molecular weight cytokeratins, ER, PR, and AR. Given these similarities, it is no surprise that the breast can also develop the entire range of tumor types encountered in the salivary glands. Although these salivary gland-type breast tumors share the morphological features and often the translocation-based molecular alterations found in their salivary gland counterparts, their clinical behavior varies.[52] Despite being triple-negative subtype, these represent tumors with low or intermediate aggressive behavior as compared with conventional triple-negative IBC and even relative to similar tumors occurring in the salivary glands. Therefore, knowledge of their site-specific behavior in the breast is important for the avoidance of over-treatment of these rare tumors.

Adenoid cystic carcinoma

Adenoid cystic carcinoma (AdCC) is a salivary gland type IBC composed of neoplastic epithelial and myoepithelial cells in tubular, cribriform, and solid patterns containing basophilic matrix and reduplicated basement membrane material. Based on architectural and cytological features, AdCC is classified as classic, solid-basaloid type, and AdCC with high-grade transformation.[52,53,133] AdCC usually presents as a mass lesion in elderly women.[50,51,53]

The characteristic molecular signature is MYB-NFIB fusion, t(6;9) translocation, and less commonly MYBL1 rearrangements or MYB amplification.[134,135] AdCCs with high-grade transformation acquire mutations in EP300, NOTCH1, ERBB2, and FGFR1 and often lack genetic alterations affecting usual TNBC.[136] The prognosis of mammary AdCC classic type is favorable compared with IBC that is TNBC; higher grade tumors have been associated with a worse prognosis.[50–53,137] Therefore, histologic features should be taken into account to guide clinical management. Of note, it remains unclear whether or not AdCC with high-grade morphology belong to the family of AdCC or a TNBC with basaloid morphology.[137]

Secretory carcinoma

Secretory carcinoma is a salivary-gland type IBC composed of epithelial cells with intracytoplasmic vacuoles and extracellular eosinophilic secretions with variable architecture and characterized by ETV6-NTRK3 fusion. Secretory carcinomas account for less than 0.05% of all invasive mammary carcinomas and occur predominantly in women, although men and children are also affected.[138–141] Patients present with a slow-growing, firm, painless, mobile mass in the retroareolar region, or with nipple discharge, and radiographical features of a circumscribed lobulated mass mimicking the appearance of a fibroadenoma.[142]

Secretory carcinomas are characterized by a t(12;15) translocation, with very low mutation burdens.[143–145] Despite a TNBC phenotype, secretory carcinomas generally have an indolent clinical course, especially in children and young adults, and only rare deaths have been reported.[138,141]

SUMMARY

Breast cancer is a heterogeneous group of tumors at the morphologic, immunohistochemical, and molecular levels. Although molecular classification continues to evolve and expand our understanding of breast cancer biology,[146] the traditional classification system still offers valuable information for clinical management. Combining the clinical presentation, radiologic findings, and use of surrogate immunohistochemical assays in conjunction with morphology, most IBC can be classified into distinct molecular subtypes in a relatively straightforward and inexpensive manner for use in clinical management. Albeit rare, it is not always possible to classify some tumors into a specific subtype due to the biologically diverse nature and these continue to be a challenge for the oncologists and the pathologists. A multidisciplinary approach will likely offer the greatest success in managing these patients.

CLINICS CARE POINTS

- The improved understanding and application of molecular classification of breast cancer has indeed paved the way for targeted therapy and immunotherapy for patients with breast cancer. However, the utilization and interpretation of molecular studies is still evolving and not practical in every patient.

- Morphologic evaluation combined with immunohistochemical studies serve as useful surrogates to understand the molecular subtype of breast cancer in routine practice. The molecular classification of breast cancer influences their appearance on imaging, including FDG and FES PET, which are useful tools to monitor patients at risk for developing metastatic diease.

- Owing to biological diversity and complex genetic factors, it is not possible to predict recurrence and determine treatment of every patient based on morphologic evaluation or molecular classification alone. Hence, it is best to pursue a multidisciplinary approach and incorporate clinical, morphological, and molecular findings to guide patient management in these cases.

DISCLOSURE

M Roy has no disclosures. A.M. Fowler receives book article royalty from Elsevier, Inc and has served on an advisory board for GE Healthcare. The Department of Radiology at the University of Wisconsin School of Medicine and Public Health receives research support from GE Healthcare. G.A. Ulaner discloses grants, consulting fees, honoraria, and/or speaker fees from Lantheus, GE Heathcare, United States, Curium, POINT, Rayze-Bio, Briacell, and ImaginAb. A. Mahajan has no disclosures.

ACKNOWLEDGMENTS

The authors would like to acknowledge Dr Paul Weisman for helpful review of this article, and Annona Martin for assistance with digital photomicrograph. They would also like to acknowledge the work of many others that could not be cited due to space limitations.

REFERENCES

1. Elston CW, Ellis IO. Pathological prognostic factors in breast cancer. I. The value of histological grade in breast cancer: experience from a large study with long-term follow-up. Histopathology 1991; 19(5):403–10.
2. Rakha EA, El-Sayed ME, Lee AH, et al. Prognostic significance of Nottingham histologic grade in invasive breast carcinoma. J Clin Oncologist 2008; 26(19):3153–8.
3. Rakha EA, El-Sayed ME, Menon S, et al. Histologic grading is an independent prognostic factor in invasive lobular carcinoma of the breast. Breast Cancer Res Treat 2008;111(1):121–7.
4. Galea MH, Blamey RW, Elston CE, et al. The Nottingham Prognostic Index in primary breast cancer. Breast Cancer Res Treat 1992;22(3):207–19.
5. Molland JG, Donnellan M, Janu NC, et al. Infiltrating lobular carcinoma–a comparison of diagnosis, management and outcome with infiltrating duct carcinoma. Breast 2004;13(5):389–96.
6. Mersin H, Yildirim E, Gülben K, et al. Is invasive lobular carcinoma different from invasive ductal carcinoma? Eur J Surg Oncol 2003;29(4):390–5.
7. Yang C, Lei C, Zhang Y, et al. Comparison of overall survival between invasive lobular breast carcinoma and invasive ductal breast carcinoma: a propensity score matching study based on SEER database. Front Oncol 2020;10:590643.
8. Korhonen T, Kuukasjärvi T, Huhtala H, et al. The impact of lobular and ductal breast cancer histology on the metastatic behavior and long term survival of breast cancer patients. Breast 2013;22(6):1119–24.
9. Dalenc F, Lusque A, De La Motte Rouge T, et al. Impact of lobular versus ductal histology on overall survival in metastatic breast cancer: a French retrospective multicentre cohort study. Eur J Cancer 2022;164:70–9.
10. Perou CM, Sorlie T, Eisen MB, et al. Molecular portraits of human breast tumours. Nature 2000; 406(6797):747–52.
11. Sorlie T, Perou CM, Tibshirani R, et al. Gene expression patterns of breast carcinomas distinguish tumor subclasses with clinical implications. Proc Natl Acad Sci U S A 2001;98(19):10869–74.
12. Sorlie T, Tibshirani R, Parker J, et al. Repeated observation of breast tumor subtypes in

independent gene expression data sets. Proc Natl Acad Sci U S A 2003;100(14):8418–23.

13. Network CGA. Comprehensive molecular portraits of human breast tumours. Nature 2012;490(7418): 61–70.

14. Houssami N, Macaskill P, von Minckwitz G, et al. Meta-analysis of the association of breast cancer subtype and pathologic complete response to neo-adjuvant chemotherapy. Eur J Cancer 2012;48(18): 3342–54.

15. Paik S, Shak S, Tang G, et al. A multigene assay to predict recurrence of tamoxifen-treated, node-negative breast cancer. N Engl J Med 2004; 351(27):2817–26.

16. van 't Veer LJ, Dai H, van de Vijver MJ, et al. Gene expression profiling predicts clinical outcome of breast cancer. Nature 2002;415(6871):530–6.

17. Sparano JA, Gray RJ, Makower DF, et al. Prospective validation of a 21-gene expression assay in breast cancer. N Engl J Med 2015;373(21):2005–14.

18. Parker JS, Mullins M, Cheang MC, et al. Supervised risk predictor of breast cancer based on intrinsic subtypes. J Clin Oncol 2009;27(8):1160–7.

19. Wallden B, Storhoff J, Nielsen T, et al. Development and verification of the PAM50-based Prosigna breast cancer gene signature assay. BMC Med Genom 2015;8:54.

20. van de Vijver MJ, He YD, van't Veer LJ, et al. A gene-expression signature as a predictor of survival in breast cancer. N Engl J Med 2002;347(25): 1999–2009.

21. Filipits M, Rudas M, Jakesz R, et al. A new molecular predictor of distant recurrence in ER-positive, HER2-negative breast cancer adds independent information to conventional clinical risk factors. Clin Cancer Res 2011;17(18):6012–20.

22. Martin M, Brase JC, Calvo L, et al. Clinical validation of the EndoPredict test in node-positive, chemotherapy-treated ER+/HER2- breast cancer patients: results from the GEICAM 9906 trial. Breast Cancer Res 2014;16(2):R38.

23. Ma XJ, Wang Z, Ryan PD, et al. A two-gene expression ratio predicts clinical outcome in breast cancer patients treated with tamoxifen. Cancer Cell 2004;5(6):607–16.

24. Ma XJ, Salunga R, Dahiya S, et al. A five-gene molecular grade index and HOXB13:IL17BR are complementary prognostic factors in early stage breast cancer. Clin Cancer Res 2008;14(9):2601–8.

25. Najjar S, Allison KH. Updates on breast biomarkers. Virchows Arch 2022;480(1):163–76.

26. Slamon DJ, Clark GM, Wong SG, et al. Human breast cancer: correlation of relapse and survival with amplification of the HER-2/neu oncogene. Science (New York, N.Y.) 1987;235(4785):177–82.

27. Modi S, Jacot W, Yamashita T, et al. Trastuzumab deruxtecan in previously treated HER2-low advanced breast cancer. N Engl J Med 2022; 387(1):9–20.

28. Schmid P, Cortes J, Pusztai L, et al. Pembrolizumab for early triple-negative breast Cancer. N Engl J Med 2020;382(9):810–21.

29. Schmid P, Salgado R, Park YH, et al. Pembrolizumab plus chemotherapy as neoadjuvant treatment of high-risk, early-stage triple-negative breast cancer: results from the phase 1b open-label, multicohort KEYNOTE-173 study. Ann Oncol 2020;31(5): 569–81.

30. Schmid P, Cortes J, Dent R, et al. Event-free survival with pembrolizumab in early triple-negative breast cancer. N Engl J Med 2022;386(6):556–67.

31. Cortes J, Rugo HS, Cescon DW, et al. Pembrolizumab plus chemotherapy in advanced triple-negative breast cancer. N Engl J Med 2022;387(3):217–26.

32. Adams S, Othus M, Patel SP, et al. A multicenter phase II trial of ipilimumab and nivolumab in unresectable or metastatic metaplastic breast cancer: cohort 36 of dual anti-CTLA-4 and anti-PD-1 blockade in rare tumors (DART, SWOG S1609). Clin Cancer Res 2022;28(2):271–8.

33. Campbell IG, Russell SE, Choong DY, et al. Mutation of the PIK3CA gene in ovarian and breast cancer. Cancer Res 2004;64(21):7678–81.

34. Bachman KE, Argani P, Samuels Y, et al. The PIK3CA gene is mutated with high frequency in human breast cancers. Cancer Biol Ther 2004;3(8): 772–5.

35. Cheang MC, Chia SK, Voduc D, et al. Ki67 index, HER2 status, and prognosis of patients with luminal B breast cancer. J Natl Cancer Inst 2009;101(10): 736–50.

36. Prat A, Cheang MC, Martín M, et al. Prognostic significance of progesterone receptor-positive tumor cells within immunohistochemically defined luminal A breast cancer. J Clin Oncol 2013;31(2):203–9.

37. Harris LN, Ismaila N, McShane LM, et al. Use of biomarkers to guide decisions on adjuvant systemic therapy for women with early-stage invasive breast cancer: American society of clinical oncology clinical practice guideline. J Clin Oncol 2016;34(10):1134–50.

38. Nielsen TO, Leung SCY, Rimm DL, et al. Assessment of Ki67 in breast cancer: updated recommendations from the international Ki67 in breast cancer working group. J Natl Cancer Inst 2021;113(7): 808–19.

39. Andre F, Ismaila N, Allison KH, et al. Biomarkers for adjuvant endocrine and chemotherapy in early-stage breast cancer: ASCO guideline update. J Clin Oncol 2022;40(16):1816–37.

40. Perou CM. Molecular stratification of triple-negative breast cancers. Oncol 2011;16(Suppl 1):61–70.

41. Weisman PS, Ng CK, Brogi E, et al. Genetic alterations of triple negative breast cancer by targeted

next-generation sequencing and correlation with tumor morphology. Mod Pathol 2016;29(5):476–88.

42. Carey LA, Perou CM, Livasy CA, et al. Race, breast cancer subtypes, and survival in the Carolina breast cancer study. JAMA 2006;295(21):2492–502.

43. Foulkes WD, Stefansson IM, Chappuis PO, et al. Germline BRCA1 mutations and a basal epithelial phenotype in breast cancer. J Natl Cancer Inst 2003;95(19):1482–5.

44. O'Brien KM, Cole SR, Tse CK, et al. Intrinsic breast tumor subtypes, race, and long-term survival in the carolina breast cancer study. Clin Cancer Res 2010;16(24):6100–10.

45. Farmer P, Bonnefoi H, Becette V, et al. Identification of molecular apocrine breast tumours by microarray analysis. Oncogene 2005;24(29):4660–71.

46. Hennessy BT, Gonzalez-Angulo AM, Stemke-Hale K, et al. Characterization of a naturally occurring breast cancer subset enriched in epithelial-to-mesenchymal transition and stem cell characteristics. Cancer Res 2009;69(10):4116–24.

47. Prat A, Parker JS, Karginova O, et al. Phenotypic and molecular characterization of the claudin-low intrinsic subtype of breast cancer. Breast Cancer Res 2010;12(5):R68.

48. Gerhard R, Ricardo S, Albergaria A, et al. Immunohistochemical features of claudin-low intrinsic subtype in metaplastic breast carcinomas. Breast 2012;21(3):354–60.

49. Taube JH, Herschkowitz JI, Komurov K, et al. Core epithelial-to-mesenchymal transition interactome gene-expression signature is associated with claudin-low and metaplastic breast cancer subtypes. Proc Natl Acad Sci U S A 2010;107(35): 15449–54.

50. Ro JY, Silva EG, Gallager HS. Adenoid cystic carcinoma of the breast. Hum Pathol 1987;18(12): 1276–81.

51. Foschini MP, Rizzo A, De Leo A, et al. Solid variant of adenoid cystic carcinoma of the breast: a case series with proposal of a new grading system. Int J Surg Pathol 2016;24(2):97–102.

52. Foschini MP, Morandi L, Asioli S, et al. The morphological spectrum of salivary gland type tumours of the breast. Pathology 2017;49(2):215–27.

53. Shin SJ, Rosen PP. Solid variant of mammary adenoid cystic carcinoma with basaloid features: a study of nine cases. Am J Surg Pathol 2002; 26(4):413–20.

54. Groheux D, Giacchetti S, Moretti JL, et al. Correlation of high 18F-FDG uptake to clinical, pathological and biological prognostic factors in breast cancer. Eur J Nucl Med Mol Imaging 2011;38(3): 426–35.

55. Arslan E, Çermik TF, Trabulus FDC, et al. Role of 18F-FDG PET/CT in evaluating molecular subtypes

and clinicopathological features of primary breast cancer. Nucl Med Commun 2018;39(7):680–90.

56. Kurland BF, Wiggins JR, Coche A, et al. Whole-body characterization of estrogen receptor status in metastatic breast cancer with 16α-18F-Fluoro-17β-Estradiol positron emission tomography: meta-analysis and recommendations for integration into clinical applications. Oncol 2020;25(10): 835–44.

57. Ulaner GA. 16α-18F-fluoro-17β-Fluoroestradiol (FES): clinical applications for patients with breast cancer. Semin Nucl Med 2022;52(5):574–83.

58. Altunay B, Morgenroth A, Beheshti M, et al. HER2-directed antibodies, affibodies and nanobodies as drug-delivery vehicles in breast cancer with a specific focus on radioimmunotherapy and radioimmunoimaging. Eur J Nucl Med Mol Imaging 2021; 48(5):1371–89.

59. Henry KE, Ulaner GA, Lewis JS. Clinical potential of human epidermal growth factor receptor 2 and human epidermal growth factor receptor 3 imaging in breast cancer. Pet Clin 2018;13(3):423–35.

60. Arpino G, Bardou VJ, Clark GM, et al. Infiltrating lobular carcinoma of the breast: tumor characteristics and clinical outcome. Breast Cancer Res 2004; 6(3):R149–56.

61. Mathew A, Rajagopal PS, Villgran V, et al. Distinct pattern of metastases in patients with invasive lobular carcinoma of the breast. Geburtshilfe Frauenheilkd 2017;77(6):660–6.

62. Cocco D, ElSherif A, Wright MD, et al. Invasive lobular breast cancer: data to support surgical decision making. Ann Surg Oncol 2021;28(10): 5723–9.

63. Cocco D, Valente SA. ASO author reflection: updating our knowledge on invasive lobular breast cancer. Ann Surg Oncol 2022;29(Suppl 3):545–6.

64. Yousef GM, Gabril MY, Al-Haddad S, et al. Invasive lobular carcinoma of the breast presenting as retroperitoneal fibrosis: a case report. J Med Case Rep 2010;4:175.

65. Hilleren DJ, Andersson IT, Lindholm K, et al. Invasive lobular carcinoma: mammographic findings in a 10-year experience. Radiology 1991;178(1): 149–54.

66. Le Gal M, Ollivier L, Asselain B, et al. Mammographic features of 455 invasive lobular carcinomas. Radiology 1992;185(3):705–8.

67. Michael M, Garzoli E, Reiner CS. Mammography, sonography and MRI for detection and characterization of invasive lobular carcinoma of the breast. Breast Dis 2008;30:21–30.

68. Lopez JK, Bassett LW. Invasive lobular carcinoma of the breast: spectrum of mammographic, US, and MR imaging findings. Radiographics 2009; 29(1):165–76.

69. Dołęga-Kozierowski B, Lis M, Marszalska-Jacak H, et al. Multimodality imaging in lobular breast cancer: differences in mammography, ultrasound, and MRI in the assessment of local tumor extent and correlation with molecular characteristics. Front Oncol 2022;12:855519.

70. Costantini M, Montella RA, Fadda MP, et al. Diagnostic challenge of invasive lobular carcinoma of the breast: what is the news? Breast magnetic resonance imaging and emerging role of contrast-enhanced spectral mammography. J Pers Med 2022;12(6):867.

71. Corso G, Figueiredo J, La Vecchia C, et al. Hereditary lobular breast cancer with an emphasis on E-cadherin genetic defect. J Med Genet 2018; 55(7):431–41.

72. Ciriello G, Gatza ML, Beck AH, et al. Comprehensive molecular portraits of invasive lobular breast cancer. Cell 2015;163(2):506–19.

73. de Groot JS, Ratze MA, van Amersfoort M, et al. αE-catenin is a candidate tumor suppressor for the development of E-cadherin-expressing lobular-type breast cancer. J Pathol 2018;245(4):456–67.

74. Simpson PT, Reis-Filho JS, Lambros MB, et al. Molecular profiling pleomorphic lobular carcinomas of the breast: evidence for a common molecular genetic pathway with classic lobular carcinomas. J Pathol 2008;215(3):231–44.

75. Vargas AC, Lakhani SR, Simpson PT. Pleomorphic lobular carcinoma of the breast: molecular pathology and clinical impact. Future Oncol 2009;5(2):233–43.

76. Petrelli F, Barni S. Response to neoadjuvant chemotherapy in ductal compared to lobular carcinoma of the breast: a meta-analysis of published trials including 1,764 lobular breast cancer. Breast Cancer Res Treat 2013;142(2):227–35.

77. Lips EH, Mukhtar RA, Yau C, et al. Lobular histology and response to neoadjuvant chemotherapy in invasive breast cancer. Breast Cancer Res Treat 2012;136(1):35–43.

78. Avril N, Menzel M, Dose J, et al. Glucose metabolism of breast cancer assessed by 18F-FDG PET: histologic and immunohistochemical tissue analysis. J Nucl Med 2001;42(1):9–16.

79. Dashevsky BZ, Goldman DA, Parsons M, et al. Appearance of untreated bone metastases from breast cancer on FDG PET/CT: importance of histologic subtype. Eur J Nucl Med Mol Imaging 2015; 42(11):1666–73.

80. Hogan MP, Goldman DA, Dashevsky B, et al. Comparison of 18F-FDG PET/CT for Systemic Staging of Newly Diagnosed Invasive Lobular Carcinoma Versus Invasive Ductal Carcinoma. J Nucl Med 2015;56(11):1674–80.

81. Ulaner GA, Goldman DA, Gonen M, et al. Initial results of a prospective clinical trial of 18F-Fluciclovine PET/CT in newly diagnosed invasive ductal and invasive lobular breast cancers. J Nucl Med 2016;57(9):1350–6.

82. Tade FI, Cohen MA, Styblo TM, et al. Anti-3-18F-FACBC (18F-Fluciclovine) PET/CT of breast cancer: an exploratory study. J Nucl Med 2016;57(9): 1357–63.

83. Ulaner GA, Jhaveri K, Chandarlapaty S, et al. Head-to-head evaluation of (18)F-FES and (18)F-FDG PET/CT in metastatic invasive lobular breast cancer. J Nucl Med 2021;62(3):326–31.

84. Eshet Y, Tau N, Apter S, et al. The Role of 68Ga-FAPI PET/CT in detection of metastatic lobular breast cancer. Clin Nucl Med 2023;48(3):228–32.

85. Rakha EA, Lee AH, Evans AJ, et al. Tubular carcinoma of the breast: further evidence to support its excellent prognosis. J Clin Oncol 2010;28(1):99–104.

86. Leibman AJ, Lewis M, Kruse B. Tubular carcinoma of the breast: mammographic appearance. AJR Am J Roentgenol 1993;160(2):263–5.

87. Günhan-Bilgen I, Oktay A. Tubular carcinoma of the breast: mammographic, sonographic, clinical and pathologic findings. Eur J Radiol 2007;61(1): 158–62.

88. Weigelt B, Horlings HM, Kreike B, et al. Refinement of breast cancer classification by molecular characterization of histological special types. J Pathol 2008;216(2):141–50.

89. Waldman FM, Hwang ES, Etzell J, et al. Genomic alterations in tubular breast carcinomas. Hum Pathol 2001;32(2):222–6.

90. Diab SG, Clark GM, Osborne CK, et al. Tumor characteristics and clinical outcome of tubular and mucinous breast carcinomas. J Clin Oncol 1999; 17(5):1442–8.

91. Louwman MW, Vriezen M, van Beek MW, et al. Uncommon breast tumors in perspective: incidence, treatment and survival in The Netherlands. Int J Cancer 2007;121(1):127–35.

92. Stolnicu S, Moldovan C, Resetkova E. Even small pure tubular carcinoma of the breast (stage T1a and T1b) can be associated with lymph node metastases - the U T MD Anderson Cancer Center experience. Eur J Surg Oncol 2016;42(6):911–2.

93. Di Saverio S, Gutierrez J, Avisar E. A retrospective review with long term follow up of 11,400 cases of pure mucinous breast carcinoma. Breast Cancer Res Treat 2008;111(3):541–7.

94. WHO Classification of Tumours Editorial Board. Breast tumours [Internet]. Lyon (France): International Agency for Research on Cancer; 2019. (WHO classification of tumours series, 5th ed.; vol. 2). Available at: https://tumourclassification.iarc. who.int/chapters/32. Accessed January 3, 21023.

95. Larribe M, Thomassin-Piana J, Jalaguier-Coudray A. Breast cancers with round lumps: correlations between imaging and anatomopathology. Diagn Interv Imaging 2014;95(1):37–46.

96. Yoo JL, Woo OH, Kim YK, et al. Can MR Imaging contribute in characterizing well-circumscribed breast carcinomas? Radiographics 2010;30(6): 1689–702.

97. Lacroix-Triki M, Suarez PH, MacKay A, et al. Mucinous carcinoma of the breast is genomically distinct from invasive ductal carcinomas of no special type. J Pathol 2010;222(3):282–98.

98. Kehr EL, Jorns JM, Ang D, et al. Mucinous breast carcinomas lack PIK3CA and AKT1 mutations. Hum Pathol 2012;43(12):2207–12.

99. Pareja F, Lee JY, Brown DN, et al. The genomic landscape of mucinous breast cancer. J Natl Cancer Inst 2019;111(7):737–41.

100. Nguyen B, Veys I, Leduc S, et al. Genomic, transcriptomic, Epigenetic, and immune profiling of mucinous breast cancer. J Natl Cancer Inst 2019; 111(7):742–6.

101. Lacroix-Triki M, Lambros MB, Geyer FC, et al. Absence of microsatellite instability in mucinous carcinomas of the breast. Int J Clin Exp Pathol 2010;4(1):22–31.

102. Paterakos M, Watkin WG, Edgerton SM, et al. Invasive micropapillary carcinoma of the breast: a prognostic study. Hum Pathol 1999;30(12):1459–63.

103. Walsh MM, Bleiweiss IJ. Invasive micropapillary carcinoma of the breast: eighty cases of an underrecognized entity. Hum Pathol 2001;32(6):583–9.

104. Chen AC, Paulino AC, Schwartz MR, et al. Prognostic markers for invasive micropapillary carcinoma of the breast: a population-based analysis. Clin Breast Cancer 2013;13(2):133–9.

105. Adrada B, Arribas E, Gilcrease M, et al. Invasive micropapillary carcinoma of the breast: mammographic, sonographic, and MRI features. AJR Am J Roentgenol 2009;193(1):W58–63.

106. Yun SU, Choi BB, Shu KS, et al. Imaging findings of invasive micropapillary carcinoma of the breast. J Breast Cancer 2012;15(1):57–64.

107. Alsharif S, Daghistani R, Kamberoğlu EA, et al. Mammographic, sonographic and MR imaging features of invasive micropapillary breast cancer. Eur J Radiol 2014;83(8):1375–80.

108. Thor AD, Eng C, Devries S, et al. Invasive micropapillary carcinoma of the breast is associated with chromosome 8 abnormalities detected by comparative genomic hybridization. Hum Pathol 2002; 33(6):628–31.

109. Marchiò C, Iravani M, Natrajan R, et al. Genomic and immunophenotypical characterization of pure micropapillary carcinomas of the breast. J Pathol 2008;215(4):398–410.

110. Marchiò C, Iravani M, Natrajan R, et al. Mixed micropapillary-ductal carcinomas of the breast: a genomic and immunohistochemical analysis of morphologically distinct components. J Pathol 2009;218(3):301–15.

111. Natrajan R, Wilkerson PM, Marchiò C, et al. Characterization of the genomic features and expressed fusion genes in micropapillary carcinomas of the breast. J Pathol 2014;232(5):553–65.

112. Dieci MV, Smutná V, Scott V, et al. Whole exome sequencing of rare aggressive breast cancer histologies. Breast Cancer Res Treat 2016;156(1): 21–32.

113. Vingiani A, Maisonneuve P, Dell'orto P, et al. The clinical relevance of micropapillary carcinoma of the breast: a case-control study. Histopathology 2013;63(2):217–24.

114. Wu Y, Zhang N, Yang Q. The prognosis of invasive micropapillary carcinoma compared with invasive ductal carcinoma in the breast: a meta-analysis. BMC Cancer 2017;17(1):839.

115. Nelson RA, Guye ML, Luu T, et al. Survival outcomes of metaplastic breast cancer patients: results from a US population-based analysis. Ann Surg Oncol 2015;22(1):24–31.

116. Schroeder MC, Rastogi P, Geyer CE, et al. Early and locally advanced metaplastic breast cancer: presentation and survival by receptor status in surveillance, epidemiology, and end results (SEER) 2010-2014. Oncol 2018;23(4):481–8.

117. Langlands F, Cornford E, Rakha E, et al. Imaging overview of metaplastic carcinomas of the breast: a large study of 71 cases. Br J Radiol 2016; 89(1064):20140644.

118. Geyer FC, Weigelt B, Natrajan R, et al. Molecular analysis reveals a genetic basis for the phenotypic diversity of metaplastic breast carcinomas. J Pathol 2010;220(5):562–73.

119. Lien HC, Lin CW, Mao TL, et al. p53 overexpression and mutation in metaplastic carcinoma of the breast: genetic evidence for a monoclonal origin of both the carcinomatous and the heterogeneous sarcomatous components. J Pathol 2004;204(2): 131–9.

120. Avigdor BE, Beierl K, Gocke CD, et al. Whole-exome sequencing of metaplastic breast carcinoma indicates monoclonality with associated ductal carcinoma component. Clin Cancer Res 2017;23(16):4875–84.

121. van Deurzen CH, Lee AH, Gill MS, et al. Metaplastic breast carcinoma: tumour histogenesis or dedifferentiation? J Pathol 2011;224(4):434–7.

122. Reis-Filho JS, Pinheiro C, Lambros MB, et al. EGFR amplification and lack of activating mutations in metaplastic breast carcinomas. J Pathol 2006; 209(4):445–53.

123. Ng CKY, Piscuoglio S, Geyer FC, et al. The landscape of somatic genetic alterations in metaplastic breast carcinomas. Clin Cancer Res 2017;23(14): 3859–70.

124. Piscuoglio S, Ng CKY, Geyer FC, et al. Genomic and transcriptomic heterogeneity in metaplastic

carcinomas of the breast. NPJ Breast Cancer 2017; 3:48.

125. Rakha EA, Coimbra ND, Hodi Z, et al. Immunoprofile of metaplastic carcinomas of the breast. Histopathology 2017;70(6):975–85.

126. Rakha EA, Tan PH, Varga Z, et al. Prognostic factors in metaplastic carcinoma of the breast: a multiinstitutional study. Br J Cancer 2015;112(2):283–9.

127. Yamaguchi R, Horii R, Maeda I, et al. Clinicopathologic study of 53 metaplastic breast carcinomas: their elements and prognostic implications. Hum Pathol 2010;41(5):679–85.

128. Paul Wright G, Davis AT, Koehler TJ, et al. Hormone receptor status does not affect prognosis in metaplastic breast cancer: a population-based analysis with comparison to infiltrating ductal and lobular carcinomas. Ann Surg Oncol 2014;21(11): 3497–503.

129. Podetta M, D'Ambrosio G, Ferrari A, et al. Lowgrade fibromatosis-like spindle cell metaplastic carcinoma: a basal-like tumor with a favorable clinical outcome. Report of two cases. Tumori 2009; 95(2):264–7.

130. Van Hoeven KH, Drudis T, Cranor ML, et al. Lowgrade adenosquamous carcinoma of the breast. A clinocopathologic study of 32 cases with ultrastructural analysis. Am J Surg Pathol 1993;17(3): 248–58.

131. Hennessy BT, Krishnamurthy S, Giordano S, et al. Squamous cell carcinoma of the breast. J Clin Oncol 2005;23(31):7827–35.

132. Hennessy BT, Giordano S, Broglio K, et al. Biphasic metaplastic sarcomatoid carcinoma of the breast. Ann Oncol 2006;17(4):605–13.

133. Massé J, Truntzer C, Boidot R, et al. Solid-type adenoid cystic carcinoma of the breast, a distinct molecular entity enriched in NOTCH and CREBBP mutations. Mod Pathol 2020;33(6):1041–55.

134. D'Alfonso TM, Mosquera JM, MacDonald TY, et al. MYB-NFIB gene fusion in adenoid cystic carcinoma of the breast with special focus paid to the solid variant with basaloid features. Hum Pathol 2014;45(11):2270–80.

135. Kim J, Geyer FC, Martelotto LG, et al. MYBL1 rearrangements and MYB amplification in breast adenoid cystic carcinomas lacking the MYB-NFIB fusion gene. J Pathol 2018;244(2):143–50.

136. Fusco N, Geyer FC, De Filippo MR, et al. Genetic events in the progression of adenoid cystic carcinoma of the breast to high-grade triple-negative breast cancer. Mod Pathol 2016;29(11):1292–305.

137. Schwartz CJ, Brogi E, Marra A, et al. The clinical behavior and genomic features of the so-called adenoid cystic carcinomas of the solid variant with basaloid features. Mod Pathol 2022;35(2): 193–201.

138. Horowitz DP, Sharma CS, Connolly E, et al. Secretory carcinoma of the breast: results from the survival, epidemiology and end results database. Breast 2012;21(3):350–3.

139. Botta G, Fessia L, Ghiringhello B. Juvenile milk protein secreting carcinoma. Virchows Arch A Pathol Anat Histol 1982;395(2):145–52.

140. McDivitt RW, Stewart FW. Breast carcinoma in children. JAMA 1966;195(5):388–90.

141. Tavassoli FA, Norris HJ. Secretory carcinoma of the breast. Cancer 1980;45(9):2404–13.

142. Mun SH, Ko EY, Han BK, et al. Secretory carcinoma of the breast: sonographic features. J Ultrasound Med 2008;27(6):947–54.

143. Tognon C, Knezevich SR, Huntsman D, et al. Expression of the ETV6-NTRK3 gene fusion as a primary event in human secretory breast carcinoma. Cancer Cell 2002;2(5):367–76.

144. Laé M, Fréneaux P, Sastre-Garau X, et al. Secretory breast carcinomas with ETV6-NTRK3 fusion gene belong to the basal-like carcinoma spectrum. Mod Pathol 2009;22(2):291–8.

145. Krings G, Joseph NM, Bean GR, et al. Genomic profiling of breast secretory carcinomas reveals distinct genetics from other breast cancers and similarity to mammary analog secretory carcinomas. Mod Pathol 2017;30(8):1086–99.

146. Thennavan A, Beca F, Xia Y, et al. Molecular analysis of TCGA breast cancer histologic types. Cell Genom 2021;1(3):100067.

Breast Cancer Screening and Diagnosis
Recent Advances in Imaging and Current Limitations

Alison R. Gegios, MD[a], Molly S. Peterson, MD[a],
Amy M. Fowler, MD, PhD[a,b,c],*

KEYWORDS

- Mammography • Digital breast tomosynthesis • Ultrasound • Breast magnetic resonance imaging
- Molecular breast imaging • Positron emission mammography • Breast cancer screening

KEY POINTS

- Mammography is the primary imaging modality used for breast cancer screening and is associated with a significant decrease in breast cancer mortality. Although screening guidelines vary by professional society, annual screening mammography starting at age 40 years for average-risk women is associated with the greatest reduction in mortality.
- Supplemental screening can be considered as an adjunct to mammography for women at high and intermediate risk for breast cancer, as well as in women with dense breasts. The 2 most prevalent modalities for supplemental screening are contrast-enhanced breast MR imaging and ultrasound.
- Molecular breast imaging also can be used to detect mammographically occult breast cancer, particularly in patients with contraindications to MR imaging, and provides functional metabolic data.

INTRODUCTION

Breast cancer detection has improved over decades with increasingly advanced technology, including digital breast tomosynthesis, breast MR imaging, and ultrasound. Breast imaging modalities with high diagnostic accuracy have a significant impact on population health, as breast cancer has surpassed lung cancer as the most commonly diagnosed nonskin cancer globally and accounts for 1 in 8 cancer diagnoses overall.[1] Breast cancer also remains the second leading cause of cancer-related mortality in women.[2]

Treatment of breast cancer has greatly improved over the past several decades, and increased emphasis has been placed on the molecular and genetic features of breast cancer. However, the size of the malignant tumor (T stage), number of nodal metastases (N stage), and presence or absence of distant metastatic disease (M stage) at the time of diagnosis also directly affects patient prognosis.[3] Imaging plays a key role in determining overall clinical stage.

This article highlights traditional breast imaging techniques, advances in imaging, as well as emerging technologies and potential future directions. Mammography, ultrasound, and breast MR imaging are the most common tools used not only for screening and diagnosis but also for preoperative locoregional staging for newly diagnosed

[a] Section of Breast Imaging and Intervention, Department of Radiology, University of Wisconsin School of Medicine and Public Health, 600 Highland Avenue, Madison, WI 53792-3252, USA; [b] University of Wisconsin Carbone Cancer Center, Madison, WI, USA; [c] Department of Medical Physics, University of Wisconsin-Madison, Madison, WI, USA
* Corresponding author. Section of Breast Imaging and Intervention, Department of Radiology, University of Wisconsin School of Medicine and Public Health, 600 Highland Avenue, Madison, WI 53792-3252.
E-mail address: afowler@uwhealth.org

PET Clin 18 (2023) 459–471
https://doi.org/10.1016/j.cpet.2023.04.003

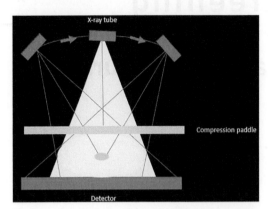

Fig. 1. During the acquisition of digital breast tomosynthesis images, the x-ray tube moves in an arc to collect images of the breast in multiple projections.

breast cancer and assessment of neoadjuvant treatment response.

MAMMOGRAPHY

Digital breast tomosynthesis (DBT) has emerged as a keystone of breast imaging. Compared with its forerunner, full-field digital mammography (FFDM), DBT examinations are associated with higher sensitivity and specificity, lower recall rates, and increased cancer detection rates.[4,5] Tomosynthesis transcends the 2-dimensional nature of FFDM by using a tomographic reconstruction algorithm in which multiple projections are obtained across an arc to minimize the effect of overlapping breast tissue and maximize the conspicuity of suspicious findings (**Fig. 1**).[6] Although DBT is associated with a slightly higher radiation dose compared with FFDM and longer interpretation times, its benefits outweigh these drawbacks for use as a screening tool.[7,8] Digital breast tomosynthesis also has been widely adopted in the diagnostic setting to evaluate patients with a finding recalled from a screening examination or patients with an area of clinical concern (eg, a palpable abnormality, nipple discharge, focal pain) (**Fig. 2**).[6,9] However, FFDM (including full-field lateral, magnification craniocaudal, and magnification mediolateral views) remains the preferred technique for evaluation of calcifications (**Fig. 3**).[10]

Contrast-enhanced mammography (CEM) recently has gained traction as a diagnostic technique that couples the use of FFDM with intravenous iodinated contrast administration to identify areas of abnormal enhancement. This technique is suitable for use in patients with a contraindication to MR imaging (eg, pacemaker, gadolinium-based contrast agent allergy, claustrophobia) although there is a potential risk that patients undergoing CEM may have an allergic reaction to iodinated contrast.[11] CEM is also faster and less costly than MR imaging, but it is associated with radiation (unlike MR imaging and ultrasound).[11] CEM has increased diagnostic accuracy compared with FFDM.[12] CEM can be used for problem-solving in the context of indeterminate imaging findings, local staging in the preoperative setting, and monitoring neoadjuvant treatment response.[11]

Screening Mammography

Screening mammography is the primary modality used for the detection of breast cancer in asymptomatic women. Breast cancer screening has been shown to reduce breast cancer mortality by at least 20% based on randomized controlled trials and up to 49% based on case-control studies.[13–17] In part, the reduction in breast cancer mortality has been attributed to the ability of mammography to detect smaller cancers than are clinically detectable.[17] Although there are variable guidelines regarding appropriate screening populations and recommended time interval between screening examinations, the American College of Radiology (ACR), Society of Breast Imaging (SBI), and National Comprehensive Cancer Network (NCCN) recommend performing screening mammography starting at age 40 years in average-risk women on a yearly basis.[18,19] In contrast, the United States Preventive Services Task Force (USPSTF) recommends screening mammograms for women between the ages of 50 and 74 years on a biennial basis.[20] The USPSTF offers a caveat that women age 40 to 49 years may discuss the age at which to start screening mammography and the frequency of screening mammography with their provider.[1,20] Screening recommendations stratified by multiple organizations, including ACR, SBI, NCCN, USPSTF, American College of Physicians, and American Association of Family Physicians, are summarized in **Table 1**.[18–24] Regardless of the age and interval at which mammography is performed, the target cancer detection rate is between 3 and 8 cancers per 1000 screening mammograms, and the target recall rate is 5% to 12% for radiologists according to the ACR.[25] Although screening mammography

---

[1]After submission of this article, the USPSTF issued a new draft recommendation statement on May 9, 2023 recommending screening mammography every other year for women ages 40 to 74 years old.

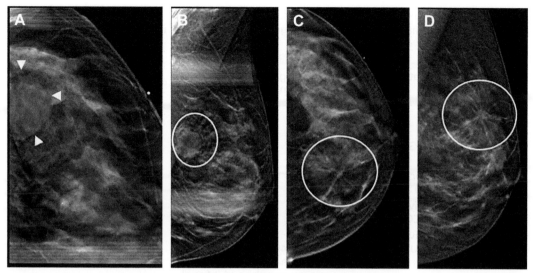

Fig. 2. Digital breast tomosynthesis views in a 48-year-old woman presenting with a palpable abnormality in the left upper outer breast. An oval mass with circumscribed margins underlies the BB marker at the area of clinical concern seen mammographically [(A) spot compression CC view (*arrowheads*); (B) spot compression MLO view (*circle*)]. Subsequent ultrasound confirmed this palpable finding was a benign cyst. However, an area of architectural distortion in the left upper inner breast (*circles*) was also seen mammographically [(C) full-field CC view; (D) full-field ML view] and corresponded to an irregular hypoechoic mass with angular margins on ultrasound (not shown). This area of architectural distortion was subsequently biopsied under ultrasound guidance and corresponded to invasive ductal carcinoma, grade 1 on pathology.

guidelines are variable, studies have shown that the maximum mortality reduction and life-years-gained benefit ensue when screening mammography begins at age 40 years.[26]

Limitations of Mammography

Despite the significant benefits of screening mammography in breast cancer mortality reduction, studies have shown that 9% to 22% of new breast cancer cases are mammographically occult or preceded by a false-negative mammogram.[27] Screening mammography is particularly limited in

women with dense breast tissue, which both reduces the sensitivity for cancer detection given its masking effect and serves as an independent risk factor for the development of breast cancer—albeit a relatively weak risk factor when compared with age, genetic mutations, and family history of breast cancer.[28,29] Nonetheless, approximately 40% of US women have dense breast tissue and may benefit from supplemental screening with ultrasound or breast MR imaging (**Fig. 4**).[30] The first breast density notification legislation was enacted in Connecticut more than a decade ago to inform patients of the limited

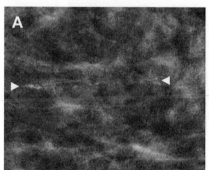
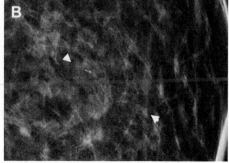

Fig. 3. Magnification CC (A) and ML (B) views were performed in a 62-year-old patient with newly diagnosed Paget disease of the nipple on punch biopsy. The 2-dimensional FFDM images demonstrate amorphous calcifications in a linear distribution (*arrowheads*), which were assessed as suspicious. Stereotactic-guided biopsy was performed, and pathology demonstrated invasive ductal carcinoma, grade 1.

Table 1
Summary of current mammography screening guidelines for average-risk women

Society	Age to Begin	Frequency
American Cancer Society (ACS)	Offer at age 40 to 45 y Recommend at age 45 y	Annual for age 40–54 y Biennial with option for annual in women ≥ 55 y
American College of Obstetricians and Gynecologists (ACOG)	40 y	Annual or biennial
American College of Radiology (ACR), Society of Breast Imaging (SBI)	40 y	Annual
National Comprehensive Cancer Network (NCCN)	40 y	Annual
United States Preventive Services Task Force (USPSTF)[1]	50 y If age 40–49 y, may discuss age at which to start screening mammography and interval with provider	Biennial
American College of Physicians (ACP)	50 y If age 40–49 y, may discuss age at which to start screening mammography; for most women, harms outweigh benefits	Biennial
American Association of Family Physicians (AAFP)	50 y If age 40–49 y, may discuss age at which to start screening mammography; for most women, harms outweigh benefits	Biennial

[1] After submission of this article, the USPSTF issued a new draft recommendation statement on May 9, 2023 recommending screening mammography every other year for women ages 40 to 74 years old.

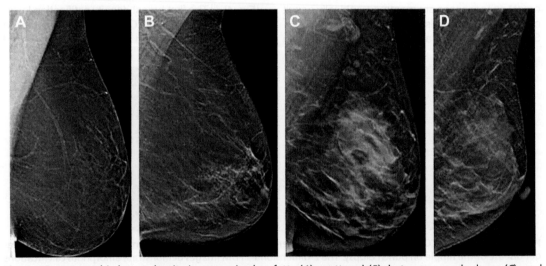

Fig. 4. Mammographic breast density is categorized as fatty (*A*), scattered (*B*), heterogeneously dense (*C*), and extremely dense (*D*).

sensitivity of mammography in the setting of dense breasts and to promote shared decision-making regarding the utility of supplemental screening based on individualized risk factors.[30] Since then, breast density notification laws have demonstrated state-specific variability in their adoption throughout the United States; some states still have no mandated notification of breast density.[30]

Overdiagnosis is often discussed as a potential limitation of screening mammography. Overdiagnosis is defined as the identification of a screen-detected malignancy that never would have resulted in clinical symptoms given its slow-growing, less aggressive nature rather than earlier detection of an aggressive, fast-growing tumor.[31] Although the rate of detection of large tumors (>2 cm) decreased after the introduction of screening mammography, some studies have attributed this to the additional detection of small tumors (<2 cm or in situ carcinoma), which increased from 36% to 68% after the introduction of screening mammography.[31] However, more recent studies have found that the incidence of breast malignancy that was fatal within 10 years of diagnosis and advanced breast cancer rate was substantially decreased in women undergoing screening mammography versus women who did not participate in screening mammography independent of advancements in treatment regimens.[32]

An additional risk of screening mammography is the anxiety that patients may experience, particularly fear of a diagnosis of breast cancer.[33] There is also a potential for false-positive imaging interpretations and, in some cases, procedures.[33] Patients may also incur burdensome costs for further diagnostic imaging, biopsies, and, occasionally, image-guided localizations and surgery. However, the anxiety women experience in regard to breast imaging is largely transient.[34] In one study, most of the women who underwent screening mammography responded that they were likely to continue to participate in screening in the future and recommend that other women do the same.[34] Based on national medical audit data, the proportion of women who are recalled from screening mammography is low (~10%), and the proportion of biopsies that are recommended in this subgroup of recalled patients is also relatively low (~20%).[35–37]

SUPPLEMENTAL SCREENING

Supplemental screening with MR imaging or, in some settings, ultrasound can be beneficial in women with an intermediate or high lifetime risk for breast cancer and in women with dense breasts.[38] Factors that contribute to increased lifetime risk of breast cancer include genetic mutations, personal or family history of breast cancer, and a history of atypia or lobular hyperplasia.[38]

It is important to understand conditions that are characterized as high, intermediate, or average risk when assessing if supplemental screening is warranted. Women with various pathogenic genetic mutations that carry a high lifetime risk of breast cancer generally benefit from supplemental screening (**Table 2**). For reference, BRCA1 and BRCA2 variants carry up to 87% and 56% estimated lifetime risk of breast cancer, respectively.[39] Women with genetic mutations that are linked to an increased risk of breast cancer have a high rate of interval cancers compared with the general population.[40] Interval cancers are defined as symptomatic cancers that are detected in the timeframe between screening examinations and generally portend a worse prognosis than screen-detected cancers.[40] Similarly, interval cancer rates are increased in patients with increased breast density and personal history of breast cancer.[40] Patients are also considered high risk if they have a lifetime risk of breast cancer greater than 20% when calculated by models such as Claus, BRCAPRO, and Tyrer-Cuzick (IBIS) that analyze various parameters that contribute to overall risk, including family history of breast cancer.[38] In addition, women with a history of mantle radiation, often in the setting of prior Hodgkin lymphoma, have a cumulative incidence of breast cancer that ranges from 13% to 20% by age 45 years.[38]

Individuals who fall into the intermediate risk category for development of breast cancer include those with a personal history of breast cancer, personal history of a high-risk lesion such as atypical ductal hyperplasia or lobular carcinoma in situ, or mammographically dense breasts.[38] Supplemental screening recommendations by the ACR and NCCN stratified by these high-risk and intermediate-risk subgroups are summarized in **Table 2**.[37,38,41–44]

Ultrasound

Studies have shown that supplemental screening with whole breast ultrasound in this intermediate-risk population increases the detection of mammographically occult, small, invasive, node-negative cancers.[45] Supplemental screening with ultrasound increases breast cancer detection by 1.8 to 4.6 cancers per 1,000 women screened.[40,46,47] Ultrasound also lacks radiation, is generally accessible across institutions, and is less costly than other supplemental screening modalities, such as MR imaging.

Table 2
Summary of current mammography screening guidelines with supplemental MR imaging for high- and intermediate-risk women

Risk Factor	ACR Guidelines	NCCN Guidelines
BRCA1, BRCA2	MG: ≥ 30 y MR imaging: ≥ 25 to 30 y	MG: 30–75 y MR imaging: >25–29 y to age 75 y After 75 y, based on individual risk
CHEK2, ATM (Ataxia telangiectasia)	MG: ≥ 30 y MR imaging: ≥ 25–30 y	MG: ≥ 40 y Consider MR imaging starting at age 30–35 y
PTEN (Cowden and Bannayan-Riley-Ruvalcaba)	MG: ≥ 30 y MR imaging: ≥ 25–30 y	MG + MR imaging: 35 y or 10 y before earliest known breast cancer diagnosis (whichever is first) to 75 y After 75 y, based on individual risk
TP53 (Li-Fraumeni)	MG: ≥ 30 y MR imaging: ≥ 25–30 y	MG: ≥ 30–75 y MR imaging: ≥ 20–75 y After 75 y, based on individual risk
NF1	Not specifically addressed	MG: ≥ 30 y Consider MR imaging from ages 30–50 y
CDH1 (hereditary diffuse gastric cancer)	MG: ≥ 30 y MR imaging: ≥ 25–30 y	MG: ≥ 30 y Consider MR imaging starting at age 30 y
PALB2 (interacts with BRCA2)	MG: ≥ 30 y MR imaging: ≥ 25–30 y	MG + MR imaging: ≥ 30 y
STK11 (Peutz-Jeghers)	MG: ≥ 30 y MR imaging: ≥ 25–30 y	MG + MR imaging: ≥ 30 y
Family history of breast cancer (>20% lifetime risk)	MG: ≥ 30 y MR imaging: ≥ 25–30 y	MG: 10 y before age at which youngest family member was diagnosed, not before age 30 y, or at age 40 y (whichever is first) MR imaging: 10 y before age at which youngest family member was diagnosed, not before age 25 y
Untested first-degree relative of mutation carrier	MG: ≥ 30 y MR imaging: ≥ 25–30 y	Not specifically addressed
Mantle radiation (age 10–30 y)	MG + MR imaging ≥ 25 y or 8 years after therapy (whichever is later)	MG: begin 8 y after radiation, but not before 30 y MR imaging: begin 8 y after radiation, but not before 25 y
ADH or lobular neoplasia (ALH/LCIS)	MG: begin at diagnosis Consider MR imaging annually starting at time of diagnosis	MG: begin at diagnosis, but not < 30 y Consider MR imaging at diagnosis, but not <25 y
Personal history of breast cancer	MG: begin at diagnosis MR imaging: at diagnosis if breast cancer diagnosed < 50 y or dense breasts at any age	MG: Annually Consider MR imaging in patients with: • Dense breasts status post-lumpectomy and radiation

(continued on next page)

Table 2 (continued)		
Risk Factor	ACR Guidelines	NCCN Guidelines
		• Patients diagnosed < 50 y • Lifetime risk of second primary cancer is >20%
Mammographically dense breasts	MG: $\geq$ 40 y MR imaging: insufficient data	MG: $\geq$ 40 y MR imaging: insufficient data

Abbreviations: ADH, atypical ductal hyperplasia; ALH, atypical lobular hyperplasia; LCIS, lobular carcinoma in situ; MG, mammography.

Adapted from Wang L, Strigel RM. Supplemental Screening for Patients at Intermediate and High Risk for Breast Cancer. *Radiol Clin North Am.* 2021;59(1):67-83.

Although supplemental screening with ultrasound has several benefits, it is important to also be cognizant of its drawbacks. The principal downside of screening whole breast ultrasound is that a large proportion of findings generate biopsies with benign results. Screening whole breast ultrasound, therefore, results in false positives and has a relatively low positive predictive value.[48] The multicenter prospective American College of Radiology Imaging Network (ACRIN) 6666 trial of supplemental whole breast ultrasound for women at elevated risk of breast cancer demonstrated a 15.1% increase in recall rate for the initial screening round and a 7.4% increase for the subsequent second and third years of screening.[49] In the ACRIN 6666 trial, the addition of physician-performed handheld screening whole breast ultrasound to mammography was associated with a 7.8% increase in the biopsy rate and a 17.8% decrease in positive predictive value (PPV3) compared with mammography alone.[49] Supplemental screening ultrasound also has been associated with a relatively large number of BI-RADS 3 (probably benign) findings and recommendations for short-interval follow-up ultrasound, which has been associated with increased patient anxiety and necessitates additional resources and costs.[48–50]

Handheld breast ultrasound is also operator-dependent and time-consuming.[51,52] However, automated whole breast ultrasound (AWBUS) increases the availability of technologists given its independent, robotic operation and decreases variability between examinations.[52] AWBUS images include axial sonographic images of the entirety of both breasts and a coronal reformatted image or cine images (**Fig. 5**). Supplemental AWBUS has a similar cancer detection rate (3.6 additional cancers per 1000 women screened) as handheld screening whole breast ultrasound and a positive predictive value for biopsies recommended at 38%.[53]

BREAST MR IMAGING

Dynamic contrast-enhanced MR imaging is the most sensitive modality for breast cancer detection with higher sensitivity than mammography, DBT, or ultrasound. In high-risk women, MR imaging and mammography combined has a sensitivity of 93% compared with 52% for ultrasound and mammography combined.[54] Thus, MR imaging is the preferred modality for supplemental breast cancer screening. There is insufficient evidence to support the use of screening MR imaging for women of average risk (<15% lifetime risk of breast cancer).[42] For intermediate-risk women (15%–20% lifetime risk of breast cancer), the ACR asserts there is insufficient evidence for or against MR imaging as an adjunct to mammography.[42] Recent studies, however, suggest some intermediate-risk women may benefit from MR imaging, including women with a history of lobular carcinoma in situ[55,56] or a personal history of breast cancer.[57,58]

Preoperative evaluation of patients with newly diagnosed breast cancer is also a common indication for breast MR imaging. MR imaging is the most accurate method for measuring tumor size, identifying pectoralis muscle or chest wall invasion, detecting the presence of multifocal and/or multicentric disease, and screening the contralateral breast for malignancy. The sensitivity of MR imaging for detecting contralateral disease is greater than 90%[59,60]; this holds prognostic significance, as patients with synchronous bilateral breast cancer or metachronous cancers diagnosed within 2 years of the primary cancer have decreased survival compared with unilateral cancers.[61] **Fig. 6** demonstrates a case of mammographically occult contralateral breast cancer detected on MR imaging.

MR imaging is also the best method for assessing tumor response to neoadjuvant therapy.[62,63] Changes in tumor size and enhancement are

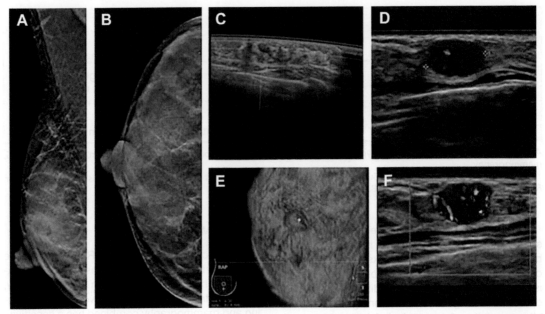

Fig. 5. A 41-year-old woman with extremely dense breasts and a negative screening mammogram [mediolateral oblique view (*A*); craniocaudal view (*B*)]. The patient subsequently underwent supplemental automated whole breast ultrasound at an outside institution [transverse view (*C*); coronal reformat (*E*)]. On diagnostic ultrasound, a suspicious subcentimeter hypoechoic mass (*D*) with internal vascularity (*F*) was identified in the right breast. The mass was biopsied and corresponded to invasive ductal carcinoma on pathology.

used to predict complete response, partial response, or nonresponse to therapy. The ACRIN 6657 trial compared MR imaging with clinical assessment and mammography and found that MR imaging was the most accurate for detecting pathologic complete response and had the strongest association with final pathologic size in patients with residual tumor burden.[64]

Other indications for breast MR imaging include axillary nodal metastasis from a breast primary that is mammographically and sonographically occult, patients with bloody nipple discharge with inconclusive findings on other imaging, and evaluation of silicone implant integrity. MR imaging protocols designed for the assessment of implant integrity rely on silicone sensitive sequences, which suppress both fat and water and are performed without intravenous contrast.

Breast MR imaging is not without limitations. Higher costs, longer scan times, and longer interpretation times have limited its widespread use. To overcome these limitations, abbreviated MR

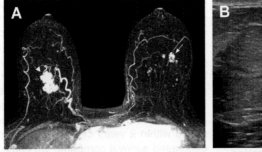
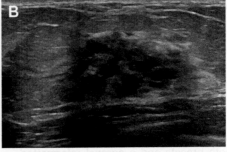

Fig. 6. A 57-year-old woman with a mammographically occult right breast cancer detected on MR imaging performed for extent of disease evaluation of a newly diagnosed left breast cancer (invasive mammary carcinoma, grade 2). (*A*) Axial maximum intensity projection image demonstrates the known biopsy-proven malignant mass in the left breast (*arrow*) as well as a small satellite mass medial to the dominant mass. An irregular enhancing mass in the right breast is also seen (*arrowhead*). (*B*) Targeted ultrasound of the right breast demonstrates an irregular mass with mixed echogenicity that correlates with the mass seen on MR imaging. Ultrasound-guided biopsy of the right breast mass revealed invasive ductal carcinoma, grade 2.

imaging protocols have been developed to shorten image acquisition and interpretation time while maintaining diagnostic accuracy. There is no universally accepted protocol, although scan time is typically less than 10 minutes. Abbreviated breast MR imaging was initially proposed and validated for breast cancer screening by Kuhl and colleagues in 2014.[65] Their abbreviated protocol consisted of a noncontrast T1-weighted sequence, a single postcontrast T1-weighted sequence, subtraction images, and a single maximum intensity projection image. With the abbreviated protocol, the acquisition time was substantially decreased (3 minutes compared with 17 minutes for the full diagnostic protocol), interpretation time of the abbreviated protocol was 28 seconds, and all 11 cancers were found with equivalent diagnostic accuracy for the abbreviated and full protocols. Subsequently, the ECOG-ACRIN Cancer Research Group conducted a multicenter, cross-sectional study (EA1141) to compare cancer detection rates of abbreviated breast MR imaging versus DBT among women with dense breasts undergoing routine screening.[66] The study enrolled 1444 average-risk women with heterogeneously dense or extremely dense breasts at 48 academic, community hospital, and private practice sites in the United States and Germany. They found that abbreviated breast MR imaging detected significantly more invasive cancers (17 women; 11.8 per 1000 women) than DBT (7 women; 4.8 per 1000 women). The cost-effectiveness of abbreviated MR imaging relative to DBT was not evaluated.

An additional limitation of breast MR imaging is its moderate pooled specificity of 71%[67]; this is attributable to the capability of both benign and malignant lesions to enhance, resulting in additional imaging and unnecessary biopsies of benign findings. MR imaging for breast cancer detection also requires the use of intravenous gadolinium-based contrast agents, which is contraindicated in patients with allergies to gadolinium and patients with severe renal impairment due to the risk of developing nephrogenic systemic fibrosis. Gadolinium should be avoided in pregnant women, as it crosses the placenta and has unknown fetal risk (pregnancy class C by the Food and Drug Administration). Furthermore, patients with ferrous aneurysm clips, known metallic foreign bodies in the eye, bionic ear implants, cardiac pacemakers, vascular filters (AAA-Zenith stent), and tissue expanders should also not have MR imaging. Other patient factors that may preclude MR imaging include inability of the patient to lie prone, extreme obesity (patients whose girth exceeds the scanner bore), and patients who are claustrophobic.

DEDICATED BREAST RADIONUCLIDE IMAGING SYSTEMS

Radionuclide-based breast imaging provides functional metabolic information to complement anatomic-based modalities discussed earlier. As an adjunct modality for breast cancer detection and characterization, dedicated breast imaging systems with high spatial resolution have been developed for single-photon emitting radiopharmaceuticals as well as positron-emitting radiopharmaceuticals. A separate article in this issue reviews dedicated breast radionuclide imaging systems in further detail (see Miral M. Patel and colleagues' article, "Molecular Breast Imaging and Positron Emission Mammography," in this issue).

Molecular breast imaging (MBI) and breast-specific gamma imaging use dual-head or single-head detectors, respectively, for detecting accumulation of ^{99m}Tc-sestamibi within the breast.[68–70] A major advantage of MBI is the detection of mammographically occult breast cancers in women with dense breasts.[71] Clinical applications for MBI include supplemental screening for women with dense breasts and increased lifetime risk of breast cancer, local staging of newly diagnosed breast cancer, evaluating response to neoadjuvant therapy, and problem solving.[72] Given similar diagnostic performance, MBI may be a suitable alternative for patients who are unable to obtain MR imaging due to contraindications and can be performed at a lower cost.

Dedicated breast imaging systems for positron-emitting radiopharmaceuticals include positron emission mammography (PEM) and dedicated breast positron emission tomography (dbPET). FDG is the major radiopharmaceutical used for dedicated breast positron imaging systems. PEM systems use a similar configuration and patient positioning as mammography with 2 opposing planar detectors. dbPET systems use a ring-type configuration with prone patient positioning. Breast-specific positron imaging systems are not widely used in clinical practice in the United States; however, there is growing clinical data and practice guidelines published by international sites.[73]

FUTURE DIRECTIONS

This review article focused on the current mainstream imaging modalities for breast cancer screening and diagnosis. Technology continues to advance in each of these areas that may eventually be incorporated into routine clinical care. Emerging imaging techniques based on mammography, ultrasound, and MR imaging have been previously reviewed by Mann and colleagues.[74] In ultrasound for example, elastography can be performed, which measures tissue stiffness and may help better characterize malignant from benign masses. Addition of elastography to conventional ultrasound may improve the positive predictive value of screening ultrasound and reduce false-positive results without missing cancers.[75] Other emerging ultrasound-based techniques include contrast-enhanced ultrasound with microbubbles,[76] optoacoustic ultrasound,[77] and ultrasound transmission tomography.[78] Hybrid imaging modalities, such as PET/MR imaging, also have been studied for breast cancer.[79] Furthermore, the addition of radiomics, artificial intelligence, and deep learning may improve diagnostic accuracy of existing breast imaging techniques and address one of the limitations of false-positive examinations.[80,81] Lastly, imaging may be combined with blood-based cancer screening tests for circulating tumor DNA.[82,83] More research is needed to validate the diagnostic accuracy and cost-effectiveness of these emerging technologies before they can be integrated into current clinical breast imaging practice.

CLINICS CARE POINTS

- Annual screening mammography starting at age 40 years for average-risk women is associated with the greatest reduction in breast cancer mortality.

- Supplemental screening with contrast-enhanced breast MRI is recommended as an adjunct to mammography for women at high-risk for breast cancer.

- Supplemental screening with ultrasound, contrast-enhanced breast MRI, or molecular breast imaging can be considered for women with mammographically dense breasts.

DISCLOSURE

A.R. Gegios and M.S. Peterson have nothing to disclose. A.M. Fowler receives book article royalty from Elsevier, Inc and has served on an advisory board for GE Healthcare. The Department of Radiology at the University of Wisconsin School of Medicine and Public Health, United States receives research support from GE Healthcare, United States.

ACKNOWLEDGMENTS

The authors acknowledge the University of Wisconsin Carbone Cancer Center Support Grant P30 CA014520 and the Department of Radiology, University of Wisconsin School of Medicine and Public Health for support. We also thank Dr Roberta Strigel for case contribution.

REFERENCES

1. Arnold M, Morgan E, Rumgay H, et al. Current and future burden of breast cancer: global statistics for 2020 and 2040. Breast 2022;66:15–23.
2. Siegel RL, Miller KD, Wagle NS, et al. Cancer statistics, 2023. CA Cancer J Clin 2023;73(1):17–48.
3. Hortobagyi GN, Edge SB, Giuliano A. New and important changes in the TNM staging system for breast cancer. Am Soc Clin Oncol Educ Book 2018;38:457–67.
4. Dang PA, Wang A, Senapati GM, et al. Comparing tumor characteristics and rates of breast cancers detected by screening digital breast tomosynthesis and full-field digital mammography. AJR Am J Roentgenol 2020;214(3):701–6.
5. Aujero MP, Gavenonis SC, Benjamin R, et al. Clinical performance of synthesized two-dimensional mammography combined with tomosynthesis in a large screening population. Radiology 2017;283(1): 70–6.
6. Chong A, Weinstein SP, McDonald ES, et al. Digital breast tomosynthesis: concepts and clinical practice. Radiology 2019;292(1):1–14.
7. Dang PA, Freer PE, Humphrey KL, et al. Addition of tomosynthesis to conventional digital mammography: effect on image interpretation time of screening examinations. Radiology 2014;270(1):49–56.
8. Gao Y, Moy L, Heller SL. Digital breast tomosynthesis: update on technology, evidence, and clinical practice. Radiographics 2021;41(2):321–37.
9. Peppard HR, Nicholson BE, Rochman CM, et al. Digital breast tomosynthesis in the diagnostic setting: indications and clinical applications. Radiographics 2015;35(4):975–90.
10. Horvat JV, Keating DM, Rodrigues-Duarte H, et al. Calcifications at digital breast tomosynthesis: imaging features and biopsy techniques. Radiographics 2019;39(2):307–18.
11. Ghaderi KF, Phillips J, Perry H, et al. Contrast-enhanced mammography: current applications and future directions. Radiographics 2019;39(7): 1907–20.
12. Jochelson MS, Lobbes MBI. Contrast-enhanced mammography: state of the art. Radiology 2021; 299(1):36–48.
13. Broeders M, Moss S, Nystrom L, et al. The impact of mammographic screening on breast cancer

mortality in Europe: a review of observational studies. J Med Screen 2012;19(Suppl 1):14–25.

14. Myers ER, Moorman P, Gierisch JM, et al. Benefits and harms of breast cancer screening: a systematic review. JAMA 2015;314(15):1615–34.

15. Nickson C, Mason KE, English DR, et al. Mammographic screening and breast cancer mortality: a case-control study and meta-analysis. Cancer Epidemiol Biomarkers Prev 2012;21(9):1479–88.

16. Niell BL, Freer PE, Weinfurtner RJ, et al. Screening for breast cancer. Radiol Clin North Am 2017; 55(6):1145–62.

17. Strandberg R, Czene K, Eriksson M, et al. Estimating distributions of breast cancer onset and growth in a Swedish mammography screening cohort. Cancer Epidemiol Biomarkers Prev 2022;31(3):569–77.

18. Monticciolo DL, Newell MS, Hendrick RE, et al. Breast cancer screening for average-risk women: recommendations from the ACR Commission on Breast Imaging. J Am Coll Radiol 2017;14(9):1137–43.

19. National Comprehensive Cancer Network. NCCN Clinical Practice Guidelines in Oncology: Breast Cancer Screening and Diagnosis (NCCN Guidelines). Version 1.2022 - June 2, 2022. Available at: https://www.nccn.org/professionals/physician_gls/pdf/breast-screening.pdf. Accessed February 27, 2023.

20. Siu AL. Screening for breast cancer: U.S. Preventive Services Task Force recommendation statement. Ann Intern Med 2016;164(4):279–96.

21. Practice bulletin number 179: breast cancer risk assessment and screening in average-risk women. Obstet Gynecol 2017;130(1):e1–16.

22. Smith RA, Andrews KS, Brooks D, et al. Cancer screening in the United States, 2019: a review of current American Cancer Society guidelines and current issues in cancer screening. CA Cancer J Clin 2019;69(3):184–210.

23. Hoover LE. Breast cancer screening: ACP releases guidance statements. Am Fam Physician 2020; 101(3):184–5.

24. Qaseem A, Lin JS, Mustafa RA, et al. Screening for breast cancer in average-risk women: a guidance statement from the American College of Physicians. Ann Intern Med 2019;170(8):547–60.

25. Lee CS, Parise C, Burleson J, et al. Assessing the recall rate for screening mammography: comparing the medicare hospital compare dataset with the national mammography database. AJR Am J Roentgenol 2018;211(1):127–32.

26. Helvie MA, Bevers TB. Screening mammography for average-risk women: the controversy and NCCN's position. J Natl Compr Cancer Netw 2018;16(11):1398–404.

27. Yang TJ, Yang Q, Haffty BG, et al. Prognosis for mammographically occult, early-stage breast cancer patients treated with breast-conservation therapy. Int J Radiat Oncol Biol Phys 2010;76(1):79–84.

28. Destounis SV, Santacroce A, Arieno A. Update on breast density, risk estimation, and supplemental screening. AJR Am J Roentgenol 2020;214(2):296–305.

29. Lee CI, Chen LE, Elmore JG. Risk-based breast cancer screening: implications of breast density. Med Clin North Am 2017;101(4):725–41.

30. Haas JS. Breast density legislation and the promise not attained. J Gen Intern Med 2019;34(2):167–8.

31. Welch HG, Prorok PC, O'Malley AJ, et al. Breast-cancer tumor size, overdiagnosis, and mammography screening effectiveness. N Engl J Med 2016; 375(15):1438–47.

32. Duffy SW, Tabár L, Yen AM, et al. Mammography screening reduces rates of advanced and fatal breast cancers: results in 549,091 women. Cancer 2020;126(13):2971–9.

33. Mack DS, Lapane KL. Screening mammography among older women: a review of United States guidelines and potential harms. J Womens Health (Larchmt) 2019;28(6):820–6.

34. Schou Bredal I, Kåresen R, Skaane P, et al. Recall mammography and psychological distress. Eur J Cancer 2013;49(4):805–11.

35. Lee CS, Bhargavan-Chatfield M, Burnside ES, et al. The national mammography database: preliminary data. AJR Am J Roentgenol 2016;206(4):883–90.

36. Lehman CD, Arao RF, Sprague BL, et al. National performance benchmarks for modern screening digital mammography: update from the Breast Cancer Surveillance Consortium. Radiology 2017; 283(1):49–58.

37. Monticciolo DL, Malak SF, Friedewald SM, et al. Breast cancer screening recommendations inclusive of all women at average risk: update from the ACR and Society of Breast Imaging. J Am Coll Radiol 2021;18(9):1280–8.

38. Wang L, Strigel RM. Supplemental screening for patients at intermediate and high risk for breast cancer. Radiol Clin North Am 2021;59(1):67–83.

39. Elezaby M, Lees B, Maturen KE, et al. BRCA mutation carriers: breast and ovarian cancer screening guidelines and imaging considerations. Radiology 2019;291(3):554–69.

40. Vourtsis A, Berg WA. Breast density implications and supplemental screening. Eur Radiol 2019; 29(4):1762–77.

41. Weinstein SP, Slanetz PJ, Lewin AA, et al. ACR Appropriateness Criteria® supplemental breast cancer screening based on breast density. J Am Coll Radiol 2021;18(11s):S456–73.

42. Mainiero MB, Moy L, Baron P, et al. ACR Appropriateness Criteria(®) breast cancer screening. J Am Coll Radiol 2017;14(11s):S383–90.

43. National Comprehensive Cancer Network. NCCN Clinical Practice Guidelines in Oncology. Genetic/Familial High-Risk Assessment: Breast, Ovarian, and

Pancreatic. Version 2.2023 - January 10, 2023. Available at: https://www.nccn.org/professionals/physician_gls/pdf/genetics_bop.pdf. Accessed February 27, 2023.

44. Monticciolo DL, Newell MS, Moy L, et al. Breast cancer screening in women at higher-than-average risk: recommendations from the ACR. J Am Coll Radiol 2018;15(3 Pt A):408–14.

45. Thigpen D, Kappler A, Brem R. The role of ultrasound in screening dense breasts-a review of the literature and practical solutions for implementation. Diagnostics 2018;8(1):20.

46. Scheel JR, Lee JM, Sprague BL, et al. Screening ultrasound as an adjunct to mammography in women with mammographically dense breasts. Am J Obstet Gynecol 2015;212(1):9–17.

47. Sprague BL, Stout NK, Schechter C, et al. Benefits, harms, and cost-effectiveness of supplemental ultrasonography screening for women with dense breasts. Ann Intern Med 2015;162(3):157–66.

48. Lee JM, Arao RF, Sprague BL, et al. Performance of screening ultrasonography as an adjunct to screening mammography in women across the spectrum of breast cancer risk. JAMA Intern Med 2019;179(5):658–67.

49. Berg WA, Zhang Z, Lehrer D, et al. Detection of breast cancer with addition of annual screening ultrasound or a single screening MRI to mammography in women with elevated breast cancer risk. JAMA 2012;307(13):1394–404.

50. Kim MJ. Medical auditing of whole-breast screening ultrasonography. Ultrasonography 2017;36(3):198–203.

51. Berg WA, Blume JD, Cormack JB, et al. Combined screening with ultrasound and mammography vs mammography alone in women at elevated risk of breast cancer. JAMA 2008;299(18):2151–63.

52. Spear GG, Mendelson EB. Automated breast ultrasound: supplemental screening for average-risk women with dense breasts. Clin Imaging 2021;76:15–25.

53. Kelly KM, Dean J, Comulada WS, et al. Breast cancer detection using automated whole breast ultrasound and mammography in radiographically dense breasts. Eur Radiol 2010;20(3):734–42.

54. Berg WA. Tailored supplemental screening for breast cancer: what now and what next? AJR Am J Roentgenol 2009;192(2):390–9.

55. Friedlander LC, Roth SO, Gavenonis SC. Results of MR imaging screening for breast cancer in high-risk patients with lobular carcinoma in situ. Radiology 2011;261(2):421–7.

56. Sung JS, Malak SF, Bajaj P, et al. Screening breast MR imaging in women with a history of lobular carcinoma in situ. Radiology 2011;261(2):414–20.

57. Lehman CD, Lee JM, DeMartini WB, et al. Screening MRI in women with a personal history of breast cancer. J Natl Cancer Inst 2016;108(3):djv349.

58. Brennan S, Liberman L, Dershaw DD, et al. Breast MRI screening of women with a personal history of breast cancer. AJR Am J Roentgenol 2010;195(2):510–6.

59. Debruhl ND, Lee SJ, Mahoney MC, et al. MRI evaluation of the contralateral breast in women with recently diagnosed breast cancer: 2-year follow-up. J Breast Imaging 2020;2(1):50–5.

60. Lehman CD, Gatsonis C, Kuhl CK, et al. MRI evaluation of the contralateral breast in women with recently diagnosed breast cancer. N Engl J Med 2007;356(13):1295–303.

61. Kollias J, Ellis IO, Elston CW, et al. Prognostic significance of synchronous and metachronous bilateral breast cancer. World J Surg 2001;25(9):1117–24.

62. Reig B, Lewin AA, Du L, et al. Breast MRI for evaluation of response to neoadjuvant therapy. Radiographics 2021;41(3):665–79.

63. Fowler AM, Mankoff DA, Joe BN. Imaging neoadjuvant therapy response in breast cancer. Radiology 2017;285(2):358–75.

64. Scheel JR, Kim E, Partridge SC, et al. MRI, clinical examination, and mammography for preoperative assessment of residual disease and pathologic complete response after neoadjuvant chemotherapy for breast cancer: ACRIN 6657 trial. AJR Am J Roentgenol 2018;210(6):1376–85.

65. Kuhl CK, Schrading S, Strobel K, et al. Abbreviated breast magnetic resonance imaging (MRI): first post-contrast subtracted images and maximum-intensity projection-a novel approach to breast cancer screening with MRI. J Clin Oncol 2014;32(22):2304–10.

66. Comstock CE, Gatsonis C, Newstead GM, et al. Comparison of abbreviated breast MRI vs digital breast tomosynthesis for breast cancer detection among women with dense breasts undergoing screening. JAMA 2020;323(8):746–56.

67. Zhang L, Tang M, Min Z, et al. Accuracy of combined dynamic contrast-enhanced magnetic resonance imaging and diffusion-weighted imaging for breast cancer detection: a meta-analysis. Acta Radiol 2016;57(6):651–60.

68. Hruska CB, O'Connor MK. Nuclear imaging of the breast: translating achievements in instrumentation into clinical use. Med Phys 2013;40(5):050901.

69. Surti S. Radionuclide methods and instrumentation for breast cancer detection and diagnosis. Semin Nucl Med 2013;43(4):271–80.

70. Hsu DF, Freese DL, Levin CS. Breast-dedicated radionuclide imaging systems. J Nucl Med 2016;57(Suppl 1):40s–5s.

71. Hunt KN. Molecular breast imaging: a scientific review. J Breast Imaging 2021;3(4):416–26.

72. Hruska CB, Corion C, de Geus-Oei L-F, et al. SNMMI procedure standard/EANM practice guideline for molecular breast imaging with dedicated γ-cameras. J Nucl Med Technol 2022;50(2):103–10.

73. Satoh Y, Kawamoto M, Kubota K, et al. Clinical practice guidelines for high-resolution breast PET, 2019 edition. Ann Nucl Med 2021;35(3):406–14.

74. Mann RM, Hooley R, Barr RG, et al. Novel approaches to screening for breast cancer. Radiology 2020;297(2):266–85.

75. Pillai A, Voruganti T, Barr R, et al. Diagnostic accuracy of shear-wave elastography for breast lesion characterization in women: a systematic review and meta-analysis. J Am Coll Radiol 2022;19(5): 625–34.e620.

76. Boca Bene I, Dudea SM, Ciurea AI. Contrast-enhanced ultrasonography in the diagnosis and treatment modulation of breast cancer. J Pers Med 2021;11(2):81.

77. Seiler SJ, Neuschler EI, Butler RS, et al. Optoacoustic imaging with decision support for differentiation of benign and malignant breast masses: a 15-reader retrospective study. AJR Am J Roentgenol 2022. https://doi.org/10.2214/AJR.2222.28470. Online ahead of print.

78. Littrup PJ, Duric N, Sak M, et al. Multicenter study of whole breast stiffness imaging by ultrasound tomography (SoftVue) for characterization of breast tissues and masses. J Clin Med 2021;10(23):5528.

79. Fowler AM, Strigel RM. Clinical advances in PET-MRI for breast cancer. Lancet Oncol 2022;23(1): e32–43.

80. Shen Y, Shamout FE, Oliver JR, et al. Artificial intelligence system reduces false-positive findings in the interpretation of breast ultrasound exams. Nat Commun 2021;12(1):5645.

81. Geras KJ, Mann RM, Moy L. Artificial intelligence for mammography and digital breast tomosynthesis: current concepts and future perspectives. Radiology 2019;293(2):246–59.

82. Lennon AM, Buchanan AH, Kinde I, et al. Feasibility of blood testing combined with PET-CT to screen for cancer and guide intervention. Science 2020; 369(6499):eabb9601.

83. Underwood JJ, Quadri RS, Kalva SP, et al. Liquid biopsy for cancer: review and implications for the radiologist. Radiology 2020;294(1):5–17.

Metabolic Positron Emission Tomography in Breast Cancer

Katherine Cecil, MD[a], Laura Huppert, MD[b,c], Rita Mukhtar, MD[c,d],
Elizabeth H. Dibble, MD[e], Sophia R. O'Brien, MD[f],
Gary A. Ulaner, MD, PhD[g,h], Courtney Lawhn-Heath, MD[a,c],*

KEYWORDS

- Fluorodeoxyglucose (FDG) • Positron emission tomography (PET) • PET/CT • Breast cancer

KEY POINTS

- The avidity of breast cancer on ^{18}F-fluorodeoxyglucose (FDG) PET/computed tomography (CT) is heavily influenced by biologic factors such as histologic subtype and receptor status.
- FDG PET/CT is superior in the evaluation of extra-axillary nodal and distant metastatic disease, with evidence of comparable overall costs between FDG PET/CT and conventional imaging, in patients with clinical stage IIB-IIIC breast cancer.
- FDG PET/CT has demonstrated value in evaluation of treatment response and detection of disease recurrence.
- Targeting amino acid metabolism with ^{18}F-fluciclovine demonstrates potential in the imaging of invasive lobular carcinoma.

INTRODUCTION

Breast cancer is the most common cancer among women in the United States and the second leading cause of cancer-related deaths; approximately 12.9% of women will be diagnosed with breast cancer at some point in their lifetime.[1] In 2023, 297,970 new cases of breast cancer were projected to be diagnosed among American women, with 43,170 projected deaths.[2] PET is a molecular imaging tool that can have a dramatic clinical impact on the care of patients with breast cancer. Depending on their molecular composition, certain

PET radiopharmaceuticals can target physiologic processes that serve as surrogate measures of cellular metabolism. Of these metabolic agents, ^{18}F-fluorodeoxyglucose (FDG) is by far the most common and has had the greatest impact on the imaging and management of patients with breast cancer. FDG PET uses cellular glucose uptake as a surrogate for cellular glucose metabolism, which is upregulated in many cancers. Amino acid transport is another metabolic process that is upregulated in many cancers and can be targeted with PET using radiolabeled synthetic amino acids such as ^{18}F-fluciclovine. Metabolic PET, especially

[a] Department of Radiology and Biomedical Imaging, University of California San Francisco, San Francisco, CA, USA; [b] Department of Medicine, University of California San Francisco, San Francisco, CA, USA; [c] Helen Diller Family Comprehensive Cancer Center, University of California San Francisco, San Francisco, CA, USA; [d] Department of Surgery, University of California San Francisco, San Francisco, CA, USA; [e] Department of Diagnostic Imaging, The Warren Alpert Medical School of Brown University/Rhode Island Hospital, Providence, RI, USA; [f] Divisions of Molecular Imaging and Therapy Breast Imaging, Department of Radiology, The Hospital of the University of Pennsylvania, Philadelphia, PA, USA; [g] Molecular Imaging and Therapy, Hoag Family Cancer Institute, Irvine, CA, USA; [h] Departments of Radiology and Translational Genomics, University of Southern California, Los Angeles, CA, USA
* Corresponding author. UCSF Medical Center, Department of Radiology and Biomedical Imaging, 505 Parnassus Avenue, S-0628, San Francisco, CA 94143.
E-mail address: courtney.lawhnheath@ucsf.edu

PET Clin 18 (2023) 473–485
https://doi.org/10.1016/j.cpet.2023.04.004
1556-8598/23/© 2023 Elsevier Inc. All rights reserved.

FDG, can have important clinical applications in appropriate patients. This article will focus on the use of metabolic PET in patients with breast cancer, including the principles of FDG and fluciclovine PET, as well as a review of literature to date evaluating when the use of FDG PET/computed tomography (CT) is appropriate, and at times preferable to conventional imaging (CT chest/abdomen/pelvis [CAP] plus bone scan).

PRINCIPLES AND TECHNIQUE OF 18F-FDG PET/CT IN BREAST CANCER

FDG is a radiopharmaceutical analog of glucose that is taken into metabolically active tumor cells via a glucose transporter (GLUT) protein and phosphorylated by the same mechanism as unlabeled deoxyglucose. However, further degradation via the glycolysis pathway is not possible for FDG-6-phosphate, and it becomes trapped in the cell until it decays or is dephosphorylated.[3] The use of FDG PET/CT in oncology is based on the principle that malignant tumors with high metabolic rates take up more glucose than surrounding tissue, and this increased uptake is thought to be due, at least in part, to increased numbers of glucose transporters (GLUT 1–3).[4,5] Increased FDG uptake is not unique to malignant cells, however, and tissues that are involved in infection, inflammation, or healing can also exhibit FDG avidity and be mistaken for malignancy.[4]

The Society of Nuclear Medicine and Molecular Imaging provides several recommendations on patient preparation, image acquisition, image processing, and interpretation of FDG PET/CT.[6] The major goals of patient preparation for oncologic PET/CT are to minimize tracer uptake in normal tissues while maintaining uptake in tumor. Recommendations include avoiding exercise the day before the examination to prevent muscular uptake, avoiding consumption of food or liquids at least 4 hours before FDG administration, keeping the patient warm to prevent physiologic brown fat uptake, and ensuring a blood glucose level less than 200 mg/dL to prevent altered tumor uptake.[6,7] The PET component of the examination is performed at least 45 minutes after radiopharmaceutical injection, ideally at a site contralateral to the site of concern.[6] The CT component of the PET/CT can be performed as a low-dose noncontrast CT for attenuation correction or as an optimized diagnostic CT scan, and this choice combined with factors such as FDG avidity, lesion size, and patient motion can influence the detection of small lesions.[7]

FDG PET/CT images are typically assessed qualitatively by visually inspecting the extent and sites of uptake, as well as in a semiquantitative manner.[4] FDG uptake is most commonly quantified using a standardized uptake value (SUV), which is a measure of tracer uptake within a lesion normalized to a distribution volume such as weight, lean body mass, or body surface area.[8] The most common clinically used PET parameter is SUVmax, the highest SUV measured within a given volume of interest. Both technical and physiologic factors can affect SUV[8] but the very high interuser reproducibility of SUVmax measurement has led to its adoption over other metrics. In breast cancer and other cancers, FDG PET SUVmax has been correlated with tumor cellularity, grade, proliferative activity, and patient prognosis.[9–13]

TUMOR HISTOLOGY, RECEPTOR STATUS, AND VISUALIZATION ON PET/CT

Breast cancer is a heterogenous disease encompassing different tumor types that are traditionally described by histologic appearance, protein expression patterns, and now increasingly molecular and genomic testing.[14] The most common histologic subtypes of breast cancer are invasive ductal carcinoma (IDC; or invasive carcinoma of no special type [NST] per the World Health Organization), which accounts for 75% to 80% of primary breast malignancies, and invasive lobular carcinoma (ILC), which accounts for 10% to 15% of primary breast malignancies.[15] Breast cancer is also classified by its receptor subtype, including estrogen receptor (ER), progesterone receptor (PR), and human epidermal growth factor-2 (HER2) status.[16] Breast cancers that express ER and/or PR are called hormone receptor positive (HR+). Breast cancers that do not express ER, PR, or HER2 are called triple negative. Evolving molecular technologies now allow tumors to be distinguished according to gene expression patterns, including luminal, HER2-positive, and basal-like tumors.[14] Tumor proliferation is currently evaluated in clinical practice by the immunohistochemical staining of Ki67, which can also help inform treatment choice.[16] For hormone receptor positive (HR+)/HER2-breast cancers, several prognostic and predictive gene expression assays have been developed that both predict risk of breast cancer recurrence and predict benefit from chemotherapy, such as the 21-gene Recurrence Score (Oncotype Dx) and the 70-gene signature (Mammaprint).[17]

In regards to FDG PET/CT, several factors including tumor grade, histologic subtype, proliferation index, hormone receptor status, and tumor phenotype influence tumoral FDG uptake.[18] Importantly, FDG avidity is lower in ILC compared with IDC at both the primary site as well as in metastatic lesions.[19–22] Therefore, when interpreting FDG PET/CT in patients with ILC, physicians should keep in mind that osseous and visceral metastases may not be well visualized on either the PET or CT portion of the examination, and in some cases may be metabolically imperceptible.[21] Given ILC is also often occult on anatomic imaging, including mammography, ultrasound, and MRI, there is a need for additional modalities including hormone receptor targeting PET tracers such as ^{18}F-fluoroestradiol (FES) for accurate visualization.[23] FES-PET will be discussed elsewhere in this issue of PET Clinics (see Gary A Ulaner and colleagues' article, "Estrogen Receptor (ER)- and Progesterone Receptor (PR)-targeted PET for Patients with Breast Cancer,"). Another factor influencing FDG uptake is grade, with grade 1 or 2 tumors showing lower FDG uptake than grade 3 tumors.[19] FDG uptake is also lower in well-differentiated ER-positive tumors than ER-negative tumors, as well as PR-positive tumors when compared with PR-negative tumors.[19] Triple negative tumors typically show significantly higher SUVs than other breast cancer subtypes.[24] Finally, FDG uptake is also weaker in breast cancers with lower proliferation rates, as evaluated by Ki67 index.[25]

^{18}F-FLUORODEOXYGLUCOSE PET PRIMARY BREAST CANCER DETECTION

The diagnostic evaluation of primary breast cancer includes dedicated breast imaging with mammography and, when indicated, ultrasound and MRI. Whole body 18F-FDG PET/CT is not indicated for most early stage breast cancers in the absence of systemic symptoms due to low sensitivity, particularly for the detection of small nonpalpable (<1.0 cm) and low-grade malignancies, with differential FDG uptake based on histologic subtype (ductal vs lobular) resulting in a lower sensitivity for ILC.[20,26] FDG PET/CT is also not specific for malignancy, as acute and chronic inflammatory changes such as postprocedural inflammation or infection, and benign breast masses such as fibroadenoma or silicone granuloma may show increased FDG activity. Even physiologic lactating breast tissue may show FDG avidity and should not be mistaken for malignancy.[26]

A significant proportion (up to 30%–40%) of incidentally discovered FDG PET-positive breast lesions represents a primary breast malignancy, such as the case shown in **Fig. 1**.[27–29] Aarstad and colleagues reported that the pooled prevalence of focal incidental breast uptake in women was 0.61% and the pooled prevalence of

malignancy of focal incidental breast uptake was 38.7%, with the most commonly detected malignancy being IDC.[27] Kang and colleagues performed a retrospective review of 48 patients with incidentally detected focal breast uptake. Malignancy was diagnosed in 37.5% of patients with statistically significant difference in malignancy rate between groups with SUVmax of less than 2 versus 2.[29] Thus, although rarely encountered, incidentally detected FDG avid foci in the breast should be correlated with earlier breast imaging and, when appropriate, further evaluated with diagnostic breast imaging such as with mammogram and ultrasound.

INITIAL STAGING

Clinical staging of breast cancer is performed using the American Joint Committee on Cancer's tumor node metastases (TNM) system, with the most recent eighth edition adopted in 2018 integrating molecular markers and disease extent for more optimal estimation of prognosis.[30] Breast cancer stage determines local and systemic treatment and affects prognosis. According to the 2023 statistics of the American Cancer Society, patients who have locoregional disease at initial staging have a 5-year survival of 86% to 99%, whereas patients presenting with de novo distant metastatic disease have a 5-year relative survival of 30%.[2] Current guidelines, including those of the National Comprehensive Cancer Network (NCCN), recommend locoregional staging workup including physical examination, mammography, sonography when appropriate, and optional breast MRI.[31] If this workup reveals regional nonaxillary lymphadenopathy (eg, internal mammary, infraclavicular, supraclavicular), chest wall or skin invasion by the primary tumor, or a primary tumor size greater than 5 cm with regional axillary lymphadenopathy, the disease is considered locally advanced breast cancer (LABC) by NCCN guidelines.[31] For LABC, systemic staging with contrast-enhanced CT of the chest, abdomen, and pelvis (CT CAP), and bone scan is recommended.[31] Per NCCN guidelines, FDG PET/CT can be used as an alternative to CT CAP and bone scan, is considered especially helpful in situations where standard imaging studies are equivocal, and "may also be helpful in identifying unsuspected regional nodal disease and/or distant metastases in LABC when used in addition to standard imaging studies."[31]

Locoregional Nodal Disease

The clinical utility of FDG PET/CT in evaluating locoregional nodal disease differs between surgically accessible axillary nodes (lateral and posterior

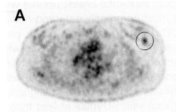
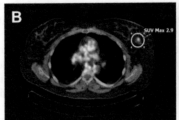
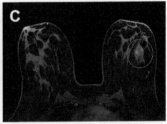

Fig. 1. Incidentally detected breast cancer on FDG PET/CT. A 38-year-old woman with history of Li-Fraumeni syndrome who underwent FDG PET/CT for further workup of abnormal liver ultrasound. (*A* and *B*) Axial FDG PET and fused axial FDG PET/CT shows incidental focal uptake in the outer left breast. (*C*) Subsequent postcontrast T1-weighted axial MRI shows nonmass enhancement in the same region. Subsequent biopsy showed high-grade ductal carcinoma in situ (DCIS), and the patient underwent bilateral mastectomy.

to pectoralis minor, or axillary levels 1–2) and regional extra-axillary nodes (including axillary level 3 [infraclavicular], supraclavicular, and internal mammary).[7] In clinically node negative patients, the current standard of care is sentinel node biopsy as the preferred technique for axillary staging, followed by axillary lymph node dissection or radiation when appropriate.[32] The sentinel node procedure has been reported to have a 97% prediction of disease status of the remaining axilla.[33] In comparison, FDG PET/CT has poor sensitivity for axillary nodal metastases, mainly attributed to spatial resolution limitations.[18,32,34,35] Kasem and colleagues recently performed a systematic review of the performance of FDG PET/CT in the assessment of axillary nodal metastases in patients with clinical stage I–III breast cancer, with sensitivities ranging from 18.5% to 85% and calculated pooled sensitivity of 52% but relatively high specificity of 91.6%.[32] Several other studies show a similarly high specificity of FDG PET/CT for axillary nodal disease.[7,18,36] Therefore, an FDG avid axillary lymph node should be considered likely to represent metastatic disease, although causes of false-positive FDG avid axillary adenopathy should also be considered. For example, in 2021 Brown and colleagues published a case series of 4 patients with reactive FDG avid axillary lymph nodes ipsilateral to site of breast malignancy following coronavirus disease 2019 vaccination.[37]

FDG PET/CT is useful in the evaluation of locoregional extra-axillary nodes, including internal mammary, infraclavicular, and supraclavicular nodes, which may not be identified by sentinel node evaluation. Unsuspected locoregional extra-axillary nodal metastases can result in upstaging and alter clinical management related to surgical extent and/or radiation therapy.[32] Groheux and colleagues prospectively compared FDG PET/CT with conventional imaging in 117 patients with LABC and found that FDG PET/CT detected unsuspected locoregional extra-

axillary nodes in 32 (27.3%) patients.[38] Several additional recent articles have reported similar findings that compared with conventional imaging, FDG PET/CT identifies all or almost all disease identified by conventional imaging with an increased sensitivity for unsuspected locoregional extra-axillary nodal metastases.[39–48]

Distant Metastases

For systemic staging, conventional imaging includes anatomic imaging with contrast enhanced CT CAP as well as functional bone imaging.[31] However, there is a growing body of recent evidence that FDG PET/CT identifies more distant metastases in a significant number of patients with LABC[18,21,39–44,46–51] and should be routinely used in initial systemic staging of breast cancer. The detection of these unsuspected metastases (eg, **Fig. 2**) has important clinical and prognostic implications, changing the patient's stage from one reflecting only locoregional disease to stage IV, and altering the treatment goal from curative to noncurative systemic therapy.[31]

The rate of detection of unsuspected distant metastases increases as pre-FDG PET/CT clinical stage increases. In a 2020 study reported in the JNCCN,[39] Ko and colleagues found that approximately 37% of patients with stage IIA–IIIC breast cancer who underwent FDG PET/CT before primary systemic therapy showed more extensive disease than was identified on conventional imaging. Out of 196 patients, the overall upstaging rate to stage IV based on FDG PET/CT findings of unsuspected distant metastases was 14%, including 0% for stage IIA, 13% for stage IIB, 22% for stage IIIA, 17% for stage IIIB, and 37% for stage IIIC.

FDG PET/CT also had similar cost when compared with conventional imaging and had lower radiation dose exposure. Several additional studies have reported similar findings, including studies focusing on male patients,[50,51] patients aged

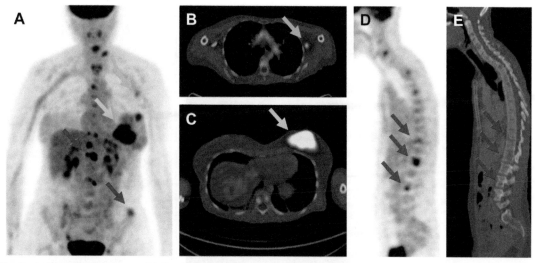

Fig. 2. A 49-year-old woman with locally advanced clinical stage IIIA breast cancer who underwent initial staging with FDG PET/CT. FDG PET MIP (*A*) and fused axial FDG PET (*B* and *C*) images show hypermetabolic left breast mass (*green arrows*), left axillary lymphadenopathy (*blue arrows*), and multiple hypermetabolic osseous lesions throughout the spine, ribs, and pelvis (*red arrows*). Sagittal FDG PET (*D*) through the spine shows several hypermetabolic vertebral body metastases, corresponding to lytic lesions on sagittal CT (*E*).

younger than 40 years,[41] patients with inflammatory breast cancer,[43] patients with triple-negative breast cancer,[47] and patients with inner quadrant primary breast tumors.[44] In 2021, Groheux reviewed the literature and concluded that FDG PET/CT is recommended for the initial systemic staging starting from clinical-stage IIB, with possible utility in patients with clinical stage IIA, although there are not enough strong data to recommend routine use in this IIA subgroup.[18] For clinical stage I patients, staging with FDG PET/CT offers no added value.[18]

When compared with conventional imaging, FDG PET/CT performs particularly well in detecting additional osseous metastases (**Fig. 3**). Morris and colleagues[52] found that in 163 patients with suspected metastatic breast cancer who underwent both bone scan and FDG PET/CT, there was discordance between FDG PET/CT and bone scan in 31 (19%) of cases. Twelve of these patients underwent pathologic examination, which provided a reference standard for the presence or absence of bone malignancy. In all 12 cases, FDG PET/CT provided a more accurate diagnosis than bone scan, matching the pathologic result. The authors conclude that FDG PET/CT may supplant bone scan for the purpose of detecting metastatic breast cancer.[52]

Another recent multicenter study published in JNCCN by Hyland and colleagues[40] also supports the routine use of FDG PET/CT in the initial systemic staging of stage IIB–IIIC breast cancer. They found that compared with conventional imaging, FDG PET/CT reduced false-positive risk

by half and decreased workup of incidental findings, allowing for earlier treatment start. FDG PET/CT was cost-effective, and at one institution was found to be cost-saving.[40]

As mentioned above, histologic subtype has an important impact on tumor visualization on FDG PET/CT. Specifically, ILC has significantly lower FDG avidity compared with IDC, and this behavior extends to metastatic disease (**Fig. 4**).[25] Hogan and colleagues[21] retrospectively identified 146 patients with stage III ILC who underwent FDG PET/CT, of which 12 (8%) were upstaged due to the presence of unsuspected distant metastases on FDG PET/CT, compared with 20 of 89 (22%) patients with stage III IDC. Additionally, 3 of 12 upstaged patients with ILC were upstaged by non-FDG avid lesions visible only on the CT images, suggesting that the impact of FDG PET/CT on systemic staging may be lower for patients with ILC than for patients with IDC.[21]

It is also important to note that ILC differs from IDC in its pattern of metastatic spread—although both IDC and ILC commonly metastasize to bones and liver, ILC demonstrates a predilection for metastases to the peritoneum, retroperitoneum, hollow viscera, and leptomeninges.[21] Detecting these sites of metastases is often challenging due to the absence of clinical symptoms until disease is extensive, as well as difficulty assessing these regions on FDG PET/CT due to physiologic and variable FDG avidity.[7,21] Dashevsky and colleagues[22] reported that untreated osseous metastases from ILC are more likely to be sclerotic and missed on FDG

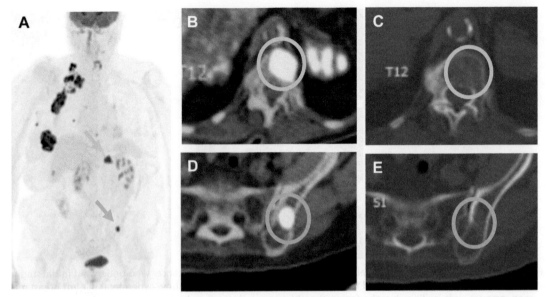

Fig. 3. Osseous lesions without CT correlate. 93 year old woman with locally advanced breast cancer. Initial staging with FDG PET/CT (*A*) revealed right axillary and supraclavicular nodal metastases, as well as hypermetabolic osseous metastases in the T12 vertebral body (*B-C, green arrow* and *green circle*) and left medial iliac bone (*D-E, blue arrow* and *blue circle*). The osseous metastases are only visible on FDG PET and do not have CT correlate.

PET due to FDG activity being no higher than background. In these cases, alternative modalities such as ER-targeted PET (discussed elsewhere in this issue) may be helpful for lesion visualization.

Thus, although there is growing and convincing evidence that FDG PET/CT detects more unsuspected distant metastatic breast cancer from clinical stages IIB–IIIC and offers possible benefit in

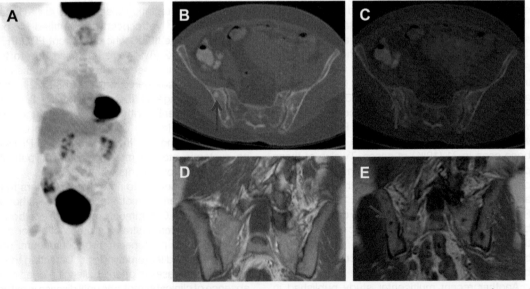

Fig. 4. Non-FDG-avid osseous metastases in a patient with ILC. MIP from FDG PET (*A*) demonstrates no abnormal foci. Axial CT and fused FDG PET/CT (*B* and *C*) demonstrate multiple sclerotic osseous (*red arrows*) lesions without FDG-avidity. Differential includes osteopoikilosis and bone metastases. On T1-weighted coronal MR 7 years before the diagnosis of breast cancer (*D*), there are no osseous lesions. MRI following diagnosis of breast cancer (*E*) demonstrates multiple new osseous lesions. Biopsy of a right ilium osseous lesion demonstrated osseous metastasis from ILC. This demonstrates the potential limitation of FDG PET for detecting ILC metastases.

stage IIA, the benefit may not be as significant in patients with ILC compared with patients with IDC, so this should be considered in future studies.[21,53] Later in this review, we will discuss ^{18}F-fluciclovine, which may be more useful in initial staging and evaluation of treatment response in patients with ILC.[53]

TREATMENT RESPONSE
Response to Neoadjuvant Chemotherapy in the Primary Breast Mass

Neoadjuvant chemotherapy (NAC) has been shown to be effective in downstaging the primary tumor and metastatic locoregional lymph nodes before surgery and is increasingly used in the management of patients with LABC to facilitate breast conservation and to assess response to systemic therapy.[54] Patients whose tumors have poor response to chemotherapy may have improved survival with the use of alternative or prolonged courses of chemotherapy, making it important to determine treatment response as early as possible to avoid ineffective therapy.[55] Several studies report a strong correlation between changes in FDG maximum SUV and pathologic response to NAC,[56–68] and some have attempted to define criteria for predicting pathologic response in tumors of varying receptor status.[69,70] If a lesion on follow-up FDG PET/CT has an SUVmax of less than or equal to 60% of the baseline SUVmax, Rousseau and colleagues reported sensitivity, specificity, and negative predictive value of FDG PET/CT in predicting pathologic response of 89%, 95%, and 85%, respectively, after 2 cycles of chemotherapy, with response defined as greater than 50% therapeutic effect as assessed by a pathologist according to the scale established by Sataloff.[68,71] Champion and colleagues reported that in patients with inflammatory breast cancer, changes in SUVmax between baseline and presurgery FDG PET/CT using a cutoff of 72% predicted distant metastasis free survival with a specificity of 80%.[70] Groheux and colleagues followed 78 patients with triple-negative breast cancer and found that the change in SUVmax after 2 cycles of chemotherapy was more pronounced in patients who achieve pathologic complete response (72% vs 42%), however, the optimal change in SUVmax for predicting pathologic complete response was specific to the treatment regimen.[67]

Although there may be a role for FDG PET/CT in metabolic evaluation of response to NAC, the current available literature lacks generalizability. The cutoff value chosen to predict response varies dramatically across studies and has been shown to differ depending on the specific treatment regimen.[67] Additionally, the definition of what constitutes a good response on FDG PET/CT varies across studies. For example, in the studies mentioned above, Rousseau and colleagues[68] defined good response as 50% therapeutic effect or greater while Champion and colleagues[70] considered pathologic complete response a satisfactory response.

Response of Metastatic Lesions

Response evaluation in metastatic breast cancer has traditionally relied on conventional imaging, namely size measurement on CT, although there is limited but growing evidence that metabolic evaluation with FDG PET/CT may be more sensitive for disease progression. FDG PET reflects metabolic changes that occur before tumor shrinking, the current CT surrogate for response.[72] Additionally, metabolic changes measured on FDG PET can be especially useful in lesions with no measurable correlate on anatomic imaging, for instance many osseous metastases. With increasing numbers of potentially effective treatments for patients with metastatic breast cancer, accurate response evaluation becomes increasingly important and can potentially affect patient survival.[73]

Reidl and colleagues[74] compared metastatic treatment response by CT and FDG PET/CT and found that among 65 patients with stage IV breast cancer, metabolic assessment by FDG PET/CT was a better predictor of progression free survival and disease-specific survival than was Response Evaluation Criteria in Solid Tumors evaluation on CT. Another recent study by Naghavi-Behzad and colleagues[75] retrospectively reviewed 300 patients with metastatic breast cancer in whom treatment response was monitored using CT, FDG PET/CT, or the combination of both modalities. In patients monitored with FDG PET/CT, the first progression leading to treatment change was detected on average 5 months earlier than in patients monitored with CT, and the 5-year overall survival rate was 42% in the FDG PET/CT group compared with 16% in the CT group and remained significant even after controlling for known risk factors.[75] Early studies of FDG PET/CT in the evaluation of breast cancer metastases showed that response versus nonresponse could be predicted after only one cycle of therapy[58]; however, more research is warranted to confirm these findings and determine optimal timing for interim FDG PET/CT imaging.

In the metastatic setting, FDG PET/CT is particularly effective in measuring response in osseous disease.[76,77] Not only is FDG PET/CT able to detect osseous metastases earlier than bone scintigraphy and CT but also is more accurate since sclerotic lesions appearing on CT after therapy may reflect osseous healing rather than new metastases, confounding interpretation.[76,78] Similarly, bone scan is affected by the phenomenon known as a flare response, in which increased avidity on bone scan may represent increased osteoblastic activity during bone healing after successful therapy and is difficult to distinguish from worsening metastatic disease.[76,78] A similar phenomenon known as metabolic flare may be seen on FDG PET, with temporarily increased FDG avidity after successful therapy; however, these changes are typically only seen in the first 1 to 2 weeks and unlikely to present on follow-up imaging, which is usually performed months after initiating therapy.[79] In fact, metabolic flare may actually be an indicator of future response to therapy.[80]

One challenge of using FDG PET/CT to assess metabolic treatment response in patients with metastatic breast cancer is the frequent display of heterogenous responses in lesions within a single patient, raising the possibility that the number of selected lesions would determine the response. However, in a study of 60 patients, Pinker and colleagues showed that the selection of either 1 or 5 lesions for response assessment did not change the prognostic value of follow-up FDG PET/CT.[81]

SUSPECTED RECURRENCE OUTSIDE THE BREAST

Current guidelines regarding follow-up after primary treatment of nonmetastatic breast cancer include clinical examination and mammography, without recommendation for cross-sectional imaging in patients who are asymptomatic.[31] When a patient is suspected of having locoregional or distant recurrence of malignancy due to a clinical symptom and/or physical examination finding, imaging can be performed for further evaluation, which may include contrast-enhanced CT CAP and/or FDG PET/CT.[82] Several studies have demonstrated that compared with CT CAP and bone scan, FDG PET/CT performs favorably in accurately detecting disease recurrence.[83–87]

Hildebrandt and colleagues followed 100 women with suspected breast cancer recurrence who were prospectively evaluated with FDG PET/ CT, contrast-enhanced CT, and bone scan.[86] They found that FDG PET/CT resulted in no false negatives and fewer false positives than the other imaging techniques, and that the diagnostic accuracy of FDG PET/CT had higher sensitivity, specificity, and superior likelihood ratios when compared with contrast-enhanced CT with or without bone scintigraphy.[86] Radan and colleagues[83] retrospectively evaluated 46 patients who presented with elevated serum tumor markers and underwent FDG PET/CT. They calculated an overall sensitivity, specificity, and accuracy of FDG PET/CT in detecting recurrent breast cancer of 90%, 71%, and 83%, respectively, compared with 70%, 47%, and 59% using contrast-enhanced CT.[83] FDG PET/CT had an impact on the management of 24 (51%) of patients.[83]

Although the accuracy of results has been the primary focus of literature evaluating FDG PET/ CT in the diagnosis of recurrent breast cancer, Holm and colleagues[87] focused on the reproducibility of FDG PET/CT versus bone scintigraphy. They found that in 100 women with suspected recurrence of breast cancer who underwent whole-body bone scintigraphy and FDG PET/CT, the proportions of agreement between readers were 93% for bone recurrence with FDG PET/CT versus 47% for planar bone scintigraphy, suggesting improved reproducibility with FDG PET/CT.[87]

Additional reviews in this issue of PET Clinics will provide further data regarding 18F-FDG for staging, restaging, and evaluation of treatment response in patients with breast cancer (see David GROHEUX article, "Breast cancer systemic staging (comparison of CT, bone scan and FDG PET/CT),"; and Saima Muzah and colleagues' article, "Evaluation of treatment response in patients with breast cancer,").

18F-FLUCICLOVINE

Amino acids are an alternate energy source to glucose and amino acid metabolism is upregulated in multiple malignancies, including breast cancers.[53] Multiple amino acid radiotracers have been used to image breast cancer with unique strengths and weaknesses. In particular, 18F-fluciclovine (anti-1-amino-3-18F-fluorocyclobutane-1-carboxylic acid) has received attention because multiple investigators have demonstrated ILC demonstrates greater 18F-fluciclovine avidity than 18F-FDG avidity, which may be valuable because 18F-FDG avidity is typically lower in ILC.[21,22,88–90]

18F-Fluciclovine is a synthetic amino acid, which was developed at Emory University. It is a leucine analog, initially proposed for imaging brain malignancies but subsequently developed and FDA-approved for imaging prostate cancer.[91] In the breast, 18F-fluciclovine demonstrates markedly increased uptake in malignant breast lesions as compared with normal breast parenchyma and benign breast lesions.[92] Uptake of 18F-fluciclovine in breast cancers correlates with tumor grade, with higher grade tumors demonstrating greater uptake.[93] 18F-Fluciclovine PET has been used to evaluate breast cancer neoadjuvant therapy response, as changes in 18F-fluciclovine correlate with decreased tumor volume on pathologic condition.[94] Although 18F-FDG uptake is greater than 18F-fluciclovine uptake in IDC tumors, 18F-fluciclovine uptake has been shown to be greater than 18F-FDG uptake in ILC tumors.[92,93] This suggests different breast cancer histologic subtypes may emphases different metabolic pathways.

Most of these initial studies emphasized local breast and nodal disease. Critical will be determining efficacy of 18F-fluciclovine for extra-axillary nodal disease and distant metastases in patients with breast cancer, where 18F-FDG has demonstrated its greatest impact. Preclinical studies of 18F-fluciclovine have demonstrated success for the detection of osseous metastases.[95,96] A drawback for 18F-fluciclovine will be physiologic avidity in the liver, a common site of metastases in patients with breast cancer.

PET/MRI

PET/MRI is a developing area of research in patients with breast cancer. In a feasibility study, Pinker and colleagues showed that FDG PET/MRI provides high sensitivity for the primary breast tumor when several MRI and PET parameters are combined and may lead to a reduction in unnecessary breast biopsies.[97] For systemic staging, at about half the radiation dose compared with FDG PET/CT, FDG PET/MRI may have better sensitivity for liver and osseous metastases,[98–101] although FDG PET/CT may by superior for lung metastases.[98,101] Additional large prospective studies will be needed to fully explore the potential of FDG PET/MRI in patients with breast cancer.

SUMMARY

The avidity of breast cancer on FDG PET/CT is heavily influenced by biologic factors such as histologic subtype and receptor status. Although FDG PET/CT has limited utility in breast cancer screening, the incidental finding of focal breast uptake on FDG PET should be further evaluated with dedicated breast imaging due to a 30% to 40% likelihood of malignancy. FDG PET/CT has demonstrated excellent value in the evaluation of extra-axillary nodal and distant metastatic disease. In fact, in patients with clinical stage IIB–IIIC breast cancer, FDG PET/CT is superior in the evaluation of extra-axillary nodal and distant metastatic disease, with evidence of comparable overall costs between FDG PET/CT and conventional imaging.

FDG PET/CT can also be used to evaluate treatment response, with retrospective evidence that FDG PET/CT is more sensitive than conventional imaging in evaluating treatment response and can accurately predict pathologic complete response or nonresponse in the early-stage setting. In the metastatic setting, FDG PET/CT can be used to detect extent of disease and response to treatment, and thus help determine whether a patient should stay on a current treatment or switch to a new treatment if there is evidence of progression. Thus, FDG PET/CT affects the management of patients with breast cancer in several clinical scenarios.

Further studies, including randomized controlled trials using FDG PET/CT, PET/MR, and other metabolic agents such as fluciclovine, will be needed to optimize the use of imaging for patients with breast cancer.

DISCLOSURE

There are no relevant disclosures.

REFERENCES

1. Cancer Stat Facts: Female Breast Cancer. Available at: https://seer.cancer.gov/statfacts/html/breast.html.
2. Siegal R, Miller K, Wagle N, et al. Cancer statistics, 2023. CA: A cancer journal for clinicians 2023; 73(1):17–48.
3. Pauwels EK, Ribeiro MJ, Stoot JK, et al. FDG accumulation and tumor biology. Nucl Med Biol 1998; 25:317–22.
4. Lim HS, Yoon W, Chung TW, et al. FDG PET/CT for the detection and evaluation of breast diseases: usefulness and limitations. Radiographics 2007; 27:S197–213.
5. Love C, Tomas MB, Thonco GG, Palestro CJ. FDG PET of infection and inflammation. Radiographics 2005;25:1357–68.
6. Delbeke D, Coleman E, Guiberteau M, et al. Procedure guideline for tumor imaging with 18F-FDG PET/CT 1.0. J Nucl Med 2006;47(5):885–95.
7. Ulaner, PET/CT for patients with breast cancer: where is the clinical impact? Am J Roentgenol 2019;213:254–65.
8. Boellard, Standards for PET image acquisition and quantitative data analysis. J Nucl Med 2009;50: 11S–20S.
9. Lee MI, Jung YJ, Kim DI, et al. Prognostic value of SUVmax in breast cancer and comparative analysis of molecular subtypes: a systematic review and meta-analysis. Medicine 2021;100:31–7.
10. Kim KH, Ryu S, Lee HY, et al. Evaluating the tumor biology of lung adenocarcinoma: a multimodal analysis. Medicine 2019;98(29):e16313.

11. Watanabe R, Tomita N, Takeuchi K, et al. SUVmax in FED-PET at the biopsy site correlates with proliferation potential of tumor cells in non-Hodgkin lymphoma. Leuk Lymphoma 2010;51(2):279–83.

12. Li D, wang Y, liu W, et al. The correlation between ^{18}F-FDG PET/CT imaging SUVmax of preoperative colon cancer primary lesions and clinicopathological factors. Journal of Oncology 2021;2021:4312296.

13. Kitajima K, Suenega Y, Minamikawa T, et al. Clinical significance of SUVmax in 18F-FDG PET/CT scan for detecting nodal metastases in patients with oral squamous cell carcinoma. SpringerPlus 2015;4:718. https://doi.org/10.1186/s40064-015-1521-6.

14. Provenazo EUG, Chin SF. Molecular Classification of Breast Cancer. PET Clinics 2018;13(3):325–38.

15. Li C AB, Anderson BO, Daling J, et al. Trends in incidence rates of invasive lobular and ductal breast carcinoma. JAMA 2003;289(11):1421–4.

16. Viale G. The current state of breast cancer classification. Ann Oncol 2012;23:x207–10.

17. vant Veer LJ, Dai H, van de Vijver MJ, et al. Gene expression profiling predicts clinical outcome of breast cancer. Nature 2002;415(6871):530–6.

18. Groheux D, Hindie E. Breast cancer: initial workup and staging with FDG PET/CT. Clinical and Translational Imaging 2021;9:221–31.

19. Groheux D, Sylvia G, Moretti JL, et al. Correlation of high 18F-FDG uptake to clinical, pathological and biological prognostic factors in breast cancer. Eur J Nucl Med Mol Imag 2011;38:426–35.

20. Avril N, Mensel M, Dose J, et al. Glucose metabolism of breast cancer assessed by 18F-FDG PET: histologic and immunohistochemical tissue analysis. J Nucl Med 2001;42(1):9–16.

21. Hogan M, Goldman D, Dashevsky B, et al. Comparison of 18F-FDG PET/CT for systemic staging of newly diagnosed invasive lobular carcinoma versus invasive ductal carcinoma. J Nucl Med 2015;56(11):1674–80.

22. Dashevsky B, Goldman D, Parsons M, et al. Appearance of untreated bone metastases from breast cancer on FDG PET/CT: importance of histologic subtype. Eur J Nucl Med Mol Imag 2015;42(11):1666–73.

23. Ulaner G, Komal J, Chandarlapaty S, et al. Head-to-Head evaluation of 18F-FES and 18F-FDG PET/CT in metastatic invasive lobular breast cancer. J Nucl Med 2021;62(3):326–31.

24. de Mooij C, Mitea C, Mottaghy F, et al. Value of 18F-FDG PET/CT for predicting axillary pathologic complete response following neoadjuvant complete response following neoadjuvant systemic therapy in breast cancer patients: emphasis on breast cancer subtype. EJNMMI Res 2021;11(1):116–27.

25. Buck A, Holger S, Kuhn T, et al. FDG uptake in breast cancer: correlation with biological and clinical prognostic parameters. Eur J Nucl Med Mol Imag 2002;29:1317–23.

26. Adejolu M, Hue L, Rohren E, et al. False-positive lesions mimicking breast cancer on FDG PET and PET/CT. Am J Roentgenol 2012;198:W304–14.

27. Aarstad E, Nordhaug P, Nadhavi-Bezhad M, et al. Prevalence of focal incidental breast uptake on FDG-PET/CT and risk of malignancy: a systematic review and meta-analysis. European Journal of Hybrid Imaging 2019;3(1):16–28.

28. Korn R, Yost A, May C, et al. Unexpected focal hypermetabolic activity in the breast: significance in patients undergoing 18F-FDG PET/CT. Am J Roentgenol 2006;187:81–5.

29. Kang BJ, Lee J, Yoo IR, et al. Clinical significance of incidental finding of focal activity in the breast at 18F-FDG PET/CT. Am J Roentgenol 2010;197:341–7.

30. Zhu H, Dogan B. American Joint committee on cancer's staging system for breast cancer, eighth edition: summary for clinicians. European Journal of Breast Health 2021;17(3):234–8.

31. Gradishar WJ, Moran MS, Abraham J, et al. Breast Cancer, Version 3.2022, NCCN Clinical Practice Guidelines in Oncology. J Natl Compr Canc Netw 2022;20(6):691–722. https://doi.org/10.6004/jnccn.2022.0030.

32. Kasem J, Wazir U, Mokbel K. Sensitivity, Specificity and the diagnostic accuracy of PET/CT for axillary staging in patients with stage I-III cancer: a systematic review of the literature. In Vivo 2021;35:23–30.

33. Krag D, Weaver D, Ashikaga T, et al. The sentinel node in breast cancer: a multicenter validation study. N Engl J Med 1998;339(14):941–6.

34. Marino M, Avendano D, Zapata P, et al. Lymph node imaging in patients with primary breast cancer: concurrent diagnostic tools. Oncol 2020;25(1):e231–42.

35. Wahl R, Siegal B, Coleman E, et al. Prospective multicenter study of axillary nodal staging by positron emission tomography in breast cancer: a report of the staging breast cancer with PET study group. J Clin Oncol 2004;22(2):277–85.

36. Veronesi U, Cicco DC, Galimberti VE, et al. A comparitive study on the value of FDG-PET and sentinel node biopsy to identify occult axillary metastases. Ann Oncol 2007;18:473–8.

37. Brown A, Sweni S, Groves A, et al. The challenge of staging breast cancer with PET/CT in the era of COVID vaccination. Clin Nucl Med 2021;46(12):1006–10.

38. Groheux D, Giachetti S, Delord M, et al. 18F-FDG PET/CT in staging patients with locally advanced or inflammatory breast cancer: comparison to conventional staging. J Nucl Med 2013;54:5–11.

39. Ko H, Baghdadi Y, Love C, et al. Clinical utility of 18F-FDG PET/CT in staging localized breast cancer before initiating preoperative systemic therapy. J Natl Compr Cancer Netw 2020;18(9):1240–6.

40. Hyland CJ, Flora V, Yau C, et al. Use of 18F-FDG PET/CT as an initial staging procedure for stage II-III breast cancer: a multicenter value analysis. JNCCN 2020;18(11):1510–7.

41. Riedl C, Slobod E, Morrow M, et al. Retrospective analysis of 18F-FDG PET/CT for staging asymptomatic breast cancer patients younger than 40 years. J Nucl Med 2014;55(10):1578–83.

42. Han S, Choi J. Impact of 18F-FDG PET, PET/CT and PET/MRI on staging and management as an initial staging modality in breast cancer: a systematic review and meta-analysis. Clin Nucl Med 2021;46(4):271–82.

43. Patel MM, Le-Petross HT. Baseline FDG PET-CT imaging is necessary for newly diagnosed inflammatory breast cancer patients: a narrative review. Chin Clin Oncol 2021;10(6):56. https://doi.org/10.21037/cco-21-82.

44. Tran A, Pio BS, Khatibi B, et al. 18F-FDG PET for staging breast cancer in patients with inner-quadrant versus outer-quadrant tuors: comparison with long-term clinical outcome. J Nucl Med 2005;49(9):1455–9.

45. Jochelson M, Lizza L, Jacobs S, et al. Detection of internal mammary adenopathy in patients with breast cancer by PET/CT and MRI. Am J Roentgenol 2015;205(4):899–904.

46. Chakraborty D, Ulaner G, Alavi A, et al. Diagnostic role of fluorodeoxyglucose PET in breast cancer. Pet Clin 2018;13:355–61.

47. Ulaner G, Goldman D, Wills J, et al. 18F-FDG-PET/CT for systemic staging of newly diagnosed triple-negative breast cancer. Eur J Nucl Med Mol Imag 2016;43:1937–44.

48. Bhoriwal S, Dio SVS, Kumar R, et al. A prospective study comparing the role of 18 FDG PET-CT with contrast-enhanced computed tomography and Tc99m bone scan for staging locally advanced breast cancer. Indian Journal of Surgical Oncology 2021;12(2):266–71.

49. Hong S, Li J, Wang S. 18FDG PET-CT for diagnosis of distant metastases in breast cancer patients. A meta-analysis. Surgical Oncology 2013;22(2):139–43.

50. Ulaner G, Juarez J, Reidl C, et al. 18F-FDG PET/CT for systemic STaging of newly diagnosed breast cancer in men. J Nucl Med 2019;60(4):472–7.

51. Piciu A, Picio D, Polocoser N, et al. Diagnostic performance of F18-FDG PET/CT in male breast cancer patients. Diagnostics 2021;11:119–29.

52. Morris P, Lynch C, Feeney J, et al. Integrated positron emission tomography/computed tomography may render bone scintigraphy unnecessary to investigate suspected metastatic breast cancer. J Clin Oncol 2010;28(19):3154–9.

53. Ulaner G, Schuster DM. Amino acid metabolism as a target for breast cancer imaging. Pet Clin 2018;13(3):437–44.

54. Moo TA, Dang C, Morrow M. Overview of breast cancer therapy. Pet Clin 2018;13(3):339–54.

55. Hobar P, Jones RC, Schouten J, et al. Multimodality treatment of locally advanced breast carcinoma. Arch Surg 1988;123(8). 951-95.

56. Keam B, Im S, Koh Y, et al. Early metabolic response using FDG PET/CT and molecular phenotypes of breast cancer treated with neoadjuvant chemotherapy. BMC Cancer 2011;11(1):452–60.

57. Avril S, Muzic JR, Plecha D, et al. 18F-FDG PET/CT for monitoring of treatment response in breast cancer. J Nucl Med 2016;57:34S–9S.

58. Dose-Schwarz J, Bader M, Jenicke L, et al. Early prediction of response to chemotherapy in metastatic breast cancer using sequential 18F-FDG PET. J Nucl Med 2005;46(1):1144–50.

59. Han S, Choi J. Prognostic value of 18F-FDG PET and PET/CT for assessment of treatment response to neoadjuvant chemotherapy in breast cancer: a systematic review and meta-analysis. Breast Cancer Res 2020;22:119–34.

60. Lee IH, Lee S, Lee JY, et al. Utility of 18F-FDG PET/CT for predicting pathologic complete response in hormone receptor-positive, HER2-negative breast cancer patients receiving neoadjuvant chemotherapy. BMC Cancer 2020;20(1):1106–15.

61. Zhang FC, Xu HY, Liu JJ, et al. 18F-FDG PET/CT for the early prediction of the response rate and survival of patients with recurrent or metastatic breast cancer. Oncol Lett 2018;16(4):4151–8.

62. Luo J, Zhirui Z, Yang Z, et al. The value of 18F-FDG PET/CT imaging combined with pretherapeutic Ki67 for early prediction of pathologic response after neoadjuvant chemotherapy in locally advanced breast cancer. Medicine 2016;95(8):e2914–21.

63. Gebhart G, Gamez C, Holmes E, et al. 18F-FDG PET/CT for early prediction of response to neoadjuvant lapatinib, trastuzumab, and their combination in HER2-positive breast cancer: results from neoALITO. J Nucl Med 2013;54(1):1862–8.

64. de Cremoux P, Biard L, Poirot B, et al. 18FDG-PET/CT and molecular markers to predict response to neoadjuvant chemotherapy and outcome in HER2-negative advanced luminal breast cancer patients. Oncotarget 2018;9(23):16343–53.

65. Ogino K, Nakajima M, Kakuta M, et al. Utility of FDG-PET/CT in the evaluation of the response of locally advanced breast cancer to neoadjuvant chemotherapy. Int Surg 2014;99(4):309–18.

66. Groheux D, Martineau A, Teixeira L, et al. 18FDG-PET/CT for predicting the outcome in ER+/HER2- breast cancer patients: comparison of clinicopathological parameters and PET image-derived indices including tumor texture analysis. Breast Cancer Res 2017;19(1):3. https://doi.org/10.1186/s13058-016-0793-2.

67. Groheux D, Biard L, Giacchetti S, et al. 18F-FDG PET/CT for the early evaluation of response to neoadjuvant treatment in triple-negative breast cancer: influence of chemotherapy regimen. J Nucl Med 2016;57(4):536–43.

68. Rousseau C, Devillers A, Sagan C, et al. Monitoring of early response to neoadjuvant chemotherapy in stage II and III breast CAncer by 18F-flourodeoxyglucose positron emission tomography. J Clin Oncol 2006;24(34):5366–72.

69. Groheux D, Hindie E, Giacchetti S, et al. Triple-negative breast cancer: early assessment with 18F-FDG PET/CT during neoadjuvant chemotherapy identifies patients who are unlikely to achieve a pathologic complete response and are at a high risk of early relapse. J Nucl Med 2012; 53(1):249–54.

70. Champion L, Lerebors F, Alberini JL, et al. 18F-FDG PET/CT to predict response to neoadjuvant chemotherapy and prognosis in inflammatory breast cancer. J Nucl Med 2015;56(9):1315–21.

71. Sataloff DM, Mason B, Prestipino AJ, et al. Pathologic response to induction chemotherapy in locally advanced carcinoma of the breast: a determinant of outcome. J Am Coll Surg 1995;180(3): 297–306.

72. Humbert O, Alexander C, Coudert B, et al. Role of positron emission tomography for the monitoring of response to therapy in breast cancer. Oncol 2015; 20(1):94–104.

73. Hildebrandt M, Naghavi-Behzad M, Vogsen M. A role of FDG-PET/CT for response evaluation in metastatic breast cancer? Semin Nucl Med 2022; 52:520–30.

74. Riedl C, Pinker K, Ulaner G, et al. Comparison of FDG-PET/CT and contrast-enhanced CT for monitoring therapy response in patients with metastatic breast cancer. Eur J Nucl Med Mol Imag 2017; 44(9):1428–37.

75. Naghavi-Behzad M, Vogsen M, Vester R, et al. Response monitoring in metastatic breast cancer: a comparison of survival times between FDG-PET/CT and CE-CT. Br J Cancer 2022;126:1271–9.

76. Du Y, Illidge T, Ell P. Fusion of metabolic function and morphology: sequential [18F]fluorodeoxyglucose positron-emission tomography/computed tomography studies yield new insights into the natural history of bone metastases in breast cancer. J Clin Oncol 2007;25:3440–7.

77. Tateishi U, Gamez C, Dawood S, et al. Bone metastases in patients with metastatic breast cancer: morphologic and metabolic monitoring of response to systemic therapy with integrated response to systemic therapy with integrated PET/CT. Radiology 2008;247(1):189–96.

78. Al-Muqbel K, Yaghan R. Effectiveness of 18F-FDG-PET/CT vs bone scintigraphy in treatment reponse assessment of bone metastases in breast cancer. Medicine (Baltim) 2016;95:e3753.

79. Quon A, Gambhir SS. FDG-PET and beyond: molecular breast cancer imaging. J Clin Oncol 2005; 23:1664–73.

80. Mortimer JE, Dehdashi F, Siegel BA, et al. Metabolic flare: indicator of hormone responsiveness in advanced breast cancer. J Clin Oncol 2001;19: 2797–803.

81. Pinker K, Riedl C, Ong L, et al. The impact that number of analyzed metastatic breast cancer lesions has on response assessment by 18F-FDG PET/CT using PERCIST. J Nucl Med 2016;57:1102–4.

82. Khatcheressian J, Hurley P, Bantug E, et al. Breast cancer follow-up and management after primary treatment: American society of clinical oncology clinical practice guideline update. J Clin Oncol 2013;31:961–5.

83. Radan L, Simona BH, Bar-Shalom R, et al. The role of FDG-PET/CT in suspected recurrence of breast cancer. Cancer 2006;107(11):2545–51.

84. Pennant M, Takwoingi Y, Pennant L, et al. A systematic review of positron emmision tomography (PET) and postiron emission tomography/ computed tomography (PET/CT) for the diagnosis of breast cancer recurrence. Health Technol Assess 2010;14(50):1–103.

85. Xiao Y, Wand L, Jiang X, et al. Diagnostic efficacy of 18F-FDG-PET or PET/CT in breast cancer with suspected recurrence: a systematic review and meta-analysis. Nucl Med Commun 2016;37(11): 1180–8.

86. Hildebrandt M, Gerke O, Baun C, et al. 18F-FDG PET/CT in suspcted recurrent breast cancer: a prospective compartive study of dual-time-point FDG PET/CT, contrast-enhanced CT, and bone scintigraphy. J Clin Oncol 2016;34(16):1889–97.

87. Holm J, Farahani Z, Gerke O, et al. Higher interrater agreement of FDG-PET/CT than bone scintigraphy in diagnosing bone recurrent breast cancer. Diagnostics 2020;10(1):1021–9.

88. Avril N, Rose A, Schelling M, et al. Breast imaging with positron emission tomography and fluorine-18 fluorodeoxyglucose: use and limitations. J Clin Oncol 2000;18(20):3495–502.

89. Bos R, van der.Hoeven J, van Der Wall E, et al. Biologic correlates of (18)fluorodeoxyglucose uptake in human breast cancer measured by positron emission tomography. J Clin Oncol 2002;20(2): 379–87.

90. Lawal I, Atinuke O, Muzahir S, et al. A tale of 3 tracers: contrasting uptake patterns of 18F-fluciclovine, 69Ga-PSMA, and 18F-FDG in the uterus and adnexa. Clin Nucl Med 2023;48(1):e26–7.

91. Savir-Baruch B, Schuster D. Prostate cancer imaging with 18F-fluciclovine. Pet Clin 2022;17(4): 607–20.

92. Tade F, Cohen M, Styblo T, et al. Anti-3-18F-FACBC (18F-fluciclovine) PET/CT of breast cancer: an exploratory study. J Nucl Med 2016;57(9):1357–63.

93. Ulaner G, Goldman D, Gonen M, et al. Initial results of a prospective clinical trial of 18F-fluciclovine PET/CT in newly diagnosed invasive ductal and invasive lobular breast cancers. J Nucl Med 2016;57(9):1350–6.

94. Ulaner G, Goldman D, Corben A, et al. Prospective clinical trial of 18F-fluciclovine PET/CT for determining the response to neoadjuvant therapy in invasive ductal and invasive lobular breast cancers. J Nucl Med 2017;58(7):1037–42.

95. Oka S, Kanagawa M, Doi Y, et al. PET tracer 18F-fluciclovine can detect histologically proven bone metastatic lesions: a preclinical study in rat osteolytic and osteoblastic bone metastasis models. Theranostics 2017;7(7):2048–64.

96. Oka S, Kanagawa M, Doi Y, et al. Fasting enhances the contrast of bone metastatic lesions in 18F-Fluciclovine-PET: preclinical study using a rat model of mixed osteolytic/osteoblastic bone metastases. Int J Mol Sci 2017;18(5):934.

97. Pinker K, Bogner W, Baltzer P, et al. Improved differentiation of benign and malignant breast tumors with multiparametric 18Fluorodeoxygluce positron emission tomography magnetic resonance imaging: a feasibility study. Clin Cancer Res 2014;20:3540–9.

98. Melsaether A, Roy R, Pujara A, et al. Comparison of whole-body 18F-FDG PET/MR imaging and whole-body 18F-FDG PET/CT in terms of lesion detection and radiation dose in patients with breast cancer. Radiology 2016;281(1):193–202.

99. Bruckmann N, Kirchner J, Umutlu L, et al. Prospective comparison of the diagnostic accuracy of 18F-FDG PET/MRI, MRI, CT, and bone scintigraphy for the detection of bone metastases in the initial staging of primary breast cancer patients. Eur Radiol 2021;31:8714–24.

100. Catalano O, Nicolia E, Rosen B, et al. Comparison of CE-FDG-PET/CT with CE-FDG-PET/MR in the evaluation of osseous metastases in breast cancer patients. Br J Cancer 2015;112(1):1452–60.

101. Maarten de Mooij C, Sunen I, Mitea C, et al. Diagnostic Performance of PET/computed tomography versus PET/MRI and diffusion-weighted imaging in the N- and M- staging of breast cancer patients. Nucl Med Commun 2020;41:995–1004.

Molecular Breast Imaging and Positron Emission Mammography

Miral M. Patel, MD[a],*, Beatriz Elena Adrada, MD, FSBI[a],
Amy M. Fowler, MD, PhD, FSBI[b,c], Gaiane M. Rauch, MD, PhD, FSBI, FSABI[d,e]

KEYWORDS

- Molecular breast imaging • Breast Specific gamma imaging • Dedicated breast PET
- Positron emission mammography • FDG • ^{99m}Tc-sestamibi

KEY POINTS

- Molecular breast imaging (MBI) is a promising adjunct breast imaging modality for breast cancer screening, staging, treatment response evaluation and problem solving, with performance similar to breast MRI.
- Current effective dose for MBI performed with 240 to 300 MBq of ^{99m}Tc-sestamibi is 2 to 2.5 mSv and can be decreased to 1.2 mSv with administration of half-dose ^{99m}Tc-sestamibi (150 MBq) and use of image-processing software, making it comparable to an effective dose of 1.2 mSv for digital mammography combined with tomosynthesis.
- Breast-specific positron imaging systems provide higher sensitivity than whole-body positron emission tomography for breast cancer detection.

INTRODUCTION

Molecular imaging methods for evaluation of breast cancer have been investigated since the 1970s, when the first report was published about accumulation of the bone imaging radiopharmaceutical technetium 99m-methyl diphosphonate (Tc99m-MDP) in the primary breast cancer of patients imaged for metastatic disease.[1] Additional reports about avid uptake of the cardiac perfusion agent ^{99m}Tc-sestamibi in breast tumors followed in the 1980s and early 1990s,[2] and led to the development of scintimammography, a nuclear medicine method for breast cancer imaging. However, scintimammography utilized large field-of-view gamma cameras used for general nuclear medicine imaging resulting in poor spatial resolution with low sensitivity for nonpalpable lesions (30%–60%).[3]

New types of dedicated single- or dual-headed nuclear medicine breast imaging systems for single photon emitting radiotracers, jointly referred to as molecular breast imaging (MBI) systems, have been developed in recent years. Additionally, there has been emergence of dedicated breast-specific imaging systems for positron emitting radiopharmaceuticals: positron emission mammography (PEM) with detectors in mammographic configuration, and dedicated breast PET (dbPET) with detectors in ring configuration. These improvements in technology led to increased utilization of both single photon and coincidence detection dedicated

[a] Department of Breast Imaging, The University of Texas MD Anderson Cancer Center, 1515 Holcombe, CPB5.3208, Houston, TX 77030, USA; [b] Department of Radiology, Section of Breast Imaging and Intervention, University of Wisconsin – Madison, 600 Highland Avenue, Madison, WI 53792-3252, USA; [c] Department of Medical Physics, University of Wisconsin Carbone Cancer Center, University of Wisconsin-Madison, 600 Highland Avenue, Madison, WI 53792-3252, USA; [d] Department of Abdominal Imaging, The University of Texas MD Anderson Cancer Center, 1515 Holcombe, Unit 1473, Houston, TX 77030, USA; [e] Department of Breast Imaging, The University of Texas MD Anderson Cancer Center, 1515 Holcombe, Unit 1473, Houston, TX 77030, USA
* Corresponding author.
E-mail address: MPatel6@mdanderson.org

PET Clin 18 (2023) 487–501
https://doi.org/10.1016/j.cpet.2023.04.005
1556-8598/23/© 2023 Elsevier Inc. All rights reserved.

breast imaging systems. They have been shown to be useful for multiple indications, such as detection of mammographically occult breast cancer, breast cancer local staging, monitoring of the response to neoadjuvant systemic therapy, and evaluating indeterminate imaging findings visualized on conventional breast imaging.[4–8] The purpose of this article is to review the available dedicated breast-specific nuclear medicine imaging modalities and discuss their role in the diagnosis and management of breast cancer.

MOLECULAR BREAST IMAGING
Equipment and Procedure

There are 2 types of MBI-dedicated gamma camera systems currently available for breast imaging. The first-generation system on the market was a single-headed gamma camera with a sodium iodide or cesium iodide detector (Eve Clear Scan e680, SmartBreast, previously known as Dilon 6800, Dilon Technologies) commonly known as breast-specific gamma imaging (BSGI). Advances in technology led to introduction of dual-headed gamma cameras with cadmium zinc telluride semiconductor detectors, usually referred as MBI, that improved spatial resolution, lesion detection, and count sensitivity: LumaGem 3200s (CMR Naviscan, Carlsbad, CA, USA); and Eve Clear Scan e750 (SmartBreast, Pittsburgh, PA, USA).[9]

Recently published Society of Nuclear Medicine and Molecular Imaging (SNMMI)/European Association of Nuclear Medicine (EANM) Procedure Standard/Practice Guidelines and American College of Radiology (ACR) Practice Parameters describe MBI technique in detail.[10,11] Therefore, we provide a brief description of the procedure in this section. Fasting for at least 3 hours and having a warm blanket around their torso is advised to patients before proceeding with the intravenous injection of the radiotracer ^{99m}Tc-sestamibi. The goal is to decrease blood flow to the liver, and increase delivery of the radiotracer to the breast.[12] The dose of ^{99m}Tc-sestamibi initially used for MBI was 740 to 1100 MBq (20–30 mCi). However, equipment optimization allowed reduction of the administered dose to 240 to 300 MBq (6.5–8 mCi).[13] The image acquisition usually starts 5 to 10 minutes after radiotracer injection. During the imaging process, the patient sits comfortably with the breast gently immobilized between 2 gamma cameras for the MBI system, or a gamma camera and a paddle for the BSGI system. The images are obtained in standard mammographic views (craniocaudal and mediolateral oblique), with an acquisition time of 10 min/view, and a total imaging time for both breasts of 40 minutes.[10]

MBI interpretation is usually performed by a fellowship-trained breast radiologist with additional training in the evaluation of MBI. MBI images are reviewed together with available standard-of-care breast imaging, such as mammogram and ultrasound. Published MBI lexicon is used for interpretation and reporting of MBI.[14,15]

Biopsy

A suspicious MBI finding should be correlated with mammography and a second look ultrasound. If conventional breast imaging does not show a correlate for the MBI finding, MBI-guided biopsy is recommended. Before the development of the MBI biopsy device, the lack of MBI biopsy capability was a barrier to the integration of MBI into the breast imaging workflow.

Direct biopsy is available for Eve Clear Scan e680 (previously Dilon 6800, Dilon), has been approved by the US Food and Drug Adminstration for Eve Clear Scan e750 (formerly Discovery NM 750b, by GE) in 2016, and is in development for the LumaGem.[16] The MBI biopsy device uses the stereotactic principle for lesion localization. The ^{99m}Tc-sestamibi dose for MBI biopsy is recommended to be increased to 600 to 800 MBq to improve lesion conspicuity. No special precautions are needed for the personnel performing the MBI biopsy procedure or when the specimen is transported and subsequently analyzed. The ability to obtain a specimen to confirm lesion retrieval during the MBI-guided biopsy is one of the main advantages over breast MRI-guided biopsy. The second advantage is the lower cost of an MBI-guided biopsy ($1500) versus MRI-guided biopsy ($3500).[17] Additional advantages of MBI-guided biopsy are the lack of contraindications to MBI, a claustrophobic-free device with good patient tolerance. Limitations of MBI-guided biopsy are comparable to the stereotactic-guided biopsy related to lesion localization in the posterior and retroareolar regions.

Clinical Indications

Screening
Mammography is the accepted gold standard for breast cancer screening. However, it has limited sensitivity in patients with dense breast tissue. Approximately three-quarters of women younger than age 50 and over one-third of women age 50 and older have dense breast tissue.[18] The presence of dense breast tissue itself also confers a 1.2 to 2 times increased risk of developing breast cancer.[19] The overall sensitivity of digital mammography has been shown to be 84%[20]; however, clinical trials in women with dense breast tissue or

increased risk of breast cancer demonstrate the sensitivity of mammography to be reduced to as low as 25% to 50%.[21] Therefore, supplemental screening modalities are recommended in these patient populations which may consist of whole breast ultrasound, MRI, or MBI, with MRI historically considered the most sensitive examination available. Unlike mammography, MBI detection of breast cancer is not affected by tissue density[22] (**Fig. 1**).

Since 2011, there have been 3 studies evaluating MBI as a supplemental screening modality in women with dense breast tissue[4,23,24] and one study evaluating BSGI detecting mammographically occult breast cancer in women at increased lifetime risk of breast cancer[25] (**Table 1**). In the initial 2011 study by Rhodes and colleagues[4] evaluating the role of supplemental screening MBI in women with dense breast tissue, MBI demonstrated an incremental cancer detection rate of 7.5 cases per 1000 women screened compared to a cancer detection rate of 3.2 cases per 1000 for patient screening with mammography alone. The addition of MBI resulted in a sensitivity increase from 27% (mammography alone) to 91% (mammography and MBI). Specificity for combined mammography and MBI was 85%. A subsequent study was performed to evaluate supplemental screening with MBI in women with dense breast tissue utilizing a lower radiation dose and demonstrated similar results with an incremental CDR of 8.8 per 1000 and increase in sensitivity from 23.8% (mammography alone) to 90.5% (mammography and MBI).[23] The recall rate was noted to increase from 11% (mammography alone) to 17.6% (mammography and MBI).[23] The 2016 study by Shermis and colleagues[24] also demonstrated a similar incremental cancer detection rate of 7.7 per 1000. The first multicenter prospective ongoing trial, Density MATTERS (Molecular Breast Imaging and Tomosynthesis to Eliminate the Reservoir of Cancers, NCT03220893), compares breast cancer detection between screening with digital breast tomosynthesis (DBT) and DBT combined with MBI. Preliminary results from this trial demonstrate a similar increase in CDR with initial MBI screening showing incremental CDR of 9.3 per 1000.[26] With recent increased emphasis on detection of *clinically significant* breast cancer, it is important to note that in the 2015 study performed by Rhodes and colleagues,[23] 80% of cancers detected by MBI alone were invasive and 82% were node negative.

To date, one retrospective review of 849 patients evaluating the incremental increase in breast cancer detection amongst high-risk women undergoing BSGI has been performed.[25] BSGI demonstrated

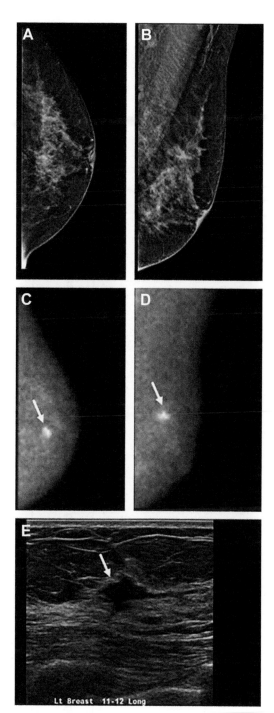

Fig. 1. A 48-year-old woman presents for routine screening. (*A, B*) CC and MLO views from screening mammogram examination demonstrate heterogeneously dense breast tissue, and the examination was read as negative. (*C, D*) CC and MLO views from subsequent MBI demonstrate 1.1 cm homogeneous mass uptake at 12:00 position 4.4 cm from the nipple (*arrow*). (*E*) US demonstrates a corresponding irregular, hypoechoic mass in the 11 to 12 o'clock position. US-guided biopsy was performed yielding invasive ductal carcinoma, low nuclear grade, ER+, PR–, HER2+.

Table 1
Molecular breast imaging and breast-specific gamma imaging performance in supplemental breast cancer screening

Study	Design	Total Enrolled	Incremental Cancer Detection Rate	Recall Rate	Sensitivity MBI		Specificity MBI		PPV1	PPV3
					MBI + Mammo		MBI + Mammo			
Rhodes et al,[4] 2011	Prospective, single academic institution	936 (dense breast)	7.5 per 1000 (7/936)	8%	82%	91%	93%	85%	12%	28%
Rhodes et al,[23] 2015	Prospective, single academic institution	1585 (dense breast)	8.8 per 1000 (14/1485)	7.5%	80%	91%	93%	83%	14.3%	33.3%
Brem et al,[25] 2016	Retrospective	849 (increased risk)	16.5 per 1000 (14/849)	25%	-	-	-	-	6.7%	14.4%
Shermis et al,[24] 2016	Retrospective, single community-based	1696 (dense breast)	7.7 per 1000 (13/1696)	8.4%	-	-	-	-	9.1%	19.4%
Maimone et al,[27] 2022	Retrospective, single institution	716 (dense breast + increased risk)	9.8 per 1000 (7/716)	13%	-	-	-	-	11.8%	27.5%

Data Source.[4,23–25]

an incremental cancer detection rate of 16.5 cancers per 1000 women screened. The most recent study published in 2022 evaluated 716 patients who underwent supplemental MBI examination for *either* dense breast tissue or increased lifetime risk and outcomes of abnormal MBI findings combining the 2 common indications for supplemental screening MBI. They reported high overall cancer detection rate of 15.4 per 1000, and 11.2 per 1000 for invasive cancers.[27]

Potential advantages for MBI compared to MRI as a supplemental screening modality include similar imaging projection to mammography (craniocaudal and mediolateral oblique views) facilitating comparison, faster interpretation time, claustrophobia-free modality, and safe in patients with renal disease, pacemakers, metallic implants, and gadolinium-based contrast agent allergies. Disadvantages include limited evaluation of lesions along the chest wall, potential difficulty with insurance coverage, and increased recall rates. An additional potential cited concern is radiation exposure which will be discussed further in subsequent sections.

Breast cancer staging

Staging of breast cancer routinely includes diagnostic mammography, ultrasound, and possibly breast MRI in certain clinical settings. The goal of complete local staging is detecting additional sites of malignancy within the ipsilateral breast or contralateral breast for accurate baseline evaluation of disease extent and surgical planning (**Fig. 2**). Although MRI demonstrates high sensitivity, it has moderate specificity and higher costs which may limit its use and lead to additional imaging evaluation and biopsies.

A meta-analysis of the use of breast MRI in staging of patients with breast cancer demonstrated that mammographically occult ipsilateral lesions were detected by MRI in 16% to 20% of women along with contralateral malignancies in 3% to 9% of women.[28] However, a high number of false positives associated with MRI require verification of MRI findings with tissue sampling which may result in treatment delays. In addition, certain patient populations including patients with claustrophobia, large body habitus, renal insufficiency, or implanted devices may not be able to undergo MRI. MBI can be especially useful for these patient populations.[29]

A 2019 prospective study compared staging of newly diagnosed breast cancer with 3 imaging modalities, MRI, contrast-enhanced mammography (CEM), and MBI. They found that all 3 modalities were effective in the local staging of breast cancer by demonstrating similar visualization of index cancers; however, MRI demonstrated a lower positive predictive value (PPV) for lesions undergoing biopsy compared to MBI and CEM (PPV MRI 28%, MBI 44%, CEM 52%).[30]

In a 2018 retrospective study published by Collarino and colleagues[6] of 287 women with biopsy-proven breast malignancy who underwent MBI for local staging, MBI detected larger tumor extent and/or additional sites of malignancy in 14% (40/287 patients). Previous studies have also demonstrated that MBI may be useful in detecting ipsilateral or contralateral malignancy with one series of 159 women with clinically suspicious breast lesions noted to have 6% additional ipsilateral foci and 5% contralateral foci detected by MBI.[31] Another study demonstrated that MBI detected larger extent of disease or additional ipsilateral of contralateral foci in 10.9% of subjects.[32]

Certain breast cancer subtypes are known to be better evaluated by MRI compared to routine staging examinations. For example, invasive lobular carcinoma (ILC) is more challenging to diagnose by mammography and ultrasound due to the infiltrative pattern of growth. For this reason, MRI is frequently used to evaluate extent of disease in patients with ILC due to its high sensitivity ranging from 77% to 100%.[33] In earlier studies, MBI has been reported to have a sensitivity of 89% to 93% and a specificity of 79% in diagnosis of ILC with Brem and colleagues[34] reporting the sensitivity of MBI to be higher than that of MRI (93% vs. 83%).[35] However, more recent studies have demonstrated limitations of MBI in detecting invasive lobular carcinoma with sensitivities for ILC noted to be 69% to 85%.[30,36] An additional limitation of MBI in staging of breast cancer is the limited ability to evaluate chest wall disease and evaluate axillary lymph nodes.

Response to neoadjuvant chemotherapy

Neoadjuvant chemotherapy (NAC; **Table 2**) is widely used in locally advanced breast cancer to reduce disease burden and potentially make a patient a candidate for breast conservation surgery as opposed to mastectomy. Imaging plays a key role by determining the baseline extent of disease, monitoring response to chemotherapy, and evaluation of residual disease after completion of therapy prior to surgery. Currently breast MRI is the primary imaging modality utilized with sensitivities for residual disease noted to be 86% to 92%, specificity 60% to 89%, and accuracy 76% to 90%.[7] MBI is a promising imaging modality for evaluation of residual disease after neoadjuvant treatment (**Fig. 3**).

A 2019 study by Hunt and colleagues[7] prospectively evaluated the accuracy of MBI and MRI to

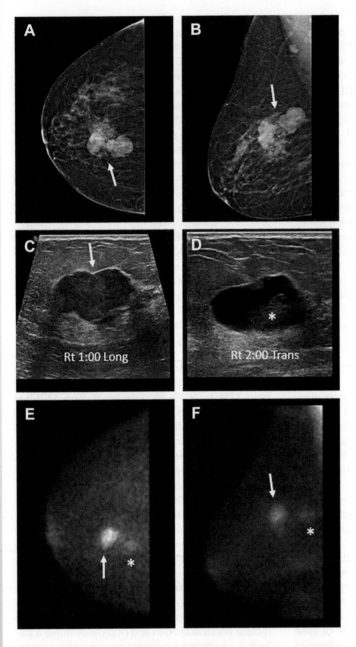

Fig. 2. A 60-year-old woman presenting with abnormal mammogram. (*A, B*) CC and MLO mammogram images demonstrate 2 adjacent masses in the upper inner quadrant of the right breast (*arrows*). (*C*) Longitudinal grayscale sonographic image demonstrates an irregular, hypoechoic mass in the right breast 1 o'clock position, 9 cm from nipple (*arrow*). Core biopsy demonstrated invasive ductal carcinoma with apocrine features, grade 2. (*D*) Transverse grayscale sonographic image demonstrates a circumscribed complex cystic and solid mass in the right breast 2 o'clock position, 12 cm from nipple. Associated increased color Doppler flow was noted in the hypoechoic component (*). Fine needle aspiration targeting the hypoechoic component demonstrated fibrocystic change versus intraductal papilloma. (*E, F*) CC and MLO MBI images demonstrate marked mass uptake in the mass at the 1 o'clock position, 9 cm from nipple (*arrow*) and moderate mass uptake in the mass at the 2 o'clock position, 12 cm from nipple (*). Given the uptake, US-guided core biopsy of the 2 o'clock position mass was recommended. Final pathology was invasive ductal carcinoma with apocrine features, grade 2.

evaluate for residual disease relative to final pathologic analysis. Although both imaging modalities in the study showed comparable measurements on baseline pre-treatment imaging, variability in prediction of residual disease post-treatment was noted with MRI demonstrating sensitivity 82.8%, specificity 69.4%, MBI sensitivity 58.9%, and specificity 82.4% and neither demonstrated high enough accuracy to replace the need to evaluate residual tumor burden on final surgical pathology specimen.

Another study by Kim and colleagues[37] in 2019 retrospectively evaluated BSGI and MRI to compare assessment of treatment response and noted similar sensitivities for both modalities (BSGI 70.2% and MRI 83.3%) with increased specificity for BSGI (BSGI 90% and MRI 60%).

A 2014 study by Lee and colleagues[38] retrospectively evaluated the performance of BSGI with MRI in the assessment of residual tumor after NAC. In the 122 patients evaluated, both modalities demonstrate similar sensitivity and specificity in residual tumor detection (MBI sensitivity and specificity 74%, 72.2% and MRI sensitivity and specificity 81.7%, 72.2%). However, there was variability in estimation of residual tumor size

Table 2
Molecular breast imaging/breast-specific gamma imaging versus MRI: evaluation of treatment response after neoadjuvant chemotherapy

Study	Patient Number	MBI Sensitivity	Specificity	MRI Sensitivity	Specificity
Lee et al,[38] 2014	122	74%	72.2%	81.7%	72.2%
Kim et al,[37] 2019	114	70.2%	90%	83.3%	60%
Hunt et al,[7] 2019	102	58.9%	82.4%	82.8%	69.4%

Data Source.[7,37,38]

based on the molecular subtype of breast cancer. Although relatively accurate measurements were noted for triple negative breast cancer, residual tumor size was underestimated by BSGI in luminal subtypes and by MRI in both luminal and HER2 subtypes.[38] Overall, no available breast imaging modality is capable of accurate evaluation of residual disease after NAC.

MBI may be utilized during NAC to predict non-responsiveness to chemotherapy. In a meta-analysis by Collarino and colleagues,[39] 3 studies investigated the ability of MBI to predict lack of response to chemotherapy before or early during NAC and demonstrated a sensitivity of 74% and a specificity of 92%. However, it was noted that there was heterogeneity amongst the study design and further investigation of MBI utilization for prediction of response was needed.[39]

Problem solving

Conventional imaging with mammogram and ultrasound is often adequate to render a final Breast Imaging Reporting and Data System (BI-RADS) category for work-up of clinical, mammographic, and ultrasound findings. In rare instances, advanced functional imaging is needed as a problem-solving imaging modality.[10,11] The role of MBI in this scenario is similar to breast MRI but at a lower cost.[40] MBI has been shown to be valuable in the resolution of complex clinical and imaging cases by mammography and ultrasound (Fig. 4). Siegal and colleagues[41] evaluated 416 patients in whom MBI was performed for problem solving of various findings including 56% for asymmetries, 14% for calcifications, 6% for mass, and 7% for evaluation of a palpable finding with negative mammography and ultrasound. A benign or negative BI-RADS was assigned in 70% of those patients helping with the resolution of the case. Sixty-eight cases (14%) resulted in biopsy. Of those, malignant pathology was present in 43%, high risk lesion in 15% and 42% were benign.[41] Only 2 cases out of 289 (0.07%) were false negatives in this study.

Weigert and colleagues[42] evaluated 1042 patients who underwent MBI for different indications. MBI was recommended in 38% of patients due to a mammographic abnormality such as asymmetry, subtle calcifications, discordant results between multiple studies, and in 11% of patients for a palpable mass with negative mammography. Comparison of the ultrasound versus MBI for workup of mammographic findings showed that MBI had higher sensitivity (80% vs. 70%), specificity (76% vs. 47%), PPV (53% vs. 32%), and negative predictive value (NPV; 92% vs. 81%) than ultrasound (US). For patients with negative or indeterminate mammographic findings, BSGI overall significantly increased detection of malignant and high-risk lesions. A retrospective study of 381 MBI results in patients with low suspicion mammographic or ultrasound findings showed the NPV of MBI to be 99.7% and false-negative rate (FNR) 2.7%, which resulted in 67.5% reduction in number of biopsies. The clinical application of the high NPV of MBI for problem solving requires further evaluation in larger patient populations.[8] Other scenarios where MBI is useful as a problem-solving imaging modality are patients with direct silicone injections, MRI incompatible implants, or with other contraindications for MRI. Approximately 15% of patients are unable to undergo breast MRI due to implantable devices, body habitus, renal insufficiency, contrast medium reaction, and claustrophobia.[40,43] MBI could be a viable option for these patients.

Radiation Dose Considerations

The misconception about the high radiation dose of MBI has been an impediment to the widespread acceptance of MBI as a breast imaging modality. The radiation dose varies among breast imaging modalities, and although the radiation during mammography is delivered directly to the breast, the ^{99m}Tc-sestamibi used for MBI is distributed systemically in the body with the highest radiation doses absorbed by the kidneys, colon, small intestine, and bladder and a smallest radiation dose to

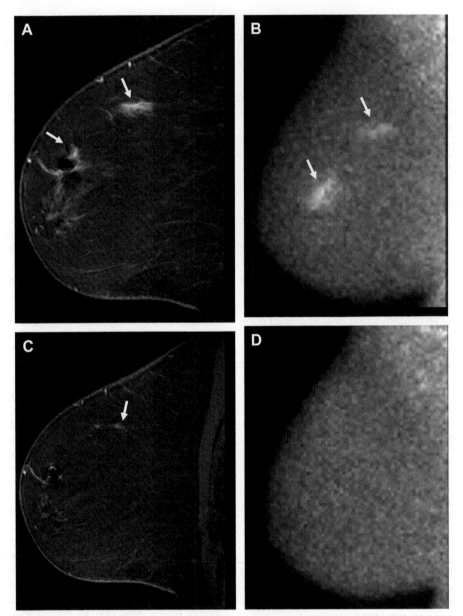

Fig. 3. A 60-year-old woman with multifocal invasive ductal breast cancer, low nuclear grade, ER-, PR-, and HER2-undergoing neoadjuvant chemotherapy. (*A*) Baseline post-contrast sagittal MR image demonstrates 2 irregular enhancing masses with associated susceptibility artifact from biopsy clips consistent with sites of biopsy-proven multifocal breast cancer. (*B*) Correlating multifocal uptake is noted on the MLO MBI image. (*C*) Post-neoadjuvant chemotherapy sagittal post-contrast MR image demonstrates residual linear non-mass enhancement (*arrow*) associated with the posterior site of biopsy-proven malignancy. (*D*) Post-neoadjuvant chemotherapy MLO MBI image demonstrates no residual uptake. Final surgical pathology demonstrated fibrosis with no invasive cancer.

the breast.[44] The effective dose equivalent, a metric reported in milliSieverts (mSv), is better suited to assess radiation to the organs and compare different imaging modalities.[45] Early gamma cameras used relatively high ^{99m}Tc-sestamibi doses of 740 to 1100 MBq (20–30 mCi), with effective doses of 5.9 to 9.4 mSv, which are above the background radiation level (3.1 mSv/y).

However, with recent equipment optimization, the ^{99m}Tc-sestamibi doses have decreased to 240 from 300 MBq (6.5–8 mCi), with an effective dose of MBI of 2 to 2.5 mSv, far lower than the background radiation level.[45] There are ongoing attempts to reduce the effective dose of MBI close to digital mammography. Tao and colleagues[46] developed an image processing algorithm which

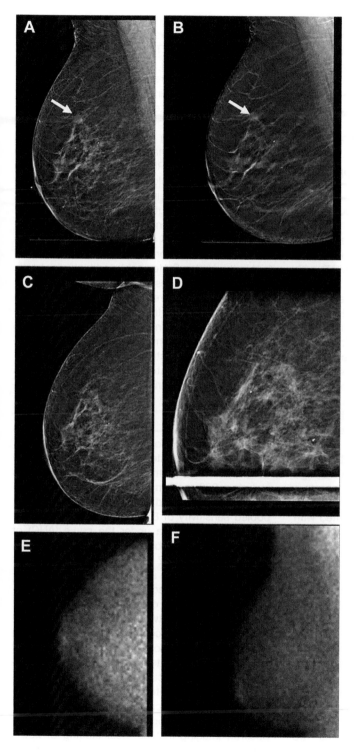

Fig. 4. A 75-year-old woman with history of left breast cancer. (*A, B*) MLO mammography 2D and 3D images demonstrate an asymmetry (*arrow*) in the superior region of the right breast. (*C, D*) Right LM and LM spot compression views demonstrate the asymmetry is not seen. Ultrasound was negative. Given her history of breast cancer, MBI was recommended for further evaluation. (*E, F*) CC and MLO MBI views show no suspicious uptake. The examination was given a BI-RADS 1: Negative for malignancy and the patient resumed annual mammogram. Subsequent mammogram follow-up (not shown) has been negative for 4 years.

provided acceptable quality MBI images with half-dose ^{99m}Tc-sestamibi (150 MBq). This resulted in an effective dose of 1.0 mSv, which is comparable to an effective dose from 2-view digital mammography combined with tomosynthesis (1.2 mSv).

The benefit-to-radiation risk ratio, defined as the ratio of estimated cancer death averted to the estimated radiation-caused cancer death per 100,000 women screened, has been shown to be lower for supplemental screening MBI than for screening mammography.[47] Brown and Covington[48] found that the benefit-to-risk ratio for MBI might overlap with mammography if variations in mammographic technique are accounted for (tomosynthesis-synthetic views, 2D full-field digital mammography), compression thickness, and age. They reported a further increase in the benefit-to-radiation risk ratio for MBI with ultra-low dose (150 MBq) of ^{99m}Tc-sestamibi as proposed by Tao and colleagues.[49]

POSITRON EMISSION MAMMOGRAPHY
Equipment and Procedure

The positron emitting radiopharmaceutical, 2-deoxy-2-[^{18}F]fluoro-D-glucose (FDG), is the most commonly used molecular imaging agent for breast cancer. Whole-body positron emission tomography/computed tomography (PET/CT) with FDG can be used clinically for initial systemic staging, restaging, and therapy response assessment for patients with breast cancer.[50] However, whole-body PET/CT is not recommended for primary breast cancer detection or for distinguishing benign from malignant breast lesions due to limited spatial resolution for subcentimeter lesions.[51,52] This technical limitation of whole-body scanners led to the development of dedicated breast imaging devices which bring the detectors closer to the breast for improved spatial resolution.[53]

There are 2 main designs for breast specific positron imaging systems.[3,54,55] The planar design consists of 2 opposing parallel planar detectors and has been termed positron emission mammography (PEM). For PEM, the patient is seated with the breast in mild compression with images acquired in the same views as conventional X-ray mammography. The other design uses a ring-shaped detector configuration in which the patient lies in the prone position. This design is typically referred to as dedicated breast PET (dbPET) and provides full tomographic images. The in plane spatial resolution of breast specific positron imaging systems is typically 1 to 2 mm compared to 4 to 6 mm with whole-body PET scanners which enables smaller lesion detection.

Clinical practice guidelines for the performance of high-resolution breast PET have been published by the Japanese Society of Nuclear Medicine.[56] As with whole-body FDG PET/CT, patients are instructed to fast for at least 4 to 6 hours. The intravenously injected activity of FDG is typically 10 mCi (370 MBq) for PEM and 3 to 5 mCi (111–185 MBq) for dbPET. Image acquisition typically begins 60 minutes after FDG injection or 90 minutes post-injection if dbPET is performed after whole-body PET. For PEM, craniocaudal and mediolateral oblique views of each breast are acquired for 10 minutes per view (40-minute total scan time). For dbPET, images are acquired for 5 to 7 minutes per ring position with the total scan time depending on breast length.

Standardized terminology has been developed to describe and interpret findings on breast-specific positron imaging.[57,58] The lexicon follows a similar organization as the American College of Radiology Breast Imaging Reporting and Data System for breast MRI.[59] Breast-specific positron imaging exams should be interpreted with other conventional breast imaging available, together with information about previous biopsy and treatment history. Experienced breast imaging radiologists who completed a 2-hour training module in PEM interpretation for a multi-institutional clinical trial in the Unites States achieved high diagnostic accuracy and interobserver agreement.[60]

An important feature of breast-specific positron imaging systems is the capability to biopsy lesions that may be only seen with PET. A PEM-guided biopsy system is commercially available that uses a stereotactic method for lesion targeting.[61–63] Biopsy systems for dbPET remain in technical development.[64]

Clinical Indications

The diagnostic performance of breast-specific positron imaging systems has been evaluated in several studies. A meta-analysis of 8 studies including 873 women with known or suspected breast cancer imaged with PEM found an overall pooled sensitivity of 85% and pooled specificity of 79% with an area under the curve (AUC) of 0.88.[65] In 2020, a subsequent meta-analysis of 5 studies including 722 women with breast cancer demonstrated better sensitivity, NPV, and accuracy of PEM compared to whole-body PET for primary breast cancer detection.[66] Specificity and PPV were similar between the 2 imaging modalities. For dbPET, recent large studies involving up to 938 women also found increased sensitivity for breast cancer detection compared to whole-body PET/CT, particularly for T1 stage tumors (<2 cm), subcentimeter tumors, lower grade tumors, and ductal carcinoma in situ.[67,68]

Potential clinical applications for breast-specific positron imaging include local staging of newly diagnosed breast cancer for surgical planning, evaluating neoadjuvant therapy response, and detecting local disease recurrence within the breast. For preoperative local staging, there have been 2 prospective studies comparing PEM with breast MRI.[5,69] Both studies showed that the sensitivity of PEM was comparable to breast MRI for detecting additional unsuspected cancers in the ipsilateral breast.[5,69] The specificity of PEM was comparable[69] or better[5] than breast MRI. For detection of residual disease after completion of neoadjuvant chemotherapy, PEM and dbPET have been shown to be more sensitive and more accurate than whole-body PET/CT.[70–72] As an early biomarker of therapy response, a decrease in FDG uptake on PEM after the first cycle of neoadjuvant chemotherapy has been shown to correlate with final pathologic response.[73] Thus, breast-specific positron imaging has similar clinical indications as breast MRI and may be a feasible alternative for patients who have contraindications for breast MRI.

In contrast to MBI, there is very limited literature regarding the use of breast-specific positron imaging as a supplemental screening modality for women with mammographically dense breasts or those with elevated lifetime risk of breast cancer. One study reported a 2.3% cancer detection rate using PEM in 265 women (165 without breast symptoms) participating in an FDG PET cancer screening program in Japan.[74]

Additional Considerations and Challenges

A barrier to the use of breast-specific positron imaging for supplemental breast cancer screening is the current radiation exposure associated with the examination (3.5 mSv effective dose equivalent from 185 MBq FDG).[56] Although this amount is comparable to natural background radiation and considered negligible risk, it is more than other breast imaging modalities, including MBI (2–2.5 mSv from 300 MBq ^{99m}Tc-sestamibi). Research efforts to reduce the radiation dose have shown clinically acceptable image quality using 25% injected FDG activity, which corresponds to a radiation dose of 0.9 mSv.[75,76]

There are additional technical and practical challenges with breast-specific positron imaging. These devices have inherently limited evaluation of the axilla and difficulty visualizing far posterior lesions near the chest wall, particularly with the prone design.[5,77,78] However, modifications to the imaging table have been shown to increase the amount of breast tissue in the field of view.[79,80] Furthermore, some indolent tumors may not have sufficient levels of glucose metabolism to be detected using FDG.[81]

SUMMARY

Recent advances in nuclear breast imaging technology with development of the dual-headed direct conversion gamma imaging systems and biopsy capability led to increased interest in this emerging nuclear medicine modality in the breast imaging community. There is a growing body of literature demonstrating similar performance of MBI in comparison with MRI for breast cancer screening, staging, treatment response assessment, and problem solving. Recently published ACR Practice Parameters and SNMMI/EANM Practice Guidelines, as well as ongoing efforts to reduce radiation dose, further support increased incorporation of MBI in the breast imaging practice. Breast-specific positron imaging systems are not widely used in clinical practice in the United States; however, there is growing clinical data published by international sites including Japan, Spain, and the Netherlands supporting its use for multiple indications. Further research is needed focused on the appropriate clinical applications for breast-specific positron imaging to provide impactful information to guide treatment decisions for patients with breast cancer. The use of radiopharmaceuticals beyond FDG may also expand the potential applications of this technology.[82,83]

CLINICS CARE POINTS

- MBI demonstrates increased incremental cancer detection rates when utilized as a supplemental screening modality in women with dense breast tissue or increased lifetime risk of breast cancer.

- MBI is a useful alternative in local staging for breast cancer demonstrating similar sensitivity to MRI and CEM and may play a role in predicting response to neoadjuvant chemotherapy.

- MBI may be used for problem-solving evaluation of mammographic asymmetries, subtle or multiple groups of calcifications, palpable findings with negative conventional imaging, discordant results between multiple studies and in patients with implants or direct silicone injections.

- Potential applications of breast-specific positron imaging are local staging, neoadjuvant treatment response evaluation, and detection of local disease recurrence in the breast.

DISCLOSURE

A.M. Fowler receives book chapter royalty from Elsevier, Inc and has served on an advisory board for GE Healthcare. The Department of Radiology at the University of Wisconsin School of Medicine and Public Health receives research support from

GE Healthcare. G.M. Rauch received research grant support from GE Healthcare.

ACKNOWLEDGMENTS

The authors acknowledge the University of Wisconsin Carbone Cancer Center Support Grant P30 CA014520 and the Department of Radiology, University of Wisconsin School of Medicine and Public Health for support. The authors acknowledge the National Institutes of Health/National Cancer Institute Cancer Center Support Grant P30 CA016672 and the Department of Breast Imaging, The University of Texas MD Anderson Cancer Center. The authors also acknowledge the work of many others that could not be discussed due to space limitations.

REFERENCES

1. Berg GR, Kalisher L, Osmond JD, et al. 99mTc-diphosphonate concentration in primary breast carcinoma. Radiology 1973;109(2):393–4.
2. Aktolun C, Bayhan H, Kir M. Clinical experience with Tc-99m MIBI imaging in patients with malignant tumors. Preliminary results and comparison with Tl-201. Clin Nucl Med 1992;17(3):171–6.
3. Hruska CB, O'Connor MK. Nuclear imaging of the breast: translating achievements in instrumentation into clinical use. Med Phys 2013;40(5):050901.
4. Rhodes DJ, Hruska CB, Phillips SW, et al. Dedicated dual-head gamma imaging for breast cancer screening in women with mammographically dense breasts. Radiology 2011;258(1):106–18.
5. Berg WA, Madsen KS, Schilling K, et al. Breast cancer: comparative effectiveness of positron emission mammography and MR imaging in presurgical planning for the ipsilateral breast. Radiology 2011;258(1):59–72.
6. Collarino A, Valdes Olmos RA, van Berkel L, et al. The clinical impact of molecular breast imaging in women with proven invasive breast cancer scheduled for breast-conserving surgery. Breast Cancer Res Treat 2018;169(3):513–22.
7. Hunt KN, Conners AL, Goetz MP, et al. Comparison of (99m)Tc-sestamibi molecular breast imaging and breast MRI in patients with invasive breast cancer receiving neoadjuvant chemotherapy. AJR Am J Roentgenol 2019;213(4):932–43.
8. Jain R, Katz DR, Kapoor AD. The clinical utility of a negative result at molecular breast imaging: initial proof of concept. Radiol Imaging Cancer 2020;2(5):e190096.
9. Hunt KN. Molecular breast imaging: a scientific review. Journal of Breast Imaging 2021;3(4):416–26.
10. Hruska CB, Corion C, de Geus-Oei L-F, et al. SNMMI procedure standard/EANM practice guideline for molecular breast imaging with dedicated γ-Cameras. J Nucl Med Technol 2022;50(2):103–10.
11. American College of Radiology. ACR practice parameter for the performance of molecular breast imaging (MBI) using a dedicated gamma camera. Available at: https://www.acr.org/-/media/ACR/Files/Practice-Parameters/MBI.pdf. Accessed January 24, 2023.
12. Swanson T, Tran TD, Ellingson L, et al. Best practices in molecular breast imaging: a guide for technologists. J Nucl Med Technol 2018. https://doi.org/10.2967/jnmt.117.204263.
13. Hruska CB, Weinmann AL, Tello Skjerseth CM, et al. Proof of concept for low-dose molecular breast imaging with a dual-head CZT gamma camera. Part II. Evaluation in patients. Med Phys 2012;39(6):3476–83.
14. Conners AL, Maxwell RW, Tortorelli CL, et al. Gamma camera breast imaging lexicon. AJR Am J Roentgenol 2012;199(6):W767–74.
15. Conners AL, Hruska CB, Tortorelli CL, et al. Lexicon for standardized interpretation of gamma camera molecular breast imaging: observer agreement and diagnostic accuracy. Eur J Nucl Med Mol Imaging 2012;39(6):971–82.
16. Hruska CB. Updates in molecular breast imaging. Semin Roentgenol 2022;57(2):134–8.
17. Adrada BE, Moseley T, Kappadath SC, et al. Molecular breast imaging-guided percutaneous biopsy of breast lesions: a new frontier on breast intervention. J Breast Imaging 2020;2(5):484–91.
18. Checka CM, Chun JE, Schnabel FR, et al. The relationship of mammographic density and age: implications for breast cancer screening. AJR Am J Roentgenol 2012;198(3):W292–5.
19. Sickles EA. The use of breast imaging to screen women at high risk for cancer. Radiol Clin North Am 2010;48(5):859–78.
20. Kerlikowske K, Hubbard RA, Miglioretti DL, et al. Comparative effectiveness of digital versus film-screen mammography in community practice in the United States: a cohort study. Ann Intern Med 2011;155(8):493–502.
21. Hruska CB. Molecular breast imaging for screening in dense breasts: state of the art and future directions. AJR Am J Roentgenol 2017;208(2):275–83.
22. Rechtman LR, Lenihan MJ, Lieberman JH, et al. Breast-specific gamma imaging for the detection of breast cancer in dense versus nondense breasts. AJR Am J Roentgenol 2014;202(2):293–8.
23. Rhodes DJ, Hruska CB, Conners AL, et al. Journal club: molecular breast imaging at reduced radiation dose for supplemental screening in mammographically dense breasts. AJR Am J Roentgenol 2015;204(2):241–51.
24. Shermis RB, Wilson KD, Doyle MT, et al. Supplemental breast cancer screening with molecular

breast imaging for women with dense breast tissue. AJR Am J Roentgenol 2016;207(2):450–7.

25. Brem RF, Ruda RC, Yang JL, et al. Breast-specific gamma-imaging for the detection of mammographically occult breast cancer in women at increased risk. J Nucl Med 2016;57(5):678–84.

26. Rhodes D, Hunt K, Conners A, et al. Abstract PD4-05: molecular breast imaging and tomosynthesis to eliminate the reservoir of undetected cancer in dense breasts: the Density MATTERS trial. Cancer Res 2019;79(4_Supplement). PD4-05-PD04-05.

27. Maimone S, Hatcher KM, Tavana A, et al. Downstream imaging following abnormal molecular breast imaging, lessons learned and suggestions for success. Clin Imaging 2022;92:44–51.

28. Plana MN, Carreira C, Muriel A, et al. Magnetic resonance imaging in the preoperative assessment of patients with primary breast cancer: systematic review of diagnostic accuracy and meta-analysis. Eur Radiol 2012;22(1):26–38.

29. Rauch GM, Adrada BE. Comparison of breast MR imaging with molecular breast imaging in breast cancer screening, diagnosis, staging, and treatment response evaluation. Magn Reson Imaging Clin N Am 2018;26(2):273–80.

30. Sumkin JH, Berg WA, Carter GJ, et al. Diagnostic performance of MRI, molecular breast imaging, and contrast-enhanced mammography in women with newly diagnosed breast cancer. Radiology 2019;293(3):531–40.

31. Brem RF, Shahan C, Rapleyea JA, et al. Detection of occult foci of breast cancer using breast-specific gamma imaging in women with one mammographic or clinically suspicious breast lesion. Acad Radiol 2010;17(6):735–43.

32. Zhou M, Johnson N, Gruner S, et al. Clinical utility of breast-specific gamma imaging for evaluating disease extent in the newly diagnosed breast cancer patient. Am J Surg 2009;197(2):159–63.

33. Mann RM. The effectiveness of MR imaging in the assessment of invasive lobular carcinoma of the breast. Magn Reson Imaging Clin N Am 2010; 18(2):259–76, ix.

34. Brem RF, Ioffe M, Rapelyea JA, et al. Invasive lobular carcinoma: detection with mammography, sonography, MRI, and breast-specific gamma imaging. AJR Am J Roentgenol 2009;192(2):379–83.

35. Kelley KA, Crawford JD, Thomas K, et al. A comparison of breast-specific gamma imaging of invasive lobular carcinomas and ductal carcinomas. JAMA Surg 2015;150(8):816–8.

36. Conners AL, Jones KN, Hruska CB, et al. Direct-conversion molecular breast imaging of invasive breast cancer: imaging features, extent of invasive disease, and comparison between invasive ductal and lobular histology. AJR Am J Roentgenol 2015; 205(3):W374–81.

37. Kim S, Plemmons J, Hoang K, et al. Breast-specific gamma imaging versus MRI: comparing the diagnostic performance in assessing treatment response after neoadjuvant chemotherapy in patients with breast cancer. AJR Am J Roentgenol 2019;212(3): 696–705.

38. Lee HS, Ko BS, Ahn SH, et al. Diagnostic performance of breast-specific gamma imaging in the assessment of residual tumor after neoadjuvant chemotherapy in breast cancer patients. Breast Cancer Res Treat 2014;145(1):91–100.

39. Collarino A, de Koster EJ, Valdes Olmos RA, et al. Is technetium-99m sestamibi imaging able to predict pathologic nonresponse to neoadjuvant chemotherapy in breast cancer? A meta-analysis evaluating current use and shortcomings. Clin Breast Cancer 2018;18(1):9–18.

40. Dibble EH, Hunt KN, Ehman EC, et al. Molecular breast imaging in clinical practice. AJR Am J Roentgenol 2020;215(2):277–84.

41. Siegal E, Angelakis E, Morris P, et al. Breast molecular imaging: a retrospective review of one institutions experience with this modality and analysis of its potential role in breast imaging decision making. Breast J 2012;18(2):111–7.

42. Weigert JM, Bertrand ML, Lanzkowsky L, et al. Results of a multicenter patient registry to determine the clinical impact of breast-specific gamma imaging, a molecular breast imaging technique. AJR Am J Roentgenol 2012;198(1):W69–75.

43. Huppe AI, Mehta AK, Brem RF. Molecular breast imaging: a comprehensive review. Semin Ultrasound CT MR 2018;39(1):60–9.

44. O'Connor MK, Li H, Rhodes DJ, et al. Comparison of radiation exposure and associated radiation-induced cancer risks from mammography and molecular imaging of the breast. Med Phys 2010;37(12):6187–98.

45. Hruska CB. Let's get real about molecular breast imaging and radiation risk. Radiol Imaging Cancer 2019;1(1):e190070.

46. Tao AT, Hruska CB, Conners AL, et al. Dose reduction in molecular breast imaging with a new image-processing algorithm. AJR Am J Roentgenol 2020; 214(1):185–93.

47. Hendrick RE, Tredennick T. Benefit to radiation risk of breast-specific gamma imaging compared with mammography in screening asymptomatic women with dense breasts. Radiology 2016;281(2):583–8.

48. Brown M, Covington MF. Comparative benefit-to-radiation risk ratio of molecular breast imaging, two-dimensional full-field digital mammography with and without tomosynthesis, and synthetic mammography with tomosynthesis. Radiol Imaging Cancer 2019; 1(1):e190005.

49. Covington MF, Brown M. Molecular breast imaging at ultra-low radiation dose. AJR Am J Roentgenol 2020;215(2):W30.

50. Fowler AM, Cho SY. PET imaging for breast cancer. Radiol Clin North Am 2021;59(5):725–35.

51. Kumar R, Chauhan A, Zhuang H, et al. Clinicopathologic factors associated with false negative FDG-PET in primary breast cancer. Breast Cancer Res Treat 2006;98(3):267–74.

52. Avril N, Rose CA, Schelling M, et al. Breast imaging with positron emission tomography and fluorine-18 fluorodeoxyglucose: use and limitations. J Clin Oncol 2000;18(20):3495–502.

53. Thompson CJ, Murthy K, Weinberg IN, et al. Feasibility study for positron emission mammography. Med Phys 1994;21(4):529–38.

54. Surti S. Radionuclide methods and instrumentation for breast cancer detection and diagnosis. Semin Nucl Med 2013;43(4):271–80.

55. Hsu DF, Freese DL, Levin CS. Breast-dedicated radionuclide imaging systems. J Nucl Med 2016;57(Suppl 1):40S–5S.

56. Satoh Y, Kawamoto M, Kubota K, et al. Clinical practice guidelines for high-resolution breast PET, 2019 edition. Ann Nucl Med 2021;35(3):406–14.

57. Narayanan D, Madsen KS, Kalinyak JE, et al. Interpretation of positron emission mammography: feature analysis and rates of malignancy. AJR Am J Roentgenol 2011;196(4):956–70.

58. Miyake KK, Kataoka M, Ishimori T, et al. A proposed dedicated breast PET lexicon: standardization of description and reporting of radiotracer uptake in the breast. Diagnostics 2021;11(7):1267.

59. Morris EA, Comstock C, Lee C, et al. ACR BI-RADS magnetic resonance imaging. In: ACR BI-RADS atlas, breast imaging reporting and data system. Reston (VA): American College of Radiology; 2013.

60. Narayanan D, Madsen KS, Kalinyak JE, et al. Interpretation of positron emission mammography and MRI by experienced breast imaging radiologists: performance and observer reproducibility. AJR Am J Roentgenol 2011;196(4):971–81.

61. Raylman RR, Majewski S, Weisenberger AG, et al. Positron emission mammography-guided breast biopsy. J Nucl Med 2001;42(6):960–6.

62. Kalinyak JE, Schilling K, Berg WA, et al. PET-guided breast biopsy. Breast J 2011;17(2):143–51.

63. Argus A, Mahoney MC. Positron emission mammography: diagnostic imaging and biopsy on the same day. AJR Am J Roentgenol 2014;202(1):216–22.

64. Hellingman D, Teixeira SC, Donswijk ML, et al. A novel semi-robotized device for high-precision (18)F-FDG-guided breast cancer biopsy. Rev Esp Med Nucl Imagen Mol 2017;36(3):158–65.

65. Caldarella C, Treglia G, Giordano A. Diagnostic performance of dedicated positron emission mammography using fluorine-18-fluorodeoxyglucose in women with suspicious breast lesions: a meta-analysis. Clin Breast Cancer 2014;14(4):241–8.

66. Keshavarz K, Jafari M, Lotfi F, et al. Positron Emission Mammography (PEM) in the diagnosis of breast cancer: a systematic review and economic evaluation. Med J Islam Repub Iran 2020;34:100.

67. Sueoka S, Sasada S, Masumoto N, et al. Performance of dedicated breast positron emission tomography in the detection of small and low-grade breast cancer. Breast Cancer Res Treat 2021;187(1):125–33.

68. Sasada S, Kimura Y, Masumoto N, et al. Breast cancer detection by dedicated breast positron emission tomography according to the World Health Organization classification of breast tumors. Eur J Surg Oncol 2021;47(7):1588–92.

69. Schilling K, Narayanan D, Kalinyak JE, et al. Positron emission mammography in breast cancer presurgical planning: comparisons with magnetic resonance imaging. Eur J Nucl Med Mol Imaging 2011;38(1):23–36.

70. Noritake M, Narui K, Kaneta T, et al. Evaluation of the response to breast cancer neoadjuvant chemotherapy using 18F-FDG positron emission mammography compared with whole-body 18F-FDG PET: a prospective observational study. Clin Nucl Med 2017;42(3):169–75.

71. Koyasu H, Goshima S, Noda Y, et al. The feasibility of dedicated breast PET for the assessment of residual tumor after neoadjuvant chemotherapy. Jpn J Radiol 2019;37(1):81–7.

72. Sasada S, Masumoto N, Goda N, et al. Dedicated breast PET for detecting residual disease after neoadjuvant chemotherapy in operable breast cancer: a prospective cohort study. Eur J Surg Oncol 2018;44(4):444–8.

73. Soldevilla-Gallardo I, Medina-Ornelas SS, Villarreal-Garza C, et al. Usefulness of positron emission mammography in the evaluation of response to neoadjuvant chemotherapy in patients with breast cancer. Am J Nucl Med Mol Imaging 2018;8(5):341–50.

74. Yamamoto Y, Tasaki Y, Kuwada Y, et al. A preliminary report of breast cancer screening by positron emission mammography. Ann Nucl Med 2016;30(2):130–7.

75. Satoh Y, Sekine T, Omiya Y, et al. Reduction of the fluorine-18-labeled fluorodeoxyglucose dose for clinically dedicated breast positron emission tomography. EJNMMI Phys 2019;6(1):21.

76. MacDonald LR, Hippe DS, Bender LC, et al. Positron emission mammography image interpretation for reduced image count levels. J Nucl Med 2016;57(3):348–54.

77. Teixeira SC, Rebolleda JF, Koolen BB, et al. Evaluation of a hanging-breast PET system for primary tumor visualization in patients with stage I-III breast cancer: comparison with standard PET/CT. AJR Am J Roentgenol 2016;206(6):1307–14.

78. Iima M, Nakamoto Y, Kanao S, et al. Clinical performance of 2 dedicated PET scanners for breast

imaging: initial evaluation. J Nucl Med 2012;53(10): 1534–42.

79. O'Connor MK, Tran TD, Swanson TN, et al. Improved visualization of breast tissue on a dedicated breast PET system through ergonomic redesign of the imaging table. EJNMMI Res 2017;7(1):100.

80. Hashimoto R, Akashi-Tanaka S, Watanabe C, et al. Diagnostic performance of dedicated breast positron emission tomography. Breast Cancer 2022; 29(6):1013–21.

81. Grana-Lopez L, Herranz M, Dominguez-Prado I, et al. Dedicated breast PET value to evaluate BI-RADS 4 breast lesions. Eur J Radiol 2018;108:201–7.

82. Jones EF, Ray KM, Li W, et al. Initial experience of dedicated breast PET imaging of ER+ breast cancers using [F-18]fluoroestradiol. NPJ Breast Cancer 2019;5:12.

83. Thakur ML, Zhang K, Berger A, et al. VPAC1 receptors for imaging breast cancer: a feasibility study. J Nucl Med 2013;54(7):1019–25.

Breast Cancer Systemic Staging (Comparison of Computed Tomography, Bone Scan, and 18F-Fluorodeoxyglucose PET/Computed Tomography)

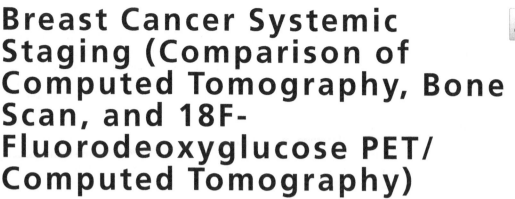

David Groheux, MD, PhD[a,b,c],*

KEYWORDS

- Breast cancer • FDG • PET/CT • CE-CT • Bone scan • Bone scintigraphy • Staging • Initial workup

KEY POINTS

- Computed tomography (CT) and 18F-fluorodeoxyglucose (FDG) PET/CT are not optimal for delineating primary tumor volume and assessing multifocality, and PET imaging is less efficient than the sentinel node biopsy to depict small axillary lymph node metastases.
- In large or locally advanced breast cancer, FDG PET/CT is useful to show lymph node involvement, especially outside of axillary level I or II (axillary level III, supraclavicular, or internal mammary chain adenopathy), which may have important implications for planned treatment.
- FDG PET/CT is more effective than bone scan and contrast-enhanced CT (CE-CT) in detecting bone and bone marrow metastases; FDG uptake is more variable in osteoblastic than in lytic or mixed metastases, and careful reading of CT data of PET/CT imaging may help detect them.
- FDG PET/CT is superior to conventional imaging techniques in detecting metastases (except for the brain) and synchronous lesions, and FDG PET/CT results in a change of treatment plan in nearly 15% of patients.
- The data support the assertion that FDG PET/CT should be used in patients with stage IIB–IIIC breast cancer; conventional imaging and CE-CT are less effective than PET/CT, especially with limited performance in patients with stage II disease.

INTRODUCTION

A lot of treatment weapons can be used in patients with breast cancer (BC): surgery, radiotherapy, chemotherapy, targeted therapy, and endocrine therapy. Treatment is tailored to the biological and histologic characteristics of the tumor and to the stage of the disease. Therefore, accurate initial workup is primordial for planning optimal treatment.[1]

Bone is the most common site of distant metastases, and whole-body planar bone scintigraphy has been a key to examination in the workup of BC.

Bone scintigraphy or bone scan (BS) historically consists in a planar whole-body acquisition [whole-body scintigraphy (WBS)]. WBS has been proved to have a high sensitivity in detecting metastasis. However, the tracer uptake not being tumor-specific, its specificity is quite low.[2] The advent of hybrid systems such as single photon

a Department of Nuclear Medicine, Saint-Louis Hospital, Paris, France; b University Paris-Diderot, INSERM U976, HIPI, Paris, France; c Centre d'Imagerie Radio-isotopique, La Rochelle, France
* Department of Nuclear Medicine, Saint-Louis Hospital, Assistance Publique-Hôpitaux de Paris, 1 avenue Claude Vellefaux, 75475 Paris Cedex 10, France.
E-mail address: dgroheux@yahoo.fr

PET Clin 18 (2023) 503–515
https://doi.org/10.1016/j.cpet.2023.04.006

emission tomography/computed tomography (SPECT/CT), has improved the performance of bone scanning.[3,4]

For the analysis of the thorax and the abdominal cavity, the thoraco-abdomino-pelvic contrast-enhanced computed tomography (CE-CT) has progressively replaced the chest X-ray and abdominal ultrasound pair. In addition to the advantage of combining 2 examinations in one, the CT scan was more efficient (especially the thoracic CT scan compared to the thoracic X-ray) and allowed a more complete analysis, for example, for the analysis of lymph nodes in the thorax.

In recent years, 18F-fluorodeoxyglucose positron emission tomography coupled with computed tomography (FDG PET/CT) has played an increasing role in the pretherapeutic staging of BC.[5-7] PET/CT has been shown to be highly accurate in detecting extra-axillary lymph nodes and distant metastases in locally advanced breast cancer (LABC) or inflammatory breast cancer (IBC)[8-14] and more recently in "intermediate risk" patients.[15-26]

The aim of this review is to evaluate the respective place of BS, thoraco-abdomino-pelvic CT, and PET/CT for the baseline staging of BC. The advantages and limitations of each technique are discussed.

TECHNICAL ASPECTS AND SPECIFICITIES OF BREAST CANCER IMAGING
Bone Scan, Computed Tomography, and 18F-Fluorodeoxyglucose PET/Computed Tomography Procedures

Whole-body planar BS is usually acquired 2 to 3 hours after injection of a technetium-labeled biphosphonate. This examination can be complemented by a SPECT/CT study for equivocal lesions, especially in the spine. Therefore, in most centers, the usual protocol for staging of bone metastases consists in a whole-body planar acquisition followed, if needed, by a targeted SPECT/CT to characterize suspicious or equivocal uptakes seen on WBS.[2] A systematic double-bed SPECT/CT of the trunk is an alternative but the added value of this strategy compared to the commonly used "WBS plus one single–bed targeted SPECT/CT" strategy is uncertain.[2]

With the advent of multidetector helicoidal CT, thoraco-abdomino-pelvic CE-CT is a quick examination, the longest time being most often the installation of the patient on the examination table. The images are recorded after the iodine injection (in the case of no contraindication), with the patient lying on her back.

PET/CT imaging usually starts 60 minutes after the intravenous injection of FDG. CT and PET data are acquired sequentially before being fused. Patients are imaged from base of skull to mid-thigh, except for specific situations. Imaging usually begins with CT acquisition. Questions remain as to whether the CT part of PET/CT should be performed as a contrast-enhanced full-dose diagnostic CT, or as a nonenhanced, low-dose CT, with additional focused segmental examination in case of inconclusive findings. Some technical constraints imposed by the PET component such as free breathing might limit the full diagnostic power of CT when performed as part of PET/CT imaging.[27]

Parameters Affecting 18F-Fluorodeoxyglucose PET/Computed Tomography Imaging in Patients with Breast Cancer

Because of partial volume effect and limited spatial resolution of the PET system, small tumor size is one of the parameters that most affect PET imaging. Modern whole-body PET systems typically have a reconstructed spatial resolution of almost 5 mm full width at half maximum, based on phantom measurements. However, detection depends not only on tumor size, but also on tumor-to-background ratio, on patients motion (respiration), and on the degree of tumor FDG avidity.[27]

FDG avidity is affected by biological characteristics of BC such as histologic subtype, proliferation, tumor grade, and hormone receptor status. FDG uptake is lower for invasive lobular carcinoma in comparison to invasive ductal carcinoma (invasive carcinoma of no specific subtype).[28] Ductal carcinoma in situ usually has lower uptake than invasive carcinomas. FDG uptake is weaker in low-proliferative tumors as assessed by the Ki67 index.[29-31] Low grade tumors have lower FDG uptake than grade 3 tumors.[28,31] In 74 patients with grade 1 to 2, estrogen receptor-positive (ER+) tumors, BC, FDG-PET findings resulted in inadequate staging in 22.9% of cases.[32] FDG avidity is lower in well-differentiated ER+ tumors than in ER– tumors and in progesterone receptor-positive (PR+) tumors than in PR– tumors.[28] FDG uptake is lower in luminal A tumors than in luminal B tumors.[33] Triple-negative tumors, that is, ER-, PR-, and having no overexpression of HER2 (ERBB2), have significantly higher standardized uptake value (SUV) values than other tumors.[28,34] High baseline SUV values of the primary tumor are associated with poorer survival, regardless of the BC subtype.[35]

BASELINE STAGING OF BREAST CANCER
Locoregional Staging

Primary tumor staging
The role of thoraco-abdomino-pelvic CT in determining the T score of the TNM classification

(Table 1) has not been well analyzed. CE-CT has better performances than CT without contrast enhancement. In 58 patients with BC, prior to breast conserving surgery, tumor was visible with CE-CT in 54 patients, doubtfully visible in 1 patient and not visible in 3 patients.[36] In comparison, performances of CT without contrast enhancement were 41, 6, and 7, respectively, for visible tumor, doubtfully visible tumor, and not visible tumor.[36] The sensitivity for tumor detection was better for CE-CT (95%) than for native CT (83%) ($P < 0.001$).[36] However, CE-CT lack performances for delineating primary tumor volume and assessing multifocality.

PET/CT has also some limitations in analyzing the primary BC tumor. Of 324 patients, 265 (81.8%) had focal uptake of FDG that corresponded with the cancerous lesion, and 21 (6.5%) had no FDG-avid findings. The remaining 38 patients had diffuse or nonspecific uptake of FDG.[37] PET is also less accurate than ultrasonography to detect primary breast tumor.[38] In 154 consecutive patients with biopsy-proven invasive BC, breast ultrasonography (USG) detected primary lesions in 153.[38] FDG PET/CT did not detect primary breast lesions in 16 (10.4%) patients. Out of 132 patients who were studied with breast MRI, the breast MRI did not detect primary breast lesions in 2 patients. The sensitivity of USG, MRI, and FDG PET/CT to detect primary breast tumor was 99.4%, 98.5%, and 89.6%, respectively. FDG PET/CT detected all primary breast lesions with the tumor size above 2 cm, but in 89 patients with a T1 lesion, FDG PET/CT detected only 73

(81.0%) primary breast lesions. When the differentiate T1 lesion was above 1 cm or below 1 cm, PET/CT detected 17 (70.8%) primary breast lesions below 1 cm and 56 (86.2%) primary breast lesion above 1 cm.[38] The postoperative histology revealed multifocal tumors in 40 cases out of 154 cases (26.0%). The sensitivity of breast USG, breast MRI, and FDG PET/CT in the detection of multiple lesions was 80.0%, 81.1%, and 12.5%, respectively, and the specificity was 92.1%, 86.3%, and 99.1%, respectively.[38]

Other studies showed that PET is less sensitive and accurate than MRI for delineating the primary tumor volume and assessing multifocality.[39,40] In a group of 40 women who underwent PET/CT and MRI,[40] MRI correctly assessed T classification in 77% and PET/CT in only 54% ($P = 0.001$). Because of the limited spatial resolution of WB PET systems, better performance is expected with PET/MRI,[41,42] as well as with high-resolution PEM imaging.[43]

In summary, CT and FDG PET/CT are not optimal for delineating primary tumor volume and assessing multifocality. USG and MRI offer greater sensitivity. There is not yet enough good data on breast-dedicated PEM and PET/MRI systems to conclude on their performance in assessing the primary tumor. Moreover, these techniques are not yet readily available in clinical routine.

Regional lymph nodes staging (axillary and extra-axillary lymph nodes staging)

There are 3 levels of axillary lymph nodes according to Berg's classification: level I, lateral to the pectoralis minor muscle; level II: posterior to the pectoralis minor muscle and level III, medial to the pectoralis minor muscle. In addition to the axilla, the breast can be drained by the supraclavicular lymphatic chain and by the internal mammary chain.[44] Lymph node dissection for BC is usually limited to levels I and II of the axillae.

CE-CT has limitations to predict lymph nodes involvement. In 235 patients with operable BC who underwent CE-CT before surgery, the size criterion of a short-axis diameter of more than 5 mm provided a sensitivity of 78%, a specificity of 75%, and an accuracy of 76% in predicting axillary lymph node (ALN) positive status.[45]

FDG PET/CT has also some limitations, especially in the case of small primary tumors. Because of partial volume effect, the sensitivity of PET is low for small lymph node metastases and micrometastases.[38,46–50] In 146 patients (51 with axilla metastases confirmed by the pathologic examination after axillary clearance), sensitivity and specificity to detect ALN metastases were respectively 41.2% and 93.7% for USG, 40.0% and 87.6% for MRI, and

Table 1
TNM stage grouping for breast cancer according to the AJCC Cancer Staging Manual[62,63]

AJCC	TNM			NCCN
Stage I	T1	N0	M0	Primary operable
Stage IIA	T0	N1	M0	breast cancer
	T1	N1	M0	
	T2	N0	M0	
Stage IIB	T2	N1	M0	
	T3	N0	M0	
Stage IIIA	T3	N1	M0	
	T0	N2	M0	Locally advanced
	T1	N2	M0	breast cancer
	T2	N2	M0	
	T3	N2	M0	
Stage IIIB	T4	N0	M0	
	T4	N1	M0	
	T4	N2	M0	
Stage IIIC	any T	N3	M0	
Stage IV	any T	any N	M1	Metastatic disease

37.3% and 95.8% for PET/CT.[38] FDG PET/CT did not detect any micrometastases.[38] In a multicenter study of 360 women with newly diagnosed invasive BC,[46] the mean sensitivity and specificity of PET for detection of axillary metastases were 61% and 80%, respectively[46]; 69.2% of primary tumor were clinical T1 BCs. In another study of 236 patients without palpable nodes, only 37% of positive sentinel nodes were detected by PET.[47]

In a meta-analysis of 19 studies (1729 patients), the sensitivity and specificity of PET to detect axillary involvement were 66% and 93%, respectively.[50] In another meta-analysis of 62 studies (10,374 patients), the sensitivity and specificity for detecting ALN metastases were, respectively, 51% and 100% for US, 83% and 85% for MRI, and 49% and 94% for PET.[51] For assessing axillary status, PET does not appear to be superior to ultrasound[52] or MRI.[53] PET/MRI may in the future outperform MRI in detecting lymph node involvement.[54,55]

However, in the staging of BC, FDG uptake by an axillary lymph node has a high positive predictive value of malignancy.[47,56,57] In 221 patients with T1-2N0 primary invasive BC who underwent breast-conserving surgery with sentinel lymph node biopsy ± ALN dissection, FDG PET/CT detected lymph node involvement with a sensitivity of 70% and a positive predictive value of 100%.[57] Inflammatory processes in the arm or shoulder, however, may decrease this positive predictive value. In particular, FDG uptake in axillary lymph nodes is typically seen within 10 days after COVID-19 vaccination.[58]

In summary, the spatial resolution of PET imaging is insufficient for depicting small axillary lymph node metastases, especially in the case of small primary tumor. FDG PET/CT is suboptimal compared with sentinel lymph node biopsy.[47] The case is different in large, advanced, or inflammatory breast tumor, especially to show lymph nodes involvement outside axillary level I or II.[8,11,20,44] The presence of FDG uptake suggestive of lymph node involvement at level III (infraclavicular area; Fig. 1) or in extra-axillary loco-regional nodes (supraclavicular area or internal mammary chain; Fig. 2) may have important implications in the management of surgery[59] and radiotherapy.[60,61] Lymph node involvement in the level III area, supraclavicular area, or internal mammary basin (in association with axillary involvement) is classified as N3 (stage IIIC) according to the AJCC classification (see Table 1).[62,63]

In the future, PET/MRI could also be of added value to detect locoregional lymph nodes in patients with newly diagnosed BC.[54,55] In 182 patients with BC, PET/MRI correctly detected significantly more nodal positive patients than MRI ($P < 0.0001$) and CT ($P < 0.0001$).[55] Subgroup analysis for different lymph node stations showed that PET/MRI detected significantly more lymph node metastases than MRI and CT in each location (axillary levels I–III, supraclavicular, mammary internal chain).[55]

Distant Staging

The presence, extent, and localization of distant metastases are key prognostic factors in patients with BC and play a central role in therapeutic decision making. The aim of the study from Mahner and colleagues,[64] published in 2008, was to compare the diagnostic performance of FDG PET (without hybrid CT images) with that of CT and conventional imaging including chest radiography, abdominal ultrasound, and BS. In a total of 119 consecutive patients (69 with newly diagnosed locally advanced disease and 50 with previous history of BC), sensitivity and specificity of imaging procedures to detect distant metastases were 43% and 98% for combined conventional imaging, 83% and 85% for CT, and 87% and 83%, for FDG PET, respectively.[64] In this preliminary work, the authors concluded that prospective studies were needed to determine whether FDG PET/CT could potentially replace the array of conventional imaging procedures.[64]

Several years later, in the study from Choi and colleagues,[38] encompassing a group of 154 consecutive patients with biopsy-proven invasive BC, the sensitivity and specificity in detecting distant metastasis were 61.5% and 99.2%, respectively, for conventional imaging and 100% and 96.4%, respectively, for FDG PET/CT.

Bone and bone marrow metastases

Bone is the most frequent site of metastases in patients with BC (see Fig. 2). In the study by Hahn and colleagues,[65] 29 consecutive women with histologically proven BC were assessed with BS and whole-body FDG PET/CT to detect bone metastases. A total of 132 lesions were detected on BS, FDG PET/CT, or both. According to the reference standard, 70/132 lesions (53%) were bone metastases, 59/132 lesions (45%) were benign, and 3 lesions (2%) remained unclear. The sensitivity of BS was 76% (53/70) compared to 96% (67/70) for FDG PET/CT. The specificity of BS and FDG PET/CT was 95% (56/59) and 92% (54/59), respectively.[65] The sensitivity was therefore lower for BS than for PET/CT, and the specificity was relatively close between the 2 imaging techniques.

In the study from van Es and colleagues,[66] baseline CE-CT, BS, and FDG PET for all patients included in the imaging patients for cancer drug selection - metastatic breast cancer (IMPACT-

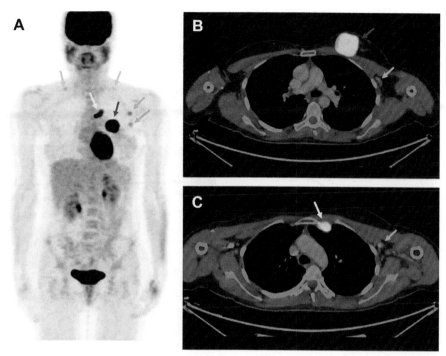

Fig. 1. A 50-year-old woman with newly diagnosed 32 mm metaplasic left breast infiltrating carcinoma, grade 3, ER–, PR–, HER2–, was referred for primary staging with FDG PET/CT (performed with contrast enhancement). The PET/CT MIP image shows the primary breast tumor (*red arrow*) and FDG foci in the axilla (*blue arrows*) and in the parasternal area (*yellow arrow*) (*A*). See also the faint FDG uptake in the supraclavicular area due to physiologic brown fat activation (*green arrows*) (*A*). Part B (fusion image, axial view) shows the primary lesion of the left breast with invasion of the pectoralis major muscle (*red arrow*) and a lymph node infiltration at level I of the axillary area (*blue arrow*). Part C (fusion image, axial view) shows another lymph node involvement of Berg's level I (*blue arrow*), and a large involvement of the internal mammary chain (*yellow arrow*). No distant metastases were seen. Following PET/CT, the disease was classified as T4 N3b M0 (stage IIIC).

MBC) study (NCT01957332) at the University Medical Center Groningen were reviewed for bone lesions. In total, 3473 unequivocal bone lesions were identified in 102 evaluated patients (39% by CE-CT, 26% by BS, and 87% by FDG PET). Additional bone lesions on FDG PET plus CE-CT compared with BS plus CE-CT led to change in MBC management recommendations in 16% of patients. BS also changed management compared with FDG PET in 1 patient (1%). In 26% of patients, an additional FDG PET examination was requested, because BS provided insufficient information.[66] In conclusion, in this exploratory analysis of newly diagnosed MBC patients, FDG PET versus BS to assess bone lesions resulted in clinically relevant management differences in 16% of patients. BS delivered insufficient information in over one-fourth of patients, resulting in an additional request for FDG PET. Based on these data, the authors stated that FDG PET should be considered a primary imaging modality for assessment of bone lesions in newly diagnosed MBC.[66]

Several other studies showed that BS is not useful when PET/CT is performed.[13,20,67] In particular, PET/CT was more sensitive and more specific than BS or CE-CT for detecting lytic or mixed bone metastases, or bone marrow involvement.[15,20,67] FDG uptake was more variable in osteoblastic metastases, and careful reading of CT data from PET/CT may help detect them.[44] In a study of 23 BC patients with bone metastases, PET/CT detected more lesions than BS (mean, 14.1 vs. 7.8 lesions, respectively, $P < 0.01$).[68] However, in the subgroup of patients with osteoblastic lesions, FDG PET/CT revealed fewer metastases than BS ($P < 0.05$). Higher SUV values were observed for osteolytic lesions compared to osteoblastic lesions (mean: 6.77 vs. 0.95, respectively, $P < 0.01$). Survival was lower in patients with osteolytic lesions than in those without ($P = 0.01$).[68] Similarly, osteoblastic lesions with no FDG uptake had a better prognosis.[68]

PET/MRI may also be of interest in the future to search for metastases in the primary staging of BC, and in particular to detect bone lesions.[54,69,70]

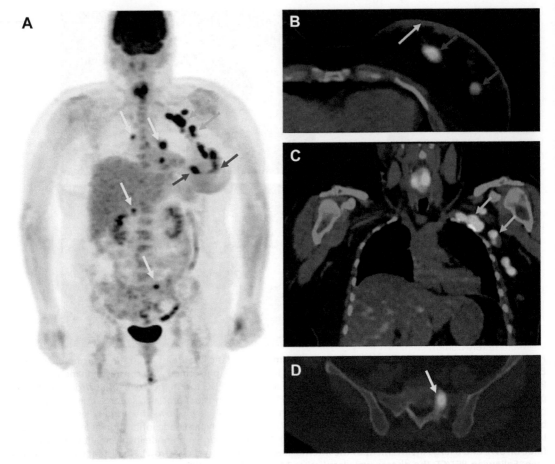

Fig. 2. A 43-year-old woman with newly diagnosed 30 mm nonspecific left breast infiltrating carcinoma, grade 2, ER+, PR+, HER2–, was referred for primary staging with FDG PET/CT. The PET/CT MIP image shows the multifocal primary breast cancer (*red arrows*) and FDG foci suggestive of regional adenopathy (*blue arrows*), as well as distant metastases (*yellow arrows*) (*A*). Part B (fusion image, axial view) shows 2 different foci of the primary lesion of the left breast (*red arrows*) with an inflammatory appearance of the breast skin (*green arrow*). Part C (fusion image, coronal view) shows an important lymph node involvement of Berg's level I, II, and III (*blue arrows*). Part D (fusion image, axial view) shows a bone metastasis of the sacrum (*yellow arrow*). Following PET/CT, the disease was classified as T4d N3a M1 (stage IV). Treatment was tailored to PET findings.

Of 154 patients with newly diagnosed BC, 7 (4,5%) had histopathologically bone metastases (41 lesions).[70] Both FDG PET/MRI and MRI alone were able to detect all of the patients with bone metastases (sensitivity 100%; specificity 100%) and did not miss any of the 41 malignant lesions (sensitivity 100%). CT detected 5/7 patients (sensitivity 71.4%; specificity 98.6%) and 23/41 lesions (sensitivity 56.1%). BS detected only 2/7 patients (sensitivity 28.6%) and 15/41 lesions (sensitivity 36.6%). Furthermore, CT and BS led to false-positive findings of bone metastases in 2 patients and in 1 patient, respectively. The sensitivity of PET/MRI and MRI alone was significantly better compared with CT ($P < 0.01$) and BS ($P < 0.01$).[70]

In summary, FDG PET/CT is more efficient than BS and CE-CT in detecting bone and bone marrow

metastases. FDG uptake is more variable in osteoblastic metastases than in lytic or mixed metastases, and careful reading of CT data from PET/CT may help detect them. PET/MRI may also be of interest in the future to search for bone metastases.

Extraskeletal distant metastases

PET/CT also performs well in detecting distant nodes, pleural, hepatic, splenic, adrenal, and pelvic metastases.[13–25] In 117 patients with LABC, we detected with PET/CT distant metastases in 43 patients (37%),[13] at the following sites: bone (n = 30), distant lymph nodes (n = 19), liver (n = 10), lungs (n = 6), and pleura (n = 2). The sensitivity and specificity of PET/CT were 100% and 97.7% for the diagnosis of bone lesions (compared with 76.7% and 94.2%, respectively, for planar BS); 100% and 99.1%, respectively, for the diagnosis of pleural metastases (vs. 50% and 100% for the dedicated CT); and 85.7% and 98.2%, respectively, for the diagnosis of pulmonary metastases (vs. 100% and 98.2% for dedicated chest CT). In this study, PET was therefore less sensitive than chest CT for the detection of small lung nodules, which could be explained by the partial volume effect and respiratory motion.[13] Regarding distant lymph node involvement, PET/CT allowed to detect supradiaphragmatic distant lymph nodes in 18 patients and infradiaphragmatic nodes in 4 patients.[13] Of the 117 patients, 10 had liver metastases. PET/CT demonstrated the 9 cases identified by abdominal CT and/or liver ultrasound and one additional patient.[13]

In another study, including 60 patients, the sensitivity and specificity of PET/CT to detect distant metastases were 100% and 98%, respectively (vs. 60% and 83% for conventional imaging).[16] PET/CT allowed to detect hepatic metastases in 2 patients.[16] The liver ultrasound showed suspicious lesions in 5 women, which were ultimately benign (3 angiomas and 2 cysts).[16]

In summary, hybrid PET/CT imaging is very effective in detecting occult distant metastases (except for the brain), with superior performances to conventional imaging.

Impact of tumor histologic and biological characteristics on the detection of metastases with 18f-fluorodeoxyglucose PET/computed tomography

FDG PET/CT has limited performance in staging lobular histologic type. Analysis of CT findings of the PET/CT images can help detect lesions with low or no FDG uptake.[71,72] In a study of 146 patients with infiltrating lobular carcinoma, PET/CT revealed distant metastases (confirmed by biopsy) in 12 cases; in 3 of these 12 patients, the metastases had no FDG uptake and were seen only on the CT component of the examination.[72]

In a prospective study of 254 patients, we investigated whether the number of metastases detected by PET/CT differed according to the grade or phenotypic subtype of the primary tumor.[20] The rates of extra-axillary lymph node metastases on FDG PET/CT were higher in grade 3 than in low grade tumors ($P = 0.004$) and in triple negative or HER2+ tumors compared to ER+/HER2- tumors ($P = 0.01$). However, the rate of distant metastases was not related to tumor grade or BC subtype,[20] which has also been found by other teams.[22,73] However, we observed that the location of metastases differed by primary tumor subtype; triple negative and HER2+ tumors had

more extraskeletal metastases than ER+/HER2- tumors.[20]

Impact of the Clinical Stage to Baseline Staging

In a meta-analysis of 29 studies (4276 patients) involving FDG PET, PET/CT, or PET/MRI, the pooled proportions of changes in stage and management were 25% and 18%, respectively. The proportion of changes increased with the clinical stage of BC.[74]

Patients with small tumor $\leq$ 2 cm (T1 of the TNM classification) are usually treated with primary surgery combined with sentinel node biopsy. PET has limited spatial resolution (approximately 5 mm) and, as discussed previously, its performance is inferior to that of the sentinel node biopsy.[50]

SUV_{max} values are lower in American Joint Commission on Cancer (AJCC) stage I than in higher stages.[75] In addition, the risk of distant metastases in T1 N0 disease (AJCC stage I) is very low and PET imaging may lead to false positive findings. In a multicenter study of 325 women with operable BC, FDG-PET (without a CT component) suggested distant metastases in 13 patients; only 3 (0.9%) were confirmed as metastatic disease and 10 (3.0%) were false positives.[48]

The situation is different in LABC and IBC.[8–14] According to the National Comprehensive Cancer Network (NCCN),[76] LABC corresponds to AJCC[63] stages IIIC, IIIB, and IIIA (except for T3N1 tumors). LABC have at least one of the following characteristics: T4 or N2 or N3[62,63,76] (see **Table 1**). IBC is classified T4d (at least stage IIB). A systematic review has shown that FDG PET/CT outperforms conventional imaging procedures for the detection of locoregional and distant metastases in the diagnostic workup of patients with IBC.[77] Several studies have also highlighted the role of FDG PET/CT in less advanced stages.[15–26]

In 254 patients classified as stage II or III (IIA, IIB, IIIA, IIIB, and IIIC) before FDG imaging, PET/CT resulted in a change in BC classification in 77 patients (30.3%).[20] It revealed unsuspected N3 disease (sub- or supraclavicular or internal mammary nodes) in 40 women and distant metastases in 53 women.[20] Distant metastases were detected in 2.3% (1/44) of patients with clinical stage IIA cancer; in 10.7% (6/56) patients with stage IIB; in 17.5% (11/63) patients with stage IIIA; in 36.5% (27/74) patients with stage IIIB and in 47.1% (8/17) patients with stage IIIC BC. Several other studies have also shown that PET/CT allows to detect metastases in a significant number of patients treated for clinical stage IIB BC or higher.[18,22,73,78] Performance in clinical stage IIA is less established. In the retrospective study by Lebon and colleagues,[79] distant metastases were detected by FDG PET/CT in 15% of stage IIB patients, and in 11% of stage IIA patients. In another retrospective study, however, PET/CT revealed distant disease in 9.8% of stage IIB patients with BC, but in only 0.8% of stage IIA patients.[80]

In a study of 196 patients with BC,[81] distant metastases were detected in 14% of patients (27/196), including 0% for stage IIA, 13% for stage IIB (10/79), 22% for stage IIIA (9/41), 17% for stage IIIB (5/30), and 37% for stage IIIC (3/8). The cost of PET/CT was comparable to that of conventional workup (based on CE-CT of the chest, abdomen, and pelvis + BS) and the radiation dose exposure was lower.[81] In another multicenter study, PET/CT baseline staging was compared to a staging by CE-CT plus BS, in 564 patients with clinical stage II–III BC (all included in the I-SPY2 trial).[82] In comparison to CE-CT plus BS modalities, FDG PET/CT reduced the risk of false positive by half (22.1% vs. 11.1%; $P = 0.0009$), and decreased work-up time for incidental findings, allowing earlier initiation of treatment. PET/CT was cost-effective and, at one institution, was shown to be cost-saving.[82]

In comparison, CE-CT has limited performance in stage II patients. In 483 patients with asymptomatic BC who underwent CE-CT, abnormal CE-CT findings, including true- and false-positive results, were detected in 65 patients (13.5%).[83] Of these, 26 patients (5.4%) showed confirmed true metastatic disease, including 18 lung metastases, 11 liver metastases, and 13 bone metastases. Upstaging to stage IV due to the results of the CE-CT scan occurred in 0 of 155 patients at stage I, 5 of 261 patients (1.9%) at stage II, and 21 of 67 patients (31.3%) at stage III.[83] The false-positive rates were 7.7%, 9.0%, and 8.7% in stages I, II, and III, respectively.[83]

In summary, data support the assertion that FDG PET/CT should be used in patients with stage IIB BC and higher. Conventional imaging and CE-CT are less efficient, especially with limited performances in stage II patients.

Impact of Imaging on Treatment Planning

In 103 women, 24 (23%) were diagnosed with distant metastases by FDG PET/CT.[84] Sensitivity and specificity for diagnosing distant metastases were 100% and 95%, respectively. On the basis of PET/CT findings, breast surgery was omitted in 18 patients and more extensive radiotherapy was performed in 16 patients.[84]

In another study of 81 patients with IBC who underwent FDG PET/CT and CE-CT prior to starting treatment, there were discordant findings in 41 patients (50.6%).[14] FDG PET/CT suggested modifications of the locoregional radiation therapy plan designed by CT alone in 15 patients and correctly characterized 5 of 7 findings equivocal for metastases on CE-CT.[14]

In 79 patients with LABC, PET/CT detected distant metastases in 36 (45.5%) patients, whereas conventional investigations (CI) (chest X-ray, abdominal sonography, and BS) could identify distant metastasis in 20 (25.3%) patients only.[85] Of the 36 patients in whom PET/CT detected distant metastases, 2 were false positive. Overall, PET/CT upstaged the disease in 38 (48.1%) patients as compared to CI: stage III to stage IV migration in 14 (17.7%) patients due to identification of additional sites of distant metastases, and within stage III upstaging in 24 (30.3%) patients due to identification of additional regional lymphadenopathy. PET/CT led to a change in management plan in 14 (17.7%) patients.[85]

In another study of 101 patients with BC, FDG PET/CT on initial staging was also compared to a CI algorithm, which included BS, chest X-ray and abdominal ultrasound.[23] PET/CT led to an upgrade of the N or M stage in overall 19 patients (19%). PET/CT findings caused a change in treatment of 11 patients (11%). The authors concluded that PET/CT has a relevant impact on initial staging and treatment of BC when compared to conventional modalities.[23]

In the study from Cochet and colleagues,[21] 142 patients with newly diagnosed BC (classification T2 and superior) were prospectively included. All patients were evaluated with complete conventional imaging procedures (mammogram and/or breast ultrasound, BS, abdominal ultrasound and/or CT, X-rays, and/or CT of the chest), followed by FDG PET/CT exploration, prior to treatment. According to CI staging, 79 patients (56%) were stage II, 46 (32%) stage III, and 17 (12%) stage IV (distant metastases). According to PET/CT findings, 30 patients (21%) were upstaged, whereas 23 (16%) were downstaged. PET/CT had a high or medium impact on management planning for 18 patients (13%). During a median follow-up of 30 months (range 9–59 months), 37 patients (26%) experienced recurrence or progression of disease and 17 (12%) died. CI staging was significantly associated with PFS ($P = 0.01$), but PET/CT staging provided stronger prognostic stratification ($P < 0.0001$). Moreover, Cox regression multivariate analysis showed that only PET/CT staging remained associated with PFS ($P < 0.0001$).

In the study from Koolen and colleagues,[19] FDG PET/CT was also superior to conventional imaging techniques in the detection of distant metastases in 154 patients with untreated stage II or III BC (sensitivity, specificity, and accuracy of PET/CT in the detection of additional distant lesions were 100%, 96%, and 97%, respectively). In 13 patients (8%), treatment was changed based on the FDG PET/CT findings; the radiation field was changed in 3 patients, an additional intervention due to synchronous tumors was performed in 4 (thyroidectomy, sigmoid resection, polypectomy, and ovariectomy), 3 patients underwent palliative radiotherapy for bone metastases, and 4 received palliative systemic therapy.

In the study from Riegger and colleagues,[86] an intravenous contrast-enhanced full-dose (CE-FD) whole-body FDG PET/CT scan was performed in 106 women. CE-FD FDG PET/CT had significantly better performances than conventional imaging to detect distances metastases (sensitivity = 75% vs. 50%, specificity = 97% vs. 98%, and accuracy = 93% vs. 90%; $P < 0.005$). CE-FD FDG PET/CT detected synchronous tumors in 3 patients (3%), including sigmoid colon cancer in 1 patient, rectal cancer in 1 patient, and an infracarinal lymph node metastasis from a bronchial carcinoma in 1 patient.[86] CE-FD FDG PET/CT findings leaded to change therapeutic management in 15 patients (14%).

In summary, FDG PET/CT is superior to conventional imaging techniques in detecting metastases and synchronous lesions, and FDG PET/CT findings lead to a change of treatment plan in nearly 15% of patients.

SUMMARY

CT and FDG PET/CT are not optimal for delineating primary tumor volume and assessing multifocality, and PET imaging is less efficient than the sentinel node biopsy to depict small axillary lymph node metastases. In large or locally advanced BC, FDG PET/CT is useful to detect lymph node involvement, especially extra-axillary adenopathy. FDG PET/CT is also more effective than BS and CE-CT in detecting bone and bone marrow metastases; FDG uptake is more variable in osteoblastic than in lytic or mixed metastases, and careful reading of CT data of PET/CT imaging may help detect them. FDG PET/CT is superior to conventional imaging techniques not only in detecting bone lesions but also in detecting extra-skeletal metastases (except for the brain) and synchronous lesions, and FDG PET/CT results in a change of treatment plan in nearly 15% of patients. Based on the available data, FDG PET/CT becomes useful for staging starting from clinical stage IIB. FDG PET/CT could be useful in patients with clinical stage IIA (T1N1 or T2N0),

but there is insufficient strong evidence to recommend routine use in this subgroup. In contrast, conventional imaging and CE-CT have limited performance in stage II patients. FDG PET/CT provides good results regardless of tumor phenotype (triple negative, luminal, or HER2+), but FDG uptake is higher in high-proliferative than in low-proliferative tumors, in high grade than in low grade tumors, in ER– than in well-differentiated ER+ tumors and FDG uptake is particularly high in triple-negative tumors. FDG uptake is lower for invasive lobular carcinoma in comparison to invasive ductal carcinoma (invasive carcinoma of no specific subtype).

CLINICS CARE POINTS

CT and FDG PET/CT are not optimal for delineating primary tumor volume and assessing multifocality. Breast MRI is more accurate

- Small lymph node axillary metastases and micrometastases are not well detected by PET and CT imaging. The sentinel node biopsy (SNB) is more efficient and FDG PET or CT imaging cannot replace the SNB procedure.
- FDG PET/CT is more effective than bone scan and CE-CT in detecting bone and bone marrow metastases. FDG uptake is more variable in osteoblastic than in lytic or mixed metastases, and careful reading of CT data of PET/CT imaging may help detect them.
- FDG PET/CT is the most efficient imaging modality to perform workup in patients with stage IIB-IIIC breast cancer. Bone scan and CE-CT are less effective.

DISCLOSURE

No conflict of interest.

REFERENCES

1. Groheux D. FDG-PET/CT for primary staging and detection of recurrence of breast cancer. Semin Nucl Med 2022;52(5):508–19.
2. Guezennec C, Keromnes N, Robin P, et al. Incremental diagnostic utility of systematic double-bed SPECT/CT for bone scintigraphy in initial staging of cancer patients. Cancer Imag 2017;17(1):16.
3. Palmedo H, Marx C, Ebert A, et al. Whole-body SPECT/CT for bone scintigraphy: diagnostic value and effect on patient management in oncological patients. Eur J Nucl Med Mol Imaging 2014;41(1):59–67.
4. Mavriopoulou E, Zampakis P, Smpiliri E, et al. Whole body bone SPET/CT can successfully replace the

conventional bone scan in breast cancer patients. A prospective study of 257 patients. Hell J Nucl Med 2018;21(2):125–33.

5. Salaün PY, Abgral R, Malard O, et al. [Update of the recommendations of good clinical practice for the use of PET in oncology]. Bull Cancer 2019;106(3): 262–74.

6. Salaün PY, Abgral R, Malard O, et al. Good clinical practice recommendations for the use of PET/CT in oncology. Eur J Nucl Med Mol Imaging 2020;47(1): 28–50.

7. Groheux D, Hindie E. Breast cancer: initial workup and staging with FDG PET/CT. Clin Transl Imaging 2021;1–11. https://doi.org/10.1007/s40336-021-00426-z.

8. Alberini JL, Lerebours F, Wartski M, et al. 18F-fluoro-deoxyglucose positron emission tomography/ computed tomography (FDG-PET/CT) imaging in the staging and prognosis of inflammatory breast cancer. Cancer 2009;115(21):5038–47.

9. Yang WT, Le-Petross HT, Macapinlac H, et al. Inflammatory breast cancer: PET/CT, MRI, mammography, and sonography findings. Breast Cancer Res Treat 2008;109(3):417–26.

10. van der Hoeven JJM, Krak NC, Hoekstra OS, et al. 18F-2-fluoro-2-deoxy-d-glucose positron emission tomography in staging of locally advanced breast cancer. J Clin Oncol 2004;22(7):1253–9.

11. Carkaci S, Macapinlac HA, Cristofanilli M, et al. Retrospective study of 18F-FDG PET/CT in the diagnosis of inflammatory breast cancer: preliminary data. J Nucl Med 2009;50(2):231–8.

12. Walker GV, Niikura N, Yang W, et al. Pretreatment staging positron emission tomography/computed tomography in patients with inflammatory breast cancer influences radiation treatment field designs. Int J Radiat Oncol Biol Phys 2012;83(5): 1381–6.

13. Groheux D, Giacchetti S, Delord M, et al. 18F-FDG PET/CT in staging patients with locally advanced or inflammatory breast cancer: comparison to conventional staging. J Nucl Med 2013;54(1):5–11.

14. Jacene HA, DiPiro PJ, Bellon J, et al. Discrepancy between FDG-PET/CT and contrast-enhanced CT in the staging of patients with inflammatory breast cancer: implications for treatment planning. Breast Cancer Res Treat 2020;181(2):383–90.

15. Groheux D, Moretti JL, Baillet G, et al. Effect of (18) F-FDG PET/CT imaging in patients with clinical Stage II and III breast cancer. Int J Radiat Oncol Biol Phys 2008;71(3):695–704.

16. Fuster D, Duch J, Paredes P, et al. Preoperative staging of large primary breast cancer with [18F]flu-orodeoxyglucose positron emission tomography/ computed tomography compared with conventional imaging procedures. J Clin Oncol 2008;26(29): 4746–51.

17. Aukema TS, Straver ME, Peeters MJTFDV, et al. Detection of extra-axillary lymph node involvement with FDG PET/CT in patients with stage II-III breast cancer. Eur J Cancer 2010;46(18):3205–10.

18. Segaert I, Mottaghy F, Ceyssens S, et al. Additional value of PET-CT in staging of clinical stage IIB and III breast cancer. Breast J 2010;16(6):617–24.

19. Koolen BB, Vrancken Peeters MJTFD, Aukema TS, et al. 18F-FDG PET/CT as a staging procedure in primary stage II and III breast cancer: comparison with conventional imaging techniques. Breast Cancer Res Treat 2012;131(1):117–26.

20. Groheux D, Hindié E, Delord M, et al. Prognostic impact of 18FDG-PET-CT findings in clinical stage III and IIB breast cancer. J Natl Cancer Inst 2012; 104(24):1879–87.

21. Cochet A, Dygai-Cochet I, Riedinger JM, et al. ^{18}F-FDG PET/CT provides powerful prognostic stratification in the primary staging of large breast cancer when compared with conventional explorations. Eur J Nucl Med Mol Imaging 2014;41(3): 428–37.

22. Riedl CC, Slobod E, Jochelson M, et al. Retrospective analysis of 18F-FDG PET/CT for staging asymptomatic breast cancer patients younger than 40 years. J Nucl Med 2014;55(10):1578–83.

23. Krammer J, Schnitzer A, Kaiser CG, et al. F-FDG PET/CT for initial staging in breast cancer patients - is there a relevant impact on treatment planning compared to conventional staging modalities? Eur Radiol 2015. https://doi.org/10.1007/s00330-015-3630-6. 18.

24. Groheux D, Giacchetti S, Espié M, et al. The Yield of 18F-FDG PET/CT in patients with clinical stage IIA, IIB, or IIIA breast cancer: a prospective study. J Nucl Med 2011;52(10):1526–34.

25. Jeong YJ, Kang DY, Yoon HJ, et al. Additional value of F-18 FDG PET/CT for initial staging in breast cancer with clinically negative axillary nodes. Breast Cancer Res Treat 2014;145(1):137–42.

26. Evangelista L, Cervino AR, Michieletto S, et al. Diagnostic and prognostic impact of fluorine-18-fluorodeoxyglucose PET/CT in preoperative and postoperative setting of breast cancer patients. Nucl Med Commun 2017;38(6):537–45.

27. Groheux D. Role of Fludeoxyglucose in breast cancer: treatment response. Pet Clin 2018;13(3): 395–414.

28. Groheux D, Giacchetti S, Moretti JL, et al. Correlation of high (18)F-FDG uptake to clinical, pathological and biological prognostic factors in breast cancer. Eur J Nucl Med Mol Imaging 2011;38(3): 426–35.

29. Buck A, Schirrmeister H, Kühn T, et al. FDG uptake in breast cancer: correlation with biological and clinical prognostic parameters. Eur J Nucl Med Mol Imaging 2002;29(10):1317–23.

30. Bos R, van Der Hoeven JJM, van Der Wall E, et al. Biologic correlates of (18)fluorodeoxyglucose uptake in human breast cancer measured by positron emission tomography. J Clin Oncol 2002;20(2):379–87.

31. Mohamadien NRA, Sayed MHM. Correlation between semiquantitative and volumetric 18F-FDG PET/computed tomography parameters and Ki-67 expression in breast cancer. Nucl Med Commun 2021;42(6):656–64.

32. Iqbal R, Mammatas LH, Aras T, et al. Diagnostic performance of [18F]FDG PET in staging Grade 1-2, estrogen receptor positive breast cancer. Diagnostics 2021;11(11):1954.

33. Humbert O, Berriolo-Riedinger A, Cochet A, et al. Prognostic relevance at 5 years of the early monitoring of neoadjuvant chemotherapy using (18)F-FDG PET in luminal HER2-negative breast cancer. Eur J Nucl Med Mol Imaging 2014;41(3):416–27.

34. Groheux D, Giacchetti S, Delord M, et al. Prognostic impact of 18F-FDG PET/CT staging and of pathological response to neoadjuvant chemotherapy in triple-negative breast cancer. Eur J Nucl Med Mol Imaging 2015;42(3):377–85.

35. Kitajima K, Miyoshi Y, Sekine T, et al. Harmonized pretreatment quantitative volume-based FDG-PET/CT parameters for prognosis of stage I-III breast cancer: multicenter study. Oncotarget 2021;12(2):95–105.

36. Boersma LJ, Hanbeukers B, Boetes C, et al. Is contrast enhancement required to visualize a known breast tumor in a pre-operative CT scan? Radiother Oncol 2011;100(2):271–5.

37. Davidson T, Shehade N, Nissan E, et al. PET/CT in breast cancer staging is useful for evaluation of axillary lymph node and distant metastases. Surg Oncol 2021;38:101567.

38. Choi YJ, Shin YD, Kang YH, et al. The effects of preoperative (18)F-FDG PET/CT in breast cancer patients in comparison to the conventional imaging study. J Breast Cancer 2012;15(4):441–8.

39. Uematsu T, Kasami M, Yuen S. Comparison of FDG PET and MRI for evaluating the tumor extent of breast cancer and the impact of FDG PET on the systemic staging and prognosis of patients who are candidates for breast-conserving therapy. Breast Cancer 2009;16(2):97–104.

40. Heusner TA, Kuemmel S, Umutlu L, et al. Breast cancer staging in a single session: whole-body PET/CT mammography. J Nucl Med 2008;49(8):1215–22.

41. Ming Y, Wu N, Qian T, et al. Progress and future Trends in PET/CT and PET/MRI Molecular imaging approaches for breast cancer. Front Oncol 2020;10:1301.

42. Taneja S, Jena A, Goel R, et al. Simultaneous whole-body (18)F-FDG PET-MRI in primary staging of breast cancer: a pilot study. Eur J Radiol 2014. https://doi.org/10.1016/j.ejrad.2014.09.008.

43. Caldarella C, Treglia G, Giordano A. Diagnostic performance of dedicated positron emission mammography using fluorine-18-fluorodeoxyglucose in women with suspicious breast lesions: a meta-analysis. Clin Breast Cancer 2014;14(4):241–8.

44. Groheux D, Espié M, Giacchetti S, et al. Performance of FDG PET/CT in the clinical management of breast cancer. Radiology 2013;266(2):388–405.

45. Shien T, Akashi-Tanaka S, Yoshida M, et al. Evaluation of axillary status in patients with breast cancer using thin-section CT. Int J Clin Oncol 2008;13(4):314–9.

46. Wahl RL, Siegel BA, Coleman RE, et al. Prospective multicenter study of axillary nodal staging by positron emission tomography in breast cancer: a report of the staging breast cancer with PET Study Group. J Clin Oncol 2004;22(2):277–85.

47. Veronesi U, De Cicco C, Galimberti VE, et al. A comparative study on the value of FDG-PET and sentinel node biopsy to identify occult axillary metastases. Ann Oncol 2007;18(3):473–8.

48. Pritchard KI, Julian JA, Holloway CMB, et al. Prospective study of 2-[18F]fluorodeoxyglucose positron emission tomography in the assessment of regional nodal spread of disease in patients with breast cancer: an Ontario clinical oncology group study. J Clin Oncol 2012;30(12):1274–9.

49. Hindié E, Groheux D, Brenot-Rossi I, et al. The sentinel node procedure in breast cancer: nuclear medicine as the starting point. J Nucl Med 2011;52(3):405–14.

50. Cooper KL, Harnan S, Meng Y, et al. Positron emission tomography (PET) for assessment of axillary lymph node status in early breast cancer: a systematic review and meta-analysis. Eur J Surg Oncol 2011;37(3):187–98.

51. Le Boulc'h M, Gilhodes J, Steinmeyer Z, et al. Pretherapeutic imaging for axillary staging in breast cancer: a systematic review and meta-analysis of ultrasound, MRI and FDG PET. J Clin Med 2021;10(7):1543.

52. Ueda S, Tsuda H, Asakawa H, et al. Utility of 18F-fluoro-deoxyglucose emission tomography/computed tomography fusion imaging (18F-FDG PET/CT) in combination with ultrasonography for axillary staging in primary breast cancer. BMC Cancer 2008;8:165.

53. Cooper KL, Meng Y, Harnan S, et al. Positron emission tomography (PET) and magnetic resonance imaging (MRI) for the assessment of axillary lymph node metastases in early breast cancer: systematic review and economic evaluation. Health Technol Assess 2011;15(4):iii–iv, 1-134.

54. Bruckmann NM, Kirchner J, Morawitz J, et al. Prospective comparison of CT and 18F-FDG PET/MRI in N and M staging of primary breast cancer patients: initial results. PLoS One 2021;16(12):e0260804.

55. Morawitz J, Bruckmann NM, Dietzel F, et al. Comparison of nodal staging between CT, MRI, and [18F]-FDG PET/MRI in patients with newly diagnosed breast cancer. Eur J Nucl Med Mol Imaging 2022; 49(3):992–1001.

56. Heusner TA, Kuemmel S, Hahn S, et al. Diagnostic value of full-dose FDG PET/CT for axillary lymph node staging in breast cancer patients. Eur J Nucl Med Mol Imaging 2009;36(10):1543–50.

57. Kong E, Choi J. The new perspective of PET/CT for axillary nodal staging in early breast cancer patients according to ACOSOG Z0011 trial PET/CT axillary staging according to Z0011. Nucl Med Commun 2021;42(12):1369–74.

58. Brown AH, Shah S, Groves AM, et al. The challenge of staging breast cancer with PET/CT in the Era of COVID vaccination. Clin Nucl Med 2021. https://doi.org/10.1097/RLU.0000000000003683.

59. Nikpayam M, Uzan C, Rivera S, et al. Impact of radical surgery on outcome in locally advanced breast cancer patients without metastasis at the time of diagnosis. Anticancer Res 2015;35(3):1729–34.

60. Borm KJ, Voppichler J, Düsberg M, et al. FDG/PET-CT-Based lymph node atlas in breast cancer patients. Int J Radiat Oncol Biol Phys 2019;103(3): 574–82.

61. Borm KJ, Oechsner M, Düsberg M, et al. Irradiation of regional lymph node areas in breast cancer - dose evaluation according to the Z0011, AMAROS, EORTC 10981-22023 and MA-20 field design. Radiother Oncol 2020;142:195–201.

62. Giuliano AE, Connolly JL, Edge SB, et al. Breast Cancer-Major changes in the American Joint Committee on Cancer eighth edition cancer staging manual. CA Cancer J Clin 2017;67(4):290–303.

63. Giuliano AE, Edge SB, Hortobagyi GN. Eighth edition of the AJCC cancer staging manual: breast cancer. Ann Surg Oncol 2018;25(7):1783–5.

64. Mahner S, Schirrmacher S, Brenner W, et al. Comparison between positron emission tomography using 2-[fluorine-18]fluoro-2-deoxy-D-glucose, conventional imaging and computed tomography for staging of breast cancer. Ann Oncol 2008;19(7):1249–54.

65. Hahn S, Heusner T, Kümmel S, et al. Comparison of FDG-PET/CT and bone scintigraphy for detection of bone metastases in breast cancer. Acta Radiol 2011;52(9):1009–14.

66. van Es SC, Velleman T, Elias SG, et al. Assessment of bone lesions with 18F-FDG PET compared with 99mTc bone scintigraphy leads to clinically relevant differences in metastatic breast cancer management. J Nucl Med 2021;62(2):177–83.

67. Morris PG, Lynch C, Feeney JN, et al. Integrated positron emission tomography/computed tomography may render bone scintigraphy unnecessary to investigate suspected metastatic breast cancer. J Clin Oncol 2010;28(19):3154–9.

68. Cook GJ, Houston S, Rubens R, et al. Detection of bone metastases in breast cancer by 18FDG PET: differing metabolic activity in osteoblastic and osteolytic lesions. J Clin Oncol 1998;16(10):3375–9.

69. Bruckmann NM, Morawitz J, Fendler WP, et al. A role of PET/MR in breast cancer? Semin Nucl Med 2022. https://doi.org/10.1053/j.semnuclmed.2022.01.003. S0001-2998(22)00003-4.

70. Bruckmann NM, Kirchner J, Umutlu L, et al. Prospective comparison of the diagnostic accuracy of 18F-FDG PET/MRI, MRI, CT, and bone scintigraphy for the detection of bone metastases in the initial staging of primary breast cancer patients. Eur Radiol 2021;31(11):8714–24.

71. Dashevsky BZ, Goldman DA, Parsons M, et al. Appearance of untreated bone metastases from breast cancer on FDG PET/CT: importance of histologic subtype. Eur J Nucl Med Mol Imaging 2015;42(11):1666–73.

72. Hogan MP, Goldman DA, Dashevsky B, et al. Comparison of 18F-FDG PET/CT for systemic staging of newly diagnosed invasive lobular carcinoma versus invasive ductal carcinoma. J Nucl Med 2015;56(11): 1674–80.

73. Ulaner GA, Castillo R, Wills J, et al. 18F-FDG-PET/CT for systemic staging of patients with newly diagnosed ER-positive and HER2-positive breast cancer. Eur J Nucl Med Mol Imaging 2017;44(9):1420–7.

74. Han S, Choi JY. Impact of 18F-FDG PET, PET/CT, and PET/MRI on staging and management as an initial staging modality in breast cancer: a systematic review and meta-analysis. Clin Nucl Med 2021;46(4):271–82.

75. Mori M, Fujioka T, Kubota K, et al. Relationship between prognostic stage in breast cancer and fluorine-18 fluorodeoxyglucose positron emission tomography/computed tomography. J Clin Med 2021; 10(14):3173.

76. NCCN Clinical Practice Guidelines in Oncology. Breast Cancer. Version 4. 2023. Available at: http://www.nccn.org/professionals/physician_gls/f_guidelines.asp. Accessed May 20, 2023.

77. van Uden DJP, Prins MW, Siesling S, et al. [18F]FDG PET/CT in the staging of inflammatory breast cancer: a systematic review. Crit Rev Oncol Hematol 2020;151:102943.

78. Ulaner GA, Castillo R, Goldman DA, et al. 18)F-FDG-PET/CT for systemic staging of newly diagnosed triple-negative breast cancer. Eur J Nucl Med Mol Imaging 2016;43(11):1937–44.

79. Lebon V, Alberini JL, Pierga JY, et al. Rate of distant metastases on 18F-FDG PET/CT at initial staging of breast cancer: comparison of women younger and older than 40 Years. J Nucl Med 2017;58(2):252–7.

80. Srour MK, Amersi F. Response to Letter to the Editor: "18FDG-PET/CT imaging in breast cancer patients with clinical stage IIB or higher. Ann Surg Oncol 2020;27(5):1710–1.

81. Ko H, Baghdadi Y, Love C, et al. Clinical utility of 18F-FDG PET/CT in staging localized breast cancer before initiating preoperative systemic therapy. J Natl Compr Canc Netw 2020;18(9): 1240–6.
82. Hyland CJ, Varghese F, Yau C, et al. Use of 18F-FDG PET/CT as an initial staging procedure for stage II-III breast cancer: a multicenter value analysis. J Natl Compr Canc Netw 2020;18(11):1510–7.
83. Tanaka S, Sato N, Fujioka H, et al. Use of contrast-enhanced computed tomography in clinical staging of asymptomatic breast cancer patients to detect asymptomatic distant metastases. Oncol Lett 2012; 3(4):772–6.

84. Vogsen M, Jensen JD, Christensen IY, et al. FDG-PET/CT in high-risk primary breast cancer-a prospective study of stage migration and clinical impact. Breast Cancer Res Treat 2020. https://doi.org/10.1007/s10549-020-05929-3.
85. Garg PK, Deo SVS, Kumar R, et al. Staging PET-CT scanning provides superior detection of lymph nodes and distant metastases than Traditional imaging in locally advanced breast cancer. World J Surg 2016;40(8):2036–42.
86. Riegger C, Herrmann J, Nagarajah J, et al. Whole-body FDG PET/CT is more accurate than conventional imaging for staging primary breast cancer patients. Eur J Nucl Med Mol Imaging 2012;39(5):852–63.

Evaluation of Treatment Response in Patients with Breast Cancer

Saima Muzahir, MD, FCPS, FRCPE[a,b,]*, Gary A. Ulaner, MD, PhD[c,d],
David M. Schuster, MD, FACR[b]

KEYWORDS

- Breast cancer • Treatment response • CT • MR imaging • FDG PET-CT • Bone scan

KEY POINTS

- In breast cancer, clinicopathologic stage and tumor biology guides the selection of appropriate imaging modalities for response assessment.
- For response monitoring FDG-PET/CT compared to CE-CT alone provides earlier detection of the first progression, leading to change or revision in treatment plans.
- FDG-PET/CT for response monitoring in patients with metastatic breast cancer may improve clinical decision-making and patient survival.

INTRODUCTION

Female breast cancer (BC) is one of the most diagnosed cancers and causes of cancer-related deaths in women, second only to lung cancer in Unites States. The American Cancer Society has estimated that 290,560 Americans will be diagnosed with BC and 43,780 will die of disease in the United States in 2022.[1] Management of BC not only depends on accurate diagnosis and staging but also on the best possible measures of response assessment. Imaging plays a vital role in the initial diagnosis and staging as well as in the response assessment to therapy, which is widely used to guide treatment decisions, although there are no specific recommendations for imaging procedures in the international metastatic breast cancer (MBC) guidelines.[2,3] In this review, we will analyze and compare the diagnostic accuracy and clinical utility of conventional and molecular imaging in the assessment of tumor response to therapy.

Locally Advanced Breast Cancer

In locally advanced BC, neoadjuvant chemotherapy (NAC) is now the standard of care.[4] The goal of NAC is to downstage primary tumors, to increase the rate of breast conservation, to eliminate micrometastatic disease, and to predict prognosis using tumor response as a parameter. Studies have shown that patients who attain pathological complete response (pCR) after NAC have a longer disease-free survival and better overall survival (OS) as compared with nonresponders.[5,6] Early and accurate assessment of response to therapy can help in making timely decisions regarding change in treatment to a more effective regimen, which can increase rates of breast conservation surgery.

NEOADJUVANT THERAPY RESPONSE ASSESSMENT

These can be broadly divided into anatomic imaging and functional imaging. Anatomic imaging

[a] Division of Nuclear Medicine and Molecular Imaging, Department of Radiology and Imaging Sciences, 1364 Clifton Road, Atlanta GA 30322, USA; [b] Division of Nuclear Medicine and Molecular Imaging, Department of Radiology and Imaging Sciences, Emory University Hospital, Room E152, 1364 Clifton Road, Atlanta, GA 30322, USA; [c] Molecular Imaging and Therapy, Hoag Family Cancer Institute, Newport Beach, CA, USA; [d] Radiology and Translational Genomics, University of Southern California, Los Angeles, CA, USA
* Corresponding author. Emory University Hospital, Division of Nuclear Medicine and Molecular Imaging, Department of Radiology and Imaging Sciences, 1364 Clifton Road, Atlanta GA 30322, USA
E-mail address: saima.muzahir@emory.edu

PET Clin 18 (2023) 517–530
https://doi.org/10.1016/j.cpet.2023.04.007
1556-8598/23/© 2023 Elsevier Inc. All rights reserved.

includes ultrasound (US), digital mammography (DM), and digital breast tomosynthesis (DBT). Functional imaging modalities include dynamic contrast-enhanced MR imaging, F-18 Fluoro-deoxyglucose positron emission tomography-computed tomography (F-18 FDG PET-CT), molecular breast imaging using 99mTc-sestamibi and newer hybrid PET-MR imaging. Currently there is lack of standard approach for the imaging evaluation and follow-up of patients undergoing NAC. According to the recent NCCN guidelines, a multidisciplinary approach should be used to determine the selection of different imaging methods before surgery.[7]

ANATOMIC IMAGING TECHNIQUES
Digital Mammography and Digital Breast Tomosynthesis

Mammography is the most used imaging modality to assess tumor size after NAC. However, the accuracy of mammography in assessing residual tumor size is highly influenced by the initial mammographic appearance of the tumor. The accuracy of mammography is higher for masses with well-circumscribed margins on pretreatment mammography compared with masses with ill-defined margins.[4] Decreases in tumor size and density are the most reliable indicators of treatment response, whereas changes in calcifications can be misleading and are considered one of the challenges in image interpretation.[8] Mammography is more sensitive than clinical examination (79% vs 49%) in the prediction of residual carcinoma; it is however not accurate enough to obviate surgical biopsy.[9] DBT has higher resolution compared with conventional DM particularly in small lesions and dense breasts.[10] It is more accurate than DM in assessing response and has a good correlation with histopathology for residual tumor size after NAC.[11] Yet, there still may be limitations related to overestimation of tumor size on DBT compared with DM.[8]

Ultrasound

US is a widely used modality in assessing response to NAC and is more accurate than mammography in assessing residual tumor size after NAC.[12,13] However, there is no difference between mammography and US in predicting complete pathologic response.[12] Several studies showed that the combined use of both mammography and US improved the accuracy of predicting a pCR to NAC compared with the use of either modality alone.[14,15] Automated breast US (ABUS) using three-dimensional images featuring high reproducibility and less operator dependence allows more appropriate evaluation of large breast

masses and architectural distortion compared with conventional breast US.[16] However, ABUS tends to underestimate residual tumor size resulting in lowest reliability compared with DM, DBT, and MR imaging.[8] US is also considered the most accurate predictor of response in axillary lymph nodes compared with mammography and physical examination.[17]

MR Imaging

MR imaging performs well in dense breasts and is the most sensitive imaging modality for detecting multifocality and monitoring patient response to NAC.[18,19] It outperforms mammography, US, and clinical examination in evaluating residual tumor after NAC with excellent correlation between macroscopic tumor size and the tumor established by MR imaging.[8] It remains as the most accurate imaging modality for NAC response assessment,[18] accurately assessing residual tumor after NAC with high sensitivity, specificity, and accuracy.[20] The multicenter American College of Radiology Imaging Network (ACRIN) 6657 study showed that not only functional tumor volume measurements are more accurate in predicting response but may also help in predicting recurrence-free survival.[21] Multiple studies using radiomic and deep learning have looked at predicting pCR from pretreatment MR images have found that separating tumors into their subtypes improves accuracy and that different features are predictive of response to therapy in different tumor subtypes.[22] MR imaging however has limited utility and can underestimate residual disease in tumors with nonmass morphology such as invasive lobular cancer and luminal tumors.[23,24] MR tends to overestimate response with taxane-based NAC.[25]

F-18 Fluorodeoxyglucose PET-CT

F-18 FDG evaluates glucose metabolism in BC cells, independent of breast density.[26] Decreased glucose metabolism within BC tissue on F-18 FDG PET-CT is a useful indicator to assess the effectiveness of NAC[27] and can provide information on tumor metabolic activity, which can help in distinguishing active tumor from posttherapeutic changes[28](Fig. 1). It is important to have knowledge about different BC histologic types because different histologic types vary in their FDG avidity and pattern of spread and key outcomes such as pathologic response and survival may vary by BC subtypes and type of treatment.[29,30] Estrogen receptor (ER)-negative tumors have statistically significantly higher FDG avidity compared with ER-positive tumors.[28,29] High-grade (grade 3) tumors have significantly higher FDG uptake than

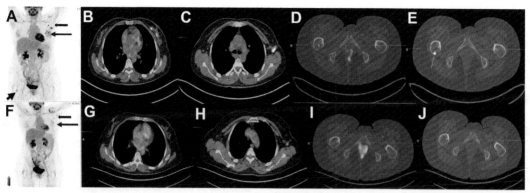

Fig. 1. A 50-year-old woman diagnosed with left breast ER-positive, HER-2-negative invasive ductal BC. (A) MIP image: Baseline FDG PET shows FDG avid multifocal left BC (*long black arrow*) with left axillary adenopathy (*thick black arrow*) and focal uptake in right proximal femur (*short black arrow*). (B) Fused transaxial FDG PET-CT image shows left primary BC, (C) fused transaxial image showing left axillary adenopathy, (D) fused transaxial image showing FDG avid right proximal femur, corresponding to a tiny lytic lesion on the CT portion of the PET examination (E, *white arrow*). (F) MIP image: Follow-up PET CT scan following chemotherapy shows favorable response to therapy with resolution of FDG uptake in left breast primary (*long black arrow*) and interval decrease in size, number, and metabolic activity in left axillary adenopathy (*short black arrow*), (G) fused transaxial image with resolution of primary lesion, (H) fused transaxial image showing response to therapy in left axillary adenopathy. (I) Fused transaxial image showing significant interval reduction in FDG uptake in right femur lytic lesion. MIP: maximal intensity projection. (J) CT portion of the PET CT exam, shows very minimal peripheral sclerosis in the right femur lytic lesion.

lower grade tumors.[31] Key outcomes such as pathologic response and survival may vary by BC subtypes and type of treatment.[32] PET parameters that best correlate with pathologic response vary based on tumor phenotype. Changes in SUVmax or total lesion glycolysis (TLG) are most adequate for triple-negative BC and for ER-positive/human epidermal growth factor receptor 2 (HER2)-negative cancers and absolute SUVmax after 2 cycles of NAC for HER2-positive BCs.[33] Schelling and colleagues showed significant differences in FDG uptake between responders and nonresponders after the first course of chemotherapy, before radiological response.[34] Large prospective multicenter evaluated changes in SUVmax at baseline and after first and second cycles of chemotherapy, their results showed that a threshold of 45% decrease in standardized uptake value (SUV) correctly identified responders, and histopathologic nonresponders were identified with a negative predictive value of 90%. Similar results were found after the second cycle when using a threshold of 55% relative decrease in SUV.[35] Another meta-analysis showed a cutoff value of SUV reduction between 55% and 65%, best correlated with pathologic condition and might potentially identify nonresponders early in the treatment course.[36] Studies have confirmed that achievement of pCR correlates with both OS and disease-free survival with the greatest benefit seen in aggressive BC subtypes.[37,38] A multicenter open label phase 2 trial in Her-2 positive early BC

assessed early metabolic responses to neoadjuvant trastuzumab and pertuzumab showed that FDG PET identified patients with HER2-positive, early-stage BC who were likely to benefit from chemotherapy-free dual HER2 blockade with trastuzumab and pertuzumab.[39] PET-CT has higher sensitivity when compared with MR as FDG has the ability to offer early metabolic response prediction when compared with MR imaging. MR imaging however has a higher specificity; therefore, a combined use of these 2 imaging modalities may have better ability to improve the diagnostic performance in assessing pCR after NAC.[40,41] Cho and colleagues in a prospective study showed that FDG PET-MR imaging can help to predict non-pCR after the first cycle of NAC.[42]

Regional Axillary Node Evaluation with F-18 Fluorodeoxyglucose Positron Emission Tomography

Regional axillary node status is the most important variable to predict prognosis. There have been very few studies assessing changes in FDG uptake in axillary lymph nodes.[43,44] Rousseau and colleagues showed that FDG PET can accurately predict the pathologic status of regional axillary lymph nodes in early-stage BC (stage II and III) after one course of NAC in 52 patients who achieved a nodal pCR. One of the limitations of the study was that not all patients had biopsy confirmed lymph node metastases at baseline; this limited the calculation of true responders.[45] The early assessment of response can help in patient management and can guide clinicians to revise their treatment plans and goals of care relative to their original plans based on FDG PET-CT imaging by avoiding ineffective chemotherapy and to continue preoperative chemotherapy in responding patients.[28]

Breast-Specific Gamma Imaging

Breast-specific gamma imaging (BSGI) using Tc-99m sestamibi 99m Tc-methoxyisobutylisonitrile (MIBI) was Food and Drug Administration (FDA) approved as a second-line breast imaging agent in dense breasts or where mammography findings are equivocal.[46,47] Breast MR imaging is considered as the modality of choice in assessing response to NAC because of superior accuracy than clinical examination, mammography, and US.[48] However, BSGI using MIBI has a potential role in assessing response to NAC in patients where breast MR imaging cannot be performed or is contraindicated.[47] In a large prospective study by Hunt and colleagues compared the size of invasive BC before and after NAC using breast MR imaging and BSGI and assessed the accuracy of post-NAC BSGI and MR imaging relative to pathologic diagnosis. The results of the study showed that both modalities show similar disease extent before NAC; however, both modalities lack sufficient accuracy in predicting pathologic complete response after NAC compared with pathologic evaluation.[49] Despite its clinical utility, BSGI is, however, not widely available.

METASTATIC BREAST CANCER THERAPY RESPONSE ASSESSMENT

MBC is now considered a chronic disease with an increase in the number of women living longer with MBC due to advancements in BC treatment. The prognosis for MBC however is still low with a 5-year OS of only 25%.[50] There have been limited studies evaluating treatment response in MBC compared with studies evaluating response to NAC. This might be because histopathologic diagnosis is almost always available after NAC but is rarely present after the treatment of metastatic disease.[51]

Contrast-Enhanced CT in Metastatic Breast Cancer

Contrast-enhanced CT (CECT) using Response Evaluation Criteria in Solid Tumors (RECIST 1.1) is widely used in response evaluation in MBC.[52,53] Most current guidelines recommend RECIST 1.1 for response evaluation, treatment, and monitoring of MBC.[3] The RECIST criteria are well defined and have a high degree of repeatability. However, it suffers from major drawback because osseous metastases are considered nonmeasurable disease and in distinguishing viable from nonviable residual tumor tissue. There is also a weak correlation between degree of response and survival.[54,55] Mandrekar and colleagues published that the RECIST criteria showed poorer correlation with survival for MBC than for other cancers (colorectal and nonsmall cell lung cancer). The results remained unchanged whether patients in the stable disease group were considered as responders, or nonresponders.[56]

F-18 Fluorodeoxyglucose Positron Emission Tomography

Accurate and early response evaluation has become more important with an increase in the number of treatment options available because it can potentially affect patient survival. The randomized clinical trials evaluating response to therapy with new drugs still use new RECIST criteria.[53] The disadvantage is that several cycles of treatment are requited before cross-sectional imaging (CT or MR imaging) can detect measurable changes in tumor size and changes in tumor do not often correlate with patient outcome. A prospective study compared FDG PET-CT with CECT showed that FDG PET-CT is superior in detecting earlier disease progression with a potentially clinically relevant median delay of 6 months for CECT.[57] Kitajima and colleagues showed that FDG PET-CT accurately assessed early response and prediction of progression after one cycle of chemotherapy in recurrent or MBC.[58] There are no specific recommendations for response monitoring for patients with MBC outside clinical trials.[3] Phase I/II clinical trials applying FDG-PET/CT to evaluate response showed that early metabolic response can predict survival and can be used as a biomarker to response evaluation, especially for molecular targeted therapies.[59,60] Riedel and colleagues showed that evaluating tumor response with FDG PET/CT seems to be a superior predictor of progression-free survival (PFS) and disease-specific survival than response on CE-CT.[54] Naghavi-Behzad and colleagues showed that there is improved patient management and a survival benefit of 14 to 24 months when FDG-PET/CT was used alone or in combination with CT.[61] A semiquantitative set of response evaluation criteria for whole-body FDG-PET/CT, Positron Emission Tomography Response Criteria in Solid Tumors (PERCIST), was proposed in 2009.[62] PERCIST has many advantages. These include high degree of repeatability, less interobserver variability than in measurements with CE-CT, the ability to differentiate between metabolically viable cancer from posttherapy changes.[54] Response assessment using PERCIST criteria is not only more sensitive in detecting progressive or responding disease response but also superior in prediction of progression-free and disease-specific survival compared with RECIST 1.1.[54,63] Several studies have shown increased sensitivity of FDG PET-CT compared with CT and bone scintigraphy (BS) in staging and response evaluation.[64,65] PERCIST-based response assessment relies on standardized uptake value (SUV) normalized by lean body mass measurement either normalized to body weight or lean body mass (SUL).[62] Ulaner and colleagues in a large multicenter trial of neratinib for rare HER2-mutant malignancies (SUMMIT) showed that using PET response criteria allowed patients with nonmeasurable disease by RECIST criteria allowed recruitment of such patients that otherwise would have been denied access to the trial.[66] Tumor heterogeneity has been associated with immune infiltration, metastasis, and drug resistance. FDG PET-CT can be used for noninvasive evaluation of tumor heterogeneity and in predicting response to chemotherapy. Patients on immunotherapy can have pseudoprogression presenting as initially increased tumor lesion size and subsequently decreased tumor burden. It is recommended to get serial FDG PET-CT scan to differentiate pseudoprogression from true progression.[67,68] Recently, a study proposed a novel method to assess intratumor and intertumor heterogeneity using FDG PET-CT in patients with triple-negative BC on immunotherapy showing that baseline intertumor heterogeneity could be a predictor for first-line immunotherapy.[69] Metabolic flare (MF) characterized by transient increase in FDG avidity of lesions after endocrine therapy is usually seen within first 2 weeks after therapy and is predictive of responsiveness to endocrine therapy.[70,71] MF however does not interfere with response assessments as FDG PET scans are usually performed no earlier than 4 to 6 weeks after initiating therapy and is generally not seen with chemotherapy. Cyclin-dependent 4/6 kinase (CDK4/6) inhibitors plus endocrine therapy is standard of care in the treatment of hormone receptor-positive HER2-negative BC. Studies have shown that FDG PET-CT can help in early response assessment in patients on CDK4/6 inhibitors and can provide prognostic information.[72,73] Groheux previously summarized the data on FDG PET/CT for monitoring treatment response in patients with MBC through 2018.[30] We expand this to now include trials through 2022 (**Table 1**), which are notable for their emphasis on prospective trials.

MR Imaging

MR imaging provides information related to the differences in the cellular density and water mobility between benign and malignant tissues with the advantage of not exposing patients to ionizing radiation.[74,] Studies have demonstrated superiority of MR imaging over BS in identifying bone metastases with a pooled sensitivity of 97% versus 79% for BS and a pooled specificity of 95% versus 82%, respectively.[75] Whole body MR imaging (WBMRI) although is not routinely used in bone dominant (BD) MBC. A retrospective study assessing the utility of WBMRI in addition to CT, BS, and FDG PET-CT in influencing anticancer treatment decisions in MBC showed that WBMRI can help in earlier identification of disease progression compared with other imaging modalities.[76] MR imaging can also help in equivocal findings on BS and can guide for local therapy in sites that were negative on a BS and can also help in management decisions through identifying complications such as cord compression associated with bone metastases.

Influence of Tumor Histology on FDG PET

The 2 most common histologic subtypes are invasive ductal carcinoma (IDC) accounting for 75% to 80% of primary BC and invasive lobular cancer (ILC), this accounts for 10% to 15% of primary BC.[77] Primary ILC and metastases from ILC have low FDG uptake compared with IDC.[33,78] Osseous metastases from ILC tend to be sclerotic and are more likely to be missed by FDG PET-CT than osseous metastases from IDC because of their low FDG uptake, which is indistinguishable from background activity.[79] The pattern of metastases in ILC is unusual with a tendency to spread to the serosal surfaces such as pleura and peritoneum, retroperitoneum and gastrointestinal, genitourinary tracts and an increased rate of leptomeningeal spread than IDC.[80] These sites of metastatic spread can be challenging to identify due to the presence of overlying physiologic FDG uptake, this most likely results in lower detection rates of ILC metastases than IDC.[80,81]

Skeletal Metastases

About 30% to 85% of patients develop bone metastases during the disease course, more commonly in ER + MBC.[82,83] Bone metastases are considered nonmeasurable by RECIST criteria[53]; therefore, clinicians usually rely on improvement in symptoms to assess response to treatment. It is challenging to evaluate changes

Table 1
Studies evaluating F-18 fluorodeoxyglucose positron emission tomography assessing response in breast cancer 2019–2022

Reference	Type	No of Patients	Site of Metastases	Timing of PET	Main Objective	Results
Ulaner et al,[66] 2019	Prospective	81	No specific site	Baseline and follow-up every 8 wk	To determine whether FDG PET can expand eligibility in biomarker-selected clinical trials by providing a means to quantitate response in patients with nonassessable disease by RECIST	PET response criteria allowed patients with non-RECIST measurable disease access to therapy and facilitated more rapid accrual of patients to this trial of a rare biomarker
Vogsen et al,[63] 2021	Retrospective	37	No specific site	Baseline and follow-up	Assessed feasibility and potential benefit of applying PERCIST for response monitoring in metastatic breast cancer using baseline PERCIST baseline and the nadir PERCIST nadir as a reference	PERCIST nadir, can be helpful in clinical decision-making and for response monitoring in MBC
Seifert et al,[72] 2021	Retrospective	8	No specific site	Baseline and 14 d after the start of treatment	Assessed feasibility of early metabolic response assessment to predict the long-term treatment response to CDK4/6 inhibitor therapy	Elevated TLG on early FDG-PET is associated with long-term treatment failure and a poor outcome in patients undergoing CDK4/6 inhibitor therapy for MBC

Study	Design	N	Site	Timing	Objective	Findings
Makhlin et al,[100] 2022	Prospective	23	Bone dominant metastases	Baseline, at 4 wk and 12 wk post-ET	To evaluate the role PET-CT early 4 wk PET-CT in predicting PFS	At the 4-wk time point PET responders had numerically longer PFS, OS and tSRE compared with nonresponders, suggesting the clinical utility of 4-wk ^{18}F-FDG PET/CT as an early predictor of treatment failure
Vogsen et al,[57] 2022	Prospective	87	No specific site	Every 9–12 wk	Compared CE-CT and FDG PET-CT or response monitoring in MBC using the standardized response evaluation criteria RECIST 1.1 and PERCIST	FDG PET-CT identified disease progression earlier than CE-CT in most patients with a potentially clinically relevant median 6-mo delay for CE-CT
Kitajima et al,[58] 2022	Prospective	33	No specific site	Before and after one cycle of systemic therapy	To evaluate the usefulness of early assessment of tumor response using FDG PET-CT after one cycle of systemic therapy in patients with recurrent and MBC	After one cycle of systemic therapy PET/CT was able to reflect early metabolic changes regardless of the lesion site and showed accuracy for early response evaluation and prediction of progression in patients with recurrent or MBC

Abbreviations: CECT, contrast-enhanced computed tomography; MBC, metastatic breast cancer; OS, overall survival; PERCIST, PET response criteria in solid tumor; PFS, progression-free survival; RECIST, response criteria in solid tumors; tSRE, time to skeletal-related event.

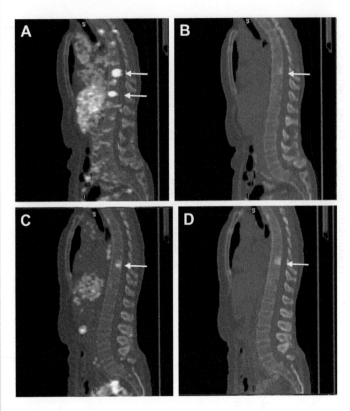

Fig. 2. A 65-year-old woman with metastatic left BC (ER positive, PR positive, HER-2 negative) with bone metastasis. (A) Fused sagittal image shows FDG avid lesions in the spine (arrows), (B) CT sagittal image shows sclerotic lesions on CT portion of the FDG PET/CT examination (arrow). (C and D) Follow-up scan, after CDK4/6 inhibitor and hormonal therapy. Sagittal fused FDG PET/CT image shows favorable response to therapy with interval decrease in metabolic activity in spine lesions (arrow). Sagittal CT image shows interval increase in sclerosis on the CT portion of the examination (arrow).

in the size of bone metastases using conventional imaging as healed sclerotic lesions do not disappear and lytic lesions can show sclerotic changes as an indicator of treatment response.[84,85]

Bone Scintigraphy

BS performed with Tc-99m labeled diphosphonate is a low cost and widely available whole-body imaging for identifying bone metastases with good sensitivity; however, it lacks specificity and this can lead to false positives.[86] Whole body BS with single photon emission computed tomography (SPECT) including a low-dose CT scan as part of SPECT-CT examination helps in improving lesion to background ratio and low-dose CT allows for anatomic lesion localization, results in increasing the diagnostic accuracy of the examination.[87] BS however has its limitations when it is used for response assessment. Coombes and colleagues assessing response to systemic therapy in patients with bone metastases showed that only 52% of responders demonstrated scintigraphic improvement and 62% of nonresponders showed scintigraphic deterioration at 6 to 8 months.[88] Flare phenomenon is usually seen in patients receiving chemotherapy or endocrine therapy between 2 weeks to 3 months

following therapy but can rarely be seen as late as 6 months after treatment.[89,90] The lag time of 3 to 6 months limits clinical utility of BS in response assessment although it has been shown that if serial bone scans confirm a flare, then it is likely to herald a favorable response to therapy.[91] Although several studies have shown the superiority of FDG PET-CT in evaluating lytic osseous metastases compared with BS; however, BS has clinical utility in assessing response if FDG exhibits minimal or no uptake.[92] Sodium fluoride PET-CT (F-18 NaF PET-CT) is similar to BS, the uptake corresponds to increased osteoblastic activity, and therefore it lacks specificity and can cause false positives; however, low-dose whole body CT acquired as part of NaF PETCT helps in improving specificity.[93] The clinical utility of F-18 NaF in monitoring response assessment is less well described in literature; however, the combined use of F-18 NaF and FDG PET-CT might be considered in selected patients with BC with suspicious sclerotic bone lesions and negative FDG PET-CT.[94]

F-18 Fluorodeoxyglucose Positron Emission Tomography

FDG PET-CT has shown superior sensitivity in the detection of bone involvement in patients with

MBC than conventional imaging and is emerging as the modality of choice for treatment monitoring of bone dominant MBC[64] (**Fig. 2**). FDG uptake in viable bone metastases acts as a tumor-specific tracer rather than reflecting altered bone microenvironment.[95] Stafford and colleagues reported a correlation between changes in 18F-FDG uptake and the overall clinical assessment of a response in patients with BD MBC.[96] Multiple studies have shown that patients with MBC who showed no change in F18 FDG uptake were twice as likely to progress than patients who showed a metabolic response.[97,98] Makhlin and colleagues showed that patients with BD MBC receiving endocrine therapy, early time point FDG PET-CT imaging at 4 weeks provides prognostic information and can help in early identification of responders versus nonresponders. The data from this study have been used to support the ongoing large multicenter EA1183 trial (FEATURE) in evaluating whether FDG-PET/CT imaging can be used to serially measure and classify the response of BD MBC to systemic therapy. The study will assess if the categories of metabolic response measured by FDG-PET/CT are predictive of key clinical endpoints: PFS, time to skeletal-related events (SRE), and OS.[99,100]

OTHER FDA-APPROVED RADIONUCLIDES
F-18 Fluoroestradiol

F18 Fluoroestradiol (18F-FES) was FDA approved in 2020 to detect ER-positive lesions in patients with recurrent or MBC as an adjunct to biopsy.[101,102] FES has additional clinical utility in imaging ILC ER + metastases that show low FDG uptake.[102] Several clinical studies have evaluated the role of 18F-FES PET/CT in not only assessing in vivo ER expression but also in predicting response to therapy, evaluation of effective ER blockade and helping the clinicians in treatment strategy decisions.[103,104] There are now published Appropriate Use Criteria for FES, which do not recommend the use of FES PET for the evaluation of treatment response at this time.[105] Estrogen Receptor-targeted PET is more fully discussed in a separate article in this issue of PET CLINICS (see Gary A Ulaner and colleagues' article, "Estrogen Receptor (ER)- and Progesterone Receptor (PR)-targeted PET for Patients with Breast Cancer,").

SUMMARY

With continued advancements in the management of BC, there will be increase in the number of women living with MBC leading to an increase in

economic burden, which includes expenses related to imaging and other diagnostic testing. It is important to appropriately select different imaging modalities that can help in accurate response assessment and help with timely treatment decision-making.

CLINICS CARE POINTS

- Digital breast tomosynthesis is more accurate than conventional digital mammography in assessing response to neoadjuvant chemotherapy with good correlation with histopathology for residual tumor size.
- Combined use of both mammography and US improves the accuracy of predicting a pathologic complete response compared to use of either modality alone.
- Breast MRI is most accurate imaging modality for assessing response to neoadjuvant chemotherapy although it has to be kept in mind that MRI tends to overestimate response with taxane based neoadjuvant chemotherapy.
- FDG PET CT can accurately predict the pathologic status of regional axillary lymph nodes in early-stage BC (stage II and III) as early as after one course of chemotherapy which can guide the oncologists in patient management however the role of FDG PET in assessing response to therapy in primary breast mass largely depends upon the tumor histology and receptor status.
- FDG PET-CT has high clinical utility in assessing response to metastatic breast cancer; using PET response criteria allows patients with non-RECIST measurable access to therapy and helps in timely clinical decision making based on response assessment. FDG PET-CT also provides prognostic information and helps to early identify responders from non-responders.
- FDG PET-CT has superior sensitivity compared to conventional imaging in the detection of osseous metastases and is emerging as the modality of choice for treatment monitoring of bone dominant metastatic breast cancer.

DISCLOSURE

GAU discloses grants, consulting fees, honoraria, and/or speaker fees from Lantheus, GE Heathcare, Curium, POINT, RayzeBio, Briacell, and ImaginAb.

REFERENCES

1. Siegel RL, Miller KD, Fuchs HE, et al. Cancer statistics, 2022. CA Cancer J Clin 2022;72(1):7–33.
2. Wockel A, Festl J, Stuber T, et al. Interdisciplinary Screening, diagnosis, therapy and follow-up of breast cancer. Guideline of the DGGG and the DKG (S3-level, AWMF Registry number 032/045OL, December 2017) - Part 1 with recommendations for the Screening, diagnosis and therapy of breast cancer. Geburtshilfe Frauenheilkd 2018; 78(10):927–48.
3. Cardoso F, Paluch-Shimon S, Senkus E, et al. 5th ESO-ESMO international consensus guidelines for advanced breast cancer (ABC 5). Ann Oncol 2020;31(12):1623–49.
4. Huber S, Wagner M, Zuna I, et al. Locally advanced breast carcinoma: evaluation of mammography in the prediction of residual disease after induction chemotherapy. Anticancer Res 2000;20(1B):553–8.
5. Fisher B, Bryant J, Wolmark N, et al. Effect of preoperative chemotherapy on the outcome of women with operable breast cancer. J Clin Oncol 1998; 16(8):2672–85.
6. Fisher ER, Wang J, Bryant J, et al. Pathobiology of preoperative chemotherapy: findings from the National surgical adjuvant breast and Bowel (NSABP) protocol B-18. Cancer 2002;95(4):681–95.
7. Gradishar WJ, Moran MS, Abraham J, et al. Breast cancer, version 3.2022, NCCN clinical practice guidelines in Oncology. J Natl Compr Canc Netw 2022;20(6):691–722.
8. Park J, Chae EY, Cha JH, et al. Comparison of mammography, digital breast tomosynthesis, automated breast ultrasound, magnetic resonance imaging in evaluation of residual tumor after neoadjuvant chemotherapy. Eur J Radiol 2018; 108:261–8.
9. Helvie MA, Joynt LK, Cody RL, et al. Locally advanced breast carcinoma: accuracy of mammography versus clinical examination in the prediction of residual disease after chemotherapy. Radiology 1996;198(2):327–32.
10. Mun HS, Kim HH, Shin HJ, et al. Assessment of extent of breast cancer: comparison between digital breast tomosynthesis and full-field digital mammography. Clin Radiol 2013;68(12):1254–9.
11. Murakami R, Tani H, Kumita S, et al. Diagnostic performance of digital breast tomosynthesis for predicting response to neoadjuvant systemic therapy in breast cancer patients: a comparison with magnetic resonance imaging, ultrasound, and full-field digital mammography. Acta Radiol Open 2021; 10(12). 20584601211063746.
12. Keune JD, Jeffe DB, Schootman M, et al. Accuracy of ultrasonography and mammography in predicting pathologic response after neoadjuvant chemotherapy for breast cancer. Am J Surg 2010;199(4):477–84.
13. Bosch AM, Kessels AG, Beets GL, et al. Preoperative estimation of the pathological breast tumour size by physical examination, mammography and ultrasound: a prospective study on 105 invasive tumours. Eur J Radiol 2003;48(3):285–92.
14. Peintinger F, Kuerer HM, Anderson K, et al. Accuracy of the combination of mammography and sonography in predicting tumor response in breast cancer patients after neoadjuvant chemotherapy. Ann Surg Oncol 2006;13(11):1443–9.
15. Makanjuola DI, Alkushi A, Al Anazi K. Defining radiologic complete response using a correlation of presurgical ultrasound and mammographic localization findings with pathological complete response following neoadjuvant chemotherapy in breast cancer. Eur J Radiol 2020;130:109146.
16. Shin HJ, Kim HH, Cha JH. Current status of automated breast ultrasonography. Ultrasonography 2015;34(3):165–72.
17. Herrada J, Iyer RB, Atkinson EN, et al. Relative value of physical examination, mammography, and breast sonography in evaluating the size of the primary tumor and regional lymph node metastases in women receiving neoadjuvant chemotherapy for locally advanced breast carcinoma. Clin Cancer Res 1997;3(9):1565–9.
18. Scheel JR, Kim E, Partridge SC, et al. MRI, clinical examination, and mammography for preoperative assessment of residual disease and pathologic complete response after neoadjuvant chemotherapy for breast cancer: ACRIN 6657 trial. AJR Am J Roentgenol 2018;210(6):1376–85.
19. Londero V, Bazzocchi M, Del Frate C, et al. Locally advanced breast cancer: comparison of mammography, sonography and MR imaging in evaluation of residual disease in women receiving neoadjuvant chemotherapy. Eur Radiol 2004;14(8):1371–9.
20. Rauch GM, Adrada BE, Kuerer HM, et al. Multimodality imaging for evaluating response to neoadjuvant chemotherapy in breast cancer. AJR Am J Roentgenol 2017;208(2):290–9.
21. Hylton NM, Blume JD, Bernreuter WK, et al. Locally advanced breast cancer: MR imaging for prediction of response to neoadjuvant chemotherapy–results from ACRIN 6657/I-SPY TRIAL. Radiology 2012;263(3):663–72.
22. Braman NM, Etesami M, Prasanna P, et al. Intratumoral and peritumoral radiomics for the pretreatment prediction of pathological complete response to neoadjuvant chemotherapy based on breast DCE-MRI. Breast Cancer Res 2017;19(1): 57.
23. Chen JH, Bahri S, Mehta RS, et al. Impact of factors affecting the residual tumor size diagnosed

by MRI following neoadjuvant chemotherapy in comparison to pathology. J Surg Oncol 2014; 109(2):158–67.

24. Mukhtar RA, Yau C, Rosen M, et al. Clinically meaningful tumor reduction rates vary by prechemotherapy MRI phenotype and tumor subtype in the I-SPY 1 TRIAL (CALGB 150007/150012; ACRIN 6657). Ann Surg Oncol 2013;20(12):3823–30.

25. Schrading S, Kuhl CK. Breast cancer: Influence of taxanes on response assessment with dynamic contrast-enhanced MR imaging. Radiology 2015; 277(3):687–96.

26. Ollivier L, Balu-Maestro C, Leclere J. Imaging in evaluation of response to neoadjuvant breast cancer treatment. Cancer Imag 2005;5(1):27–31.

27. Wahl RL, Zasadny K, Helvie M, et al. Metabolic monitoring of breast cancer chemohormonotherapy using positron emission tomography: initial evaluation. J Clin Oncol 1993;11(11):2101–11.

28. Avril S, Muzic RF Jr, Plecha D, et al. (1)(8)F-FDG PET/CT for monitoring of treatment response in breast cancer. J Nucl Med 2016;57(Suppl 1): 34S–9S.

29. Groheux D, Majdoub M, Sanna A, et al. Early metabolic response to neoadjuvant treatment: FDG PET/CT criteria according to breast cancer subtype. Radiology 2015;277(2):358–71.

30. Groheux D. Role of Fludeoxyglucose in breast cancer: treatment response. Pet Clin 2018;13(3): 395–414.

31. Ueda S, Tsuda H, Asakawa H, et al. Clinicopathological and prognostic relevance of uptake level using 18F-fluorodeoxyglucose positron emission tomography/computed tomography fusion imaging (18F-FDG PET/CT) in primary breast cancer. Jpn J Clin Oncol 2008;38(4):250–8.

32. Schneider-Kolsky ME, Hart S, Fox J, et al. The role of chemotherapeutic drugs in the evaluation of breast tumour response to chemotherapy using serial FDG-PET. Breast Cancer Res 2010;12(3):R37.

33. Bos R, van Der Hoeven JJ, van Der Wall E, et al. Biologic correlates of (18)fluorodeoxyglucose uptake in human breast cancer measured by positron emission tomography. J Clin Oncol 2002;20(2): 379–87.

34. Schelling M, Avril N, Nahrig J, et al. Positron emission tomography using [(18)F]Fluorodeoxyglucose for monitoring primary chemotherapy in breast cancer. J Clin Oncol 2000;18(8):1689–95.

35. Schwarz-Dose J, Untch M, Tiling R, et al. Monitoring primary systemic therapy of large and locally advanced breast cancer by using sequential positron emission tomography imaging with [18F]fluorodeoxyglucose. J Clin Oncol 2009;27(4):535–41.

36. Wang Y, Zhang C, Liu J, et al. Is 18F-FDG PET accurate to predict neoadjuvant therapy response in breast cancer? A meta-analysis. Breast Cancer Res Treat 2012;131(2):357–69.

37. van der Hage JA, van de Velde CJ, Julien JP, et al. Preoperative chemotherapy in primary operable breast cancer: results from the European Organization for Research and Treatment of Cancer trial 10902. J Clin Oncol 2001;19(22):4224–37.

38. von Minckwitz G, Untch M, Blohmer JU, et al. Definition and impact of pathologic complete response on prognosis after neoadjuvant chemotherapy in various intrinsic breast cancer subtypes. J Clin Oncol 2012;30(15):1796–804.

39. Perez-Garcia JM, Gebhart G, Ruiz Borrego M, et al. Chemotherapy de-escalation using an (18)F-FDG-PET-based pathological response-adapted strategy in patients with HER2-positive early breast cancer (PHERGain): a multicentre, randomised, open-label, non-comparative, phase 2 trial. Lancet Oncol 2021;22(6):858–71.

40. Kwong MS, Chung GG, Horvath LJ, et al. Postchemotherapy MRI overestimates residual disease compared with histopathology in responders to neoadjuvant therapy for locally advanced breast cancer. Cancer J 2006;12(3):212–21.

41. Liu Q, Wang C, Li P, et al. Corrigendum to "the role of (18)F-FDG PET/CT and MRI in assessing pathological complete response to neoadjuvant chemotherapy in patients with breast cancer: a Systematic review and meta-analysis". BioMed Res Int 2016;2016:1235429.

42. Cho N, Im SA, Cheon GJ, et al. Integrated (18)F-FDG PET/MRI in breast cancer: early prediction of response to neoadjuvant chemotherapy. Eur J Nucl Med Mol Imaging 2018;45(3):328–39.

43. Bassa P, Kim EE, Inoue T, et al. Evaluation of preoperative chemotherapy using PET with fluorine-18-fluorodeoxyglucose in breast cancer. J Nucl Med 1996;37(6):931–8.

44. Mankoff DA, Dunnwald LK, Gralow JR, et al. Changes in blood flow and metabolism in locally advanced breast cancer treated with neoadjuvant chemotherapy. J Nucl Med 2003;44(11):1806–14.

45. Rousseau C, Devillers A, Campone M, et al. FDG PET evaluation of early axillary lymph node response to neoadjuvant chemotherapy in stage II and III breast cancer patients. Eur J Nucl Med Mol Imaging 2011;38(6):1029–36.

46. O'Connor M, Rhodes D, Hruska C. Molecular breast imaging. Expert Rev Anticancer Ther 2009; 9(8):1073–80.

47. Muzahir S. Molecular breast cancer imaging in the Era of Precision Medicine. AJR Am J Roentgenol 2020;215(6):1512–9.

48. Bouzon A, Acea B, Soler R, et al. Diagnostic accuracy of MRI to evaluate tumour response and residual tumour size after neoadjuvant chemotherapy in breast cancer patients. Radiol Oncol 2016;50(1):73–9.

49. Hunt KN, Conners AL, Goetz MP, et al. Comparison of (99m)Tc-sestamibi molecular breast imaging and breast MRI in patients with invasive breast cancer receiving neoadjuvant chemotherapy. AJR Am J Roentgenol 2019;213(4):932–43.

50. Lim B, Hortobagyi GN. Current challenges of metastatic breast cancer. Cancer Metastasis Rev 2016;35(4):495–514.

51. Ulaner GA. PET/CT for patients with breast cancer: where is the clinical impact? AJR Am J Roentgenol 2019;213(2):254–65.

52. Bensch F, van Kruchten M, Lamberts LE, et al. Molecular imaging for monitoring treatment response in breast cancer patients. Eur J Pharmacol 2013; 717(1–3):2–11.

53. Eisenhauer EA, Therasse P, Bogaerts J, et al. New response evaluation criteria in solid tumours: revised RECIST guideline (version 1.1). Eur J Cancer 2009;45(2):228–47.

54. Riedl CC, Pinker K, Ulaner GA, et al. Comparison of FDG-PET/CT and contrast-enhanced CT for monitoring therapy response in patients with metastatic breast cancer. Eur J Nucl Med Mol Imaging 2017; 44(9):1428–37.

55. Fojo AT, Noonan A. Why RECIST works and why it should stay–counterpoint. Cancer Res 2012; 72(20):5151–7 [discussion: 5158].

56. Mandrekar SJ, An MW, Meyers J, et al. Evaluation of alternate categorical tumor metrics and cut points for response categorization using the RECIST 1.1 data warehouse. J Clin Oncol 2014; 32(8):841–50.

57. Vogsen M, Harbo F, Jakobsen NM, et al. Response monitoring in metastatic breast cancer - a prospective study comparing (18)F-FDG PET/CT with conventional CT. J Nucl Med 2023;64(3):355–61.

58. Kitajima K, Higuchi T, Yamakado K, et al. Early assessment of tumor response using (18)F-FDG PET/CT after one cycle of systemic therapy in patients with recurrent and metastatic breast cancer. Hell J Nucl Med 2022;25(2):155–62.

59. Lin NU, Guo H, Yap JT, et al. Phase II study of Lapatinib in combination with trastuzumab in patients with human epidermal growth factor receptor 2-positive metastatic breast cancer: clinical outcomes and predictive value of early [18F]fluorodeoxyglucose positron emission tomography imaging (TBCRC 003). J Clin Oncol 2015;33(24): 2623–31.

60. Mayer IA, Abramson VG, Isakoff SJ, et al. Stand up to cancer phase Ib study of pan-phosphoinositide-3-kinase inhibitor buparlisib with letrozole in estrogen receptor-positive/human epidermal growth factor receptor 2-negative metastatic breast cancer. J Clin Oncol 2014;32(12):1202–9.

61. Naghavi-Behzad M, Vogsen M, Vester RM, et al. Response monitoring in metastatic breast cancer: a comparison of survival times between FDG-PET/CT and CE-CT. Br J Cancer 2022;126(9):1271–9.

62. Wahl RL, Jacene H, Kasamon Y, et al. From RECIST to PERCIST: Evolving Considerations for PET response criteria in solid tumors. J Nucl Med 2009;50(Suppl 1):122S–50S.

63. Vogsen M, Bulow JL, Ljungstrom L, et al. FDG-PET/CT for response monitoring in metastatic breast cancer: the Feasibility and benefits of applying PERCIST. Diagnostics 2021;11(4):723.

64. Hansen JA, Naghavi-Behzad M, Gerke O, et al. Diagnosis of bone metastases in breast cancer: lesion-based sensitivity of dual-time-point FDG-PET/CT compared to low-dose CT and bone scintigraphy. PLoS One 2021;16(11):e0260066.

65. Hildebrandt MG, Lauridsen JF, Vogsen M, et al. FDG-PET/CT for response monitoring in metastatic breast cancer: Today, Tomorrow, and beyond. Cancers 2019;11(8):1190.

66. Ulaner GA, Saura C, Piha-Paul SA, et al. Impact of FDG PET imaging for expanding patient Eligibility and measuring treatment response in a Genome-Driven Basket trial of the pan-HER kinase inhibitor, neratinib. Clin Cancer Res 2019;25(24):7381–7.

67. Ma Y, Wang Q, Dong Q, et al. How to differentiate pseudoprogression from true progression in cancer patients treated with immunotherapy. Am J Cancer Res 2019;9(8):1546–53.

68. Costa LB, Queiroz MA, Barbosa FG, et al. Reassessing patterns of response to immunotherapy with PET: from morphology to metabolism. Radiographics 2021;41(1):120–43.

69. Xie Y, Liu C, Zhao Y, et al. Heterogeneity derived from (18) F-FDG PET/CT predicts immunotherapy outcome for metastatic triple-negative breast cancer patients. Cancer Med 2022;11(9):1948–55.

70. Dehdashti F, Mortimer JE, Trinkaus K, et al. PET-based estradiol challenge as a predictive biomarker of response to endocrine therapy in women with estrogen-receptor-positive breast cancer. Breast Cancer Res Treat 2009;113(3):509–17.

71. Mortimer JE, Dehdashti F, Siegel BA, et al. Metabolic flare: indicator of hormone responsiveness in advanced breast cancer. J Clin Oncol 2001; 19(11):2797–803.

72. Seifert R, Kuper A, Tewes M, et al. [18F]-Fluorodeoxyglucose positron emission tomography/CT to assess the early metabolic response in patients with hormone receptor-positive HER2-negative Metastasized breast cancer treated with Cyclin-dependent 4/6 kinase inhibitors. Oncol Res Treat 2021;44(7–8):400–7.

73. Taralli S, Lorusso M, Scolozzi V, et al. Response evaluation with (18)F-FDG PET/CT in metastatic breast cancer patients treated with Palbociclib: first experience in clinical practice. Ann Nucl Med 2019;33(3):193–200.

74. Miles A, Evans RE, Halligan S, et al. Predictors of patient preference for either whole body magnetic resonance imaging (WB-MRI) or CT/PET-CT for staging colorectal or lung cancer. J Med Imaging Radiat Oncol 2020;64(4):537–45.

75. Shen G, Deng H, Hu S, et al. Comparison of choline-PET/CT, MRI, SPECT, and bone scintigraphy in the diagnosis of bone metastases in patients with prostate cancer: a meta-analysis. Skeletal Radiol 2014;43(11):1503–13.

76. Bhaludin BN, Tunariu N, Koh DM, et al. A review on the added value of whole-body MRI in metastatic lobular breast cancer. Eur Radiol 2022;32(9):6514–25.

77. Li CI, Anderson BO, Daling JR, et al. Trends in incidence rates of invasive lobular and ductal breast carcinoma. JAMA 2003;289(11):1421–4.

78. Buck A, Schirrmeister H, Kuhn T, et al. FDG uptake in breast cancer: correlation with biological and clinical prognostic parameters. Eur J Nucl Med Mol Imaging 2002;29(10):1317–23.

79. Dashevsky BZ, Goldman DA, Parsons M, et al. Appearance of untreated bone metastases from breast cancer on FDG PET/CT: importance of histologic subtype. Eur J Nucl Med Mol Imaging 2015; 42(11):1666–73.

80. He H, Gonzalez A, Robinson E, et al. Distant metastatic disease manifestations in infiltrating lobular carcinoma of the breast. AJR Am J Roentgenol 2014;202(5):1140–8.

81. Hogan MP, Goldman DA, Dashevsky B, et al. Comparison of 18F-FDG PET/CT for systemic staging of newly diagnosed invasive lobular carcinoma versus invasive ductal carcinoma. J Nucl Med 2015;56(11):1674–80.

82. van Uden DJP, van Maaren MC, Strobbe LJA, et al. Metastatic behavior and overall survival according to breast cancer subtypes in stage IV inflammatory breast cancer. Breast Cancer Res 2019;21(1):113.

83. Yang H, Wang R, Zeng F, et al. Impact of molecular subtypes on metastatic behavior and overall survival in patients with metastatic breast cancer: a single-center study combined with a large cohort study based on the Surveillance, Epidemiology and End Results database. Oncol Lett 2020; 20(4):87.

84. Morris PG, Lynch C, Feeney JN, et al. Integrated positron emission tomography/computed tomography may render bone scintigraphy unnecessary to investigate suspected metastatic breast cancer. J Clin Oncol 2010;28(19):3154–9.

85. Morris PG, Ulaner GA, Eaton A, et al. Standardized uptake value by positron emission tomography/computed tomography as a prognostic variable in metastatic breast cancer. Cancer 2012;118(22): 5454–62.

86. Brenner AI, Koshy J, Morey J, et al. The bone scan. Semin Nucl Med 2012;42(1):11–26.

87. Buck AK, Nekolla S, Ziegler S, et al. Spect/ct. J Nucl Med 2008;49(8):1305–19.

88. Coombes RC, Dady P, Parsons C, et al. Assessment of response of bone metastases to systemic treatment in patients with breast cancer. Cancer 1983;52(4):610–4.

89. Schneider JA, Divgi CR, Scott AM, et al. Flare on bone scintigraphy following Taxol chemotherapy for metastatic breast cancer. J Nucl Med 1994; 35(11):1748–52.

90. Vogel CL, Schoenfelder J, Shemano I, et al. Worsening bone scan in the evaluation of antitumor response during hormonal therapy of breast cancer. J Clin Oncol 1995;13(5):1123–8.

91. Coleman RE, Mashiter G, Whitaker KB, et al. Bone scan flare predicts successful systemic therapy for bone metastases. J Nucl Med 1988;29(8):1354–9.

92. Koolen BB, Vegt E, Rutgers EJ, et al. FDG-avid sclerotic bone metastases in breast cancer patients: a PET/CT case series. Ann Nucl Med 2012; 26(1):86–91.

93. Cook GJR, Goh V. Molecular imaging of bone metastases and their response to therapy. J Nucl Med 2020;61(6):799–806.

94. Taralli S, Caldarella C, Lorusso M, et al. Comparison between 18F-FDG and 18F-NaF PET imaging for assessing bone metastases in breast cancer patients: a literature review. Clinical and Translational Imaging 2020;8(2):65–78.

95. Cook GJ, Azad GK, Goh V. Imaging bone metastases in breast cancer: staging and response assessment. J Nucl Med 2016;57(Suppl 1): 27S–33S.

96. Stafford SE, Gralow JR, Schubert EK, et al. Use of serial FDG PET to measure the response of bone-dominant breast cancer to therapy. Acad Radiol 2002;9(8):913–21.

97. Specht JM, Tam SL, Kurland BF, et al. Serial 2-[18F] fluoro-2-deoxy-D-glucose positron emission tomography (FDG-PET) to monitor treatment of bone-dominant metastatic breast cancer predicts time to progression (TTP). Breast Cancer Res Treat 2007;105(1):87–94.

98. Peterson LM, O'Sullivan J, Wu QV, et al. Prospective study of serial (18)F-FDG PET and (18)F-Fluoride PET to predict time to skeletal-related events, time to progression, and survival in patients with bone-dominant metastatic breast cancer. J Nucl Med 2018;59(12):1823–30.

99. Using FDG pet ct to assess response of bone dominant metastatic breast. cancer 2020. NCT04316117.

100. Makhlin I, Korhonen KE, Martin ML, et al. (18)F-FDG PET/CT for the evaluation of therapy response in hormone receptor-positive bone-dominant metastatic breast cancer. Radiol Imaging Cancer 2022; 4(6):e220032.

101. Ulaner GA, Jhaveri K, Chandarlapaty S, et al. Head-to-Head evaluation of (18)F-FES and (18)F-FDG PET/CT in metastatic invasive lobular breast cancer. J Nucl Med 2021;62(3):326–31.

102. Chae SY, Son HJ, Lee DY, et al. Comparison of diagnostic sensitivity of [(18)F]fluoroestradiol and [(18)F]fluorodeoxyglucose positron emission tomography/computed tomography for breast cancer recurrence in patients with a history of estrogen receptor-positive primary breast cancer. EJNMMI Res 2020;10(1):54.

103. Linden HM, Kurland BF, Peterson LM, et al. Fluoroestradiol positron emission tomography reveals differences in pharmacodynamics of aromatase inhibitors, tamoxifen, and fulvestrant in patients with metastatic breast cancer. Clin Cancer Res 2011; 17(14):4799–805.

104. Liao GJ, Clark AS, Schubert EK, et al. 18F-Fluoroestradiol PET: current status and potential Future clinical applications. J Nucl Med 2016;57(8): 1269–75.

105. Ulaner GA, Mankoff DA, Clark AS, et al. Appropriate use criteria for estrogen receptor–targeted PET imaging with 16α-^{18}F-Fluoro-17β-Fluoroestradiol. J Nuc Med 2023;64(3):351–4.

Estrogen Receptor-Targeted and Progesterone Receptor-Targeted PET for Patients with Breast Cancer

Gary A. Ulaner, MD, PhD[a,b],*, Amy M. Fowler, MD, PhD[c], Amy S. Clark, MD[d], Hannah Linden, MD[e]

KEYWORDS

- Estrogen receptor • Progesterone receptor • Position emission tomography • Breast cancer

KEY POINTS

- 16α-^{18}F-fluoro-17β-fluoroestradiol (^{18}F-FES) is a PET radiotracer that targets estrogen receptor (ER) and is FDA-approved for patients with ER-positive recurrent or metastatic breast cancer.
- Because there are few benign lesions that express sufficient ER to demonstrate ^{18}F-FES-avidity on PET, a positive ^{18}F-FES PET has high specificity for ER-positive malignancy.
- Clinical applications of ^{18}F-FES include assisting in the selection of patients to receive (or not receive) endocrine therapies, assessing ER status in lesions that are difficult to biopsy, and resolving inconclusive findings on other imaging modalities.
- Newer progesterone receptor-targeted PET tracers are now in clinical trials, with early but impressive results.

INTRODUCTION

Molecular imaging has become a powerful force in radiology and medicine, with multiple somatostatin receptor-targeting imaging and therapy agents for patients with neuroendocrine cancers[1,2] and prostate-specific membrane antigen-targeting agents for patients with prostate cancer[3-5] receiving FDA-approval since 2016. Somewhat less known is the impact of molecular imaging on patients with breast cancer. Multiple PET tracers have been developed for estrogen receptor (ER), progesterone receptor (PR), and human epidermal growth factor (HER)-targeted PET imaging for patients with breast cancer.[6-8] This review article focused on ER and PR-targeted steroid PET tracers. A separate article in this issue reviews HER-targeted PET tracers (see Ducharme and colleagues' article, "HER2/HER3 PET Imaging: Challenges and Opportunities," in this issue).[9]

ESTROGEN RECEPTOR-TARGETED IMAGING

ER is highly expressed in 70% to 80% of breast cancers.[10] ER status is both a prognostic and predictive biomarker because it both distinguishes tumors with favorable and unfavorable prognosis, as well as determines effective treatment regimens.[11-13] Although ER status on immunohistochemistry (IHC) helps predict which patients will respond to endocrine therapy, still up to 50% of ER-positive breast cancers will not respond to

[a] Molecular Imaging and Therapy, Hoag Family Cancer Institute, Newport Beach, CA, USA; [b] Radiology and Translational Genomics, University of Southern California, Los Angeles, CA, USA; [c] Radiology, University of Wisconsin School of Medicine and Public Health, Madison, WI, USA; [d] Division of Hematology/Oncology, University of Pennsylvania, Philadelphia, PA, USA; [e] Medical Oncology, University of Washington, Seattle, WA, USA
* Corresponding author. Molecular Imaging and Therapy, Hoag Family Cancer Institute, 16105 Sand Canyon, Suite 215, Irvine, CA.
E-mail address: gary.ulaner@hoag.org

PET Clin 18 (2023) 531–542
https://doi.org/10.1016/j.cpet.2023.04.008
1556-8598/23/© 2023 Elsevier Inc. All rights reserved.

endocrine therapy.[14] Better biomarkers for selecting patients for endocrine therapy are needed.

16α-[18F]-fluoro-17β-fluoroestradiol ([18F]-FES) is a radiolabeled form of estradiol (**Fig. 1**) that binds to ER and allows noninvasive, whole-body evaluation of ER, which is functional for binding ligand. [18F]-FES has demonstrated strong sensitivity (78%, 95% confidence interval [CI] of 65%–88%) and outstanding specificity (98%, 95% CI 65%–100%) for the detection of ER-positive malignancy,[15] with a positive predictive value of 90% (95% CI 83%–94%) and a negative predictive value of 71% (95% CI 55%–83%).[16] The success of [18F]-FES has led to it becoming the first FDA-approved ER-targeting PET agent in 2020, under the brand name Cerianna (GE Healthcare, Chicago, IL, USA). Recently, the Society of Nuclear Medicine and Molecular Imaging has published Appropriate Use Criteria for [18F]-FES.[17]

[18F]-FES is intravenously administered, and it demonstrates rapid blood clearance with physiologic uptake and excretion through the liver and kidneys. Normal physiologic distribution of [18F]-FES is depicted in **Fig. 2**. Low physiologic uptake in the breasts, lymph nodes, bone, lung, and brain allows for sensitive imaging of many of the most common sites of breast cancer spread. However, a notable limitation is the liver, where there is high physiologic background, which prevents optimal evaluation using [18F]-FES.

There are few known false positives on [18F]-FES PET. Normal uterus and ovaries may be [18F]-FES-avid.[18] Meningiomas may be [18F]-FES-avid[19] and brain MR may be needed to distinguish benign

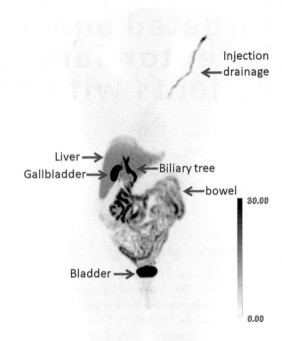

Fig. 2. Maximum intensity projection (MIP) image demonstrates the normal biodistribution of [18F]-FES. Physiologic excretion is seen in the liver (with the biliary tree, gallbladder, and bowel) and urine/bladder. Retained [18F]-FES is seen in the veins of the injected extremity. Physiologic [18F]-FES may also be seen in the uterus and ovaries.

meningiomas from intracranial malignancy. Rare benign metastasizing leiomyomas may be [18F]-FES-avid.[20] Endometriosis and radiation changes in the lung have also been noted to be [18F]-FES-avid.[21,22] Other than these exceptions, a positive [18F]-FES PET has a high specificity for ER-positive malignancy, such as breast, ovarian, and uterine cancers.[15,22,23]

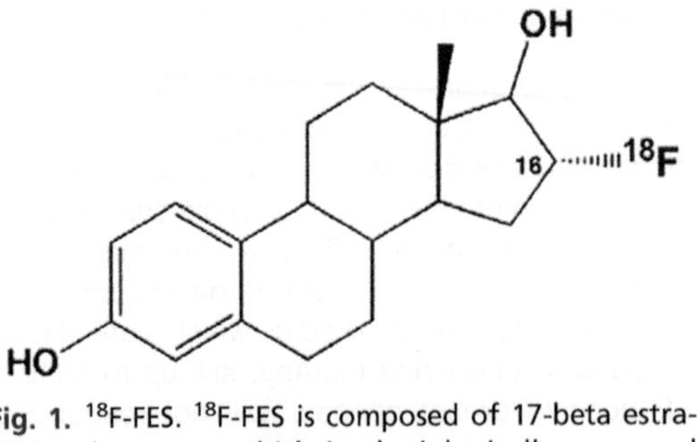

Substantial data have been accumulated on the use of [18F]-FES PET in patients with breast cancer. The FDA label for [18F]-FES states it is "indicated for use with position emission tomography (PET) imaging for the detection of estrogen receptor (ER)-positive lesions as an adjunct to biopsy in patients with recurrent or metastatic breast cancer".[24] This broad label allows for multiple potential clinical applications in patients with estrogen receptor (ER)-positive breast cancer. To appreciate the potential clinical applications [18F]-FES PET can have on patient care, it must be recognized that [18F]-FES is a distinct radiotracer from the more commonly used [18F]-FDG PET. [18F]-FDG PET has demonstrated clinical impact in patients with breast cancer through systemic staging of patients with locally advanced breast cancer, where [18F]-FDG PET

Fig. 1. [18F]-FES. [18F]-FES is composed of 17-beta estradiol, a hormone, which is physiologically expressed in all humans, radiolabeled with fluorine-18, a positron emitter. [18F]-FES is used as a PET radiotracer, allowing for whole body in vivo localization of ER, which is available for ligand binding. (*Adapted from* Katzenellenbogen JA. The quest for improving the management of breast cancer by functional imaging: The discovery and development of 16α-[(18)F]fluoroestradiol (FES), a PET radiotracer for the estrogen receptor, a historical review. *Nuclear medicine and biology*. Jan 2021;92:24-37. https://doi.org/10.1016/j.nucmedbio.2020.02.007.)

can detect previously unsuspected extra-axillary and distant metastases,[24–29] as well as through measuring response to systemic therapy, where criteria for measuring therapy response by ^{18}F-FDG PET[24] may surpass measurement by anatomic criteria such as Response Criteria in Solid Tumors.[30,31] ^{18}F-FES PET has yet to demonstrate value in either of these common clinical scenarios. Instead, ^{18}F-FES PET has demonstrated clinical value for its own unique, but no less important, clinical applications.

Potentially the most impactful clinical application of ^{18}F-FES PET is helping to select patients with metastatic ER-positive breast cancer who are most appropriate for receiving (or not receiving) endocrine axis therapies. The 70% to 80% of patients with metastatic breast cancers that are ER-positive on IHC are generally treated in the first and often second or third line with endocrine therapies that decrease available estrogens, decrease ER signal transduction, or decrease downstream effects of ER activation.[32,33] Single agent endocrine therapy was used first line until the development of cyclin-dependent kinase 4/6 inhibitors showed improved outcomes, including response rate and survival.[34,35] These modern therapies are now standard of care. However, many patients with tumors that are ER-positive on IHC do not respond to these endocrine axis therapies.[36,37] This may be due to the fact that not all ER visualized by IHC is available or functional for binding to its estrogen ligand.[6,15,38–40] Thus, the presence of ER on IHC may not be the optimal method of selecting patients for endocrine therapies. Molecular imaging with ^{18}F-FES PET may be more able to distinguish tumors with ER capable of binding its estrogen ligand, and thus better to predict which tumors will and will not respond to endocrine-based therapies. Eighteen prospective trials,[36,41–57] including 603 individual subjects, have demonstrated ^{18}F-FES PET as a successful predictive biomarker for identifying patients with metastatic breast cancer that will not respond to endocrine therapy despite ER-positivity on IHC (reviewed in ref[23]). These trials have most commonly been performed in the setting of initial diagnosis of metastatic disease and progression of metastatic disease during treatment with a first-line or subsequent-line endocrine therapy, with fewer trials involving patients at initial diagnosis of primary breast cancer. In these trials, positivity on ^{18}F-FES PET did not guarantee response to endocrine therapy, however, disease that was negative on ^{18}F-FES PET nearly always failed to respond to hormonal therapy. Of note, the first prospective trial examining ^{18}F-FES for patients with metastatic ER + breast cancer

receiving first-line endocrine therapy (NCT02398773) has just completed enrollment and should help elucidate its utility in this setting. By identifying patients with metastatic breast cancer who will not respond to endocrine therapy despite ER-positivity on IHC, a single ^{18}F-FES PET examination could prevent a patient from undergoing an ineffective line of therapy, as well as the costs and side effects of that therapy, and a delay in receiving a more effective line of therapy. Given the large numbers of patients with metastatic breast cancer who are candidates for endocrine therapies,[58] this single application of ^{18}F-FES PET can impact the lives of thousands of women a year in the United States alone.

An example of using ^{18}F-FES PET to help identify a patient with metastatic ER-positive breast cancer that is unlikely to respond to hormonal therapy is shown in **Fig. 3**. In this case, despite the presence of progressing metastatic disease visualized on ^{18}F-FDG PET, the disease was not ^{18}F-FES-avid, suggesting the disease lacked ER that was functional for binding estrogen, and thus ER signaling was likely not relevant for tumor growth in this patient. Published trials suggest this patient would have a very low likelihood of responding to a subsequent round of endocrine therapy; thus, the patient was treated with chemotherapy. An example of using ^{18}F-FES PET to help identify a patient with metastatic ER-positive breast cancer that is appropriate for hormonal therapy is shown in **Fig. 4**. In this case, the metastatic disease was ^{18}F-FES-avid, confirming the presence of ER able to bind estrogen. Although published trials demonstrate this does not guarantee response to endocrine therapy, the likelihood of success is high, and this patient did receive endocrine therapy, which resulted in a treatment response. The ^{18}F-FES PET in this patient also demonstrated intracranial foci, which subsequent brain MR confirmed were previously unknown brain metastases. The low physiologic uptake of ^{18}F-FES in the brain makes it amenable for the detection of brain metastases, in contrast to ^{18}F-FDG.

Another opportunity for clinical usage of ^{18}F-FES PET is solving clinical dilemmas caused by inconclusive or nondiagnostic results from other imaging studies. These dilemmas may occur because of the limitations of other imaging modalities; for instance, lesions on CT or MR may not have characteristics that are definitively malignant or benign, or occur because of a unique situation in the patient, for instance, the presence of 2 or more primary malignancies with different ER status. At least 4 studies have demonstrated value of ^{18}F-FES PET when other imaging modalities are inconclusive,[59–62] with a recent trial

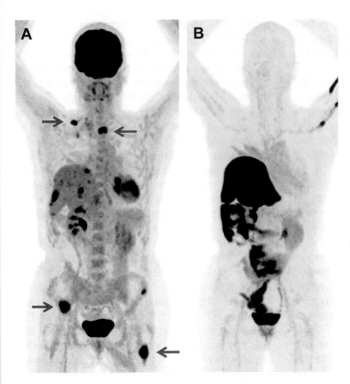

Fig. 3. Using ¹⁸F-FES PET to identify a patient with metastatic ER-positive breast cancer that will likely not respond to endocrine therapy. (*A*) MIP image from an ¹⁸F-FDG PET/CT in a 60-year-old woman with ER-positive, HER2-negative metastatic breast cancer with disease progression on first-line endocrine therapy, demonstrates multiple ¹⁸F-FDG-avid osseous (*arrows*) and hepatic metastases. A clinical decision was to be made whether to start a second-line endocrine therapy agent or defer to chemotherapy. To help with this decision, an ¹⁸F-FES PET/CT was performed. (*B*) MIP image from the ¹⁸F-FES PET/CT demonstrates the known osseous disease on the ¹⁸F-FDG PET is not ¹⁸F-FES-avid. This suggests ER is not able to bind its estrogen ligand and subsequent endocrine-based therapy will not be efficacious. Treatment was shifted to chemotherapy.

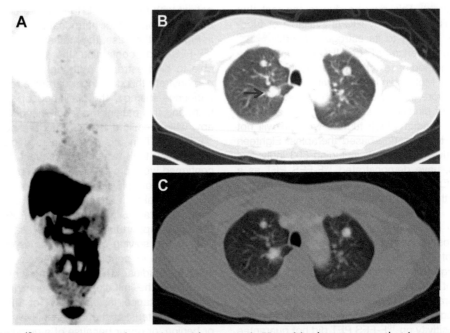

Fig. 4. Using ¹⁸F-FES PET to identify a patient with metastatic ER-positive breast cancer that is appropriate for endocrine therapy. (*A*) MIP image from an ¹⁸F-FES PET/CT in a 53-year-old woman with ER-positive, HER2-negative metastatic breast cancer and progressing lung metastases on CT demonstrates foci in the lungs (*arrow*) and brain. (*B*) Axial CT on lung window and (*C*) axial fused ¹⁸F-FES PET/CT on lung window demonstrate the lung metastases are ¹⁸F-FES-avid. Endocrine therapy was chosen for this patient. In addition, a brain MR was recommended to evaluate the cranial foci, which confirmed brain metastases (not shown).

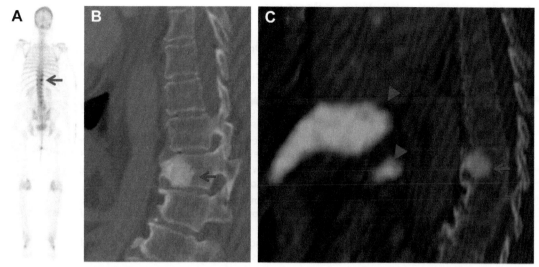

Fig. 5. Using ^{18}F-FES PET to further evaluate an inconclusive finding on other imaging modalities. (*A*) Posterior planar image from a ^{99m}Tc-MDP bone scan in a 69-year-old woman with history of ER-positive, HER2-negative breast cancer and new mid back pain demonstrates a focus in the T11 vertebra (*arrow*). (*B*) Sagittal image on bone windows from a corresponding CT scan demonstrates a sclerotic lesion in the T11 vertebra (*arrow*). A differential of metastatic disease and benign degenerative disease was given. An ^{18}F-FES PET/CT was performed for further evaluation. (*C*) Sagittal fused ^{18}F-FES PET/CT image from the ^{18}F-FES PET/CT demonstrates the sclerotic focus is not ^{18}F-FES-avid. Physiologic ^{18}F-FES-avidity was seen in the liver and bowel (*arrowheads*). The T11 vertebra lesion was called probably benign, and the patient was placed on a watch and wait strategy. The lesion remained stable on CT and MR for 13 months, then a new oncologist ordered a biopsy of the lesion. Pathology from CT-guided biopsy was benign, demonstrating only bone and bone marrow.

determining that ^{18}F-FES PET could solve an unanswered question in more than 80% of cases[62] and another determining an ^{18}F-FES PET in this clinical scenario could lead to changes in management in nearly 50% of cases.[59]

An example of utilizing ^{18}F-FES PET to resolve inconclusive findings from a CT and bone scan is shown in **Fig. 5**. This patient with a history of ER-positive breast cancer underwent CT and bone scan according to National Comprehensive Cancer Network (NCCN) guidelines[24] for suspicion of disease recurrence. These 2 imaging modalities demonstrated findings that might be attributable to malignancy or benign degenerative changes, and an ^{18}F-FES PET was ordered for further evaluation. The osseous lesion was not ^{18}F-FES-avid and thus probably not an ER-positive osseous metastasis. Indeed, the lesion remained stable for 13 months without treatment, supporting benignity. When the patient saw a new oncologist, the lesion was biopsied, providing a definite benign diagnosis. In this case, ^{18}F-FES PET provided reassurance that the abnormalities on CT and bone scan were not malignant and treatment could be deferred. Of note, ^{18}F-FDG PET would likely not be valuable in this scenario because both malignancy and degenerative changes may be hypermetabolic and thus ^{18}F-FDG-avid.

A third opportunity for clinical impact of ^{18}F-FES PET is the assessment of ER status in lesions that are difficult to biopsy. Although biopsy with IHC is the most common method for determination of lesional ER status, some lesions may be difficult to biopsy and may pose substantial risk to the patient (such as brain lesions). In addition, the most common site of ER + metastasis is bone, and these lesions may be challenging to sample; as such, many patients do not have histologically confirmed metastatic disease. Patient frailty may also contribute to the desire to avoid biopsy. In such cases, noninvasive evaluation by ^{18}F-FES PET can help determine ER status.[15] The threshold for using ^{18}F-FES PET in this manner will depend on the individual lesion under investigation and the availability of skilled interventional radiology practitioners.

A fourth opportunity for impact with ^{18}F-FES PET lies in its use as a pharmcodynamic biomarker as part of clinical trials for novel ER-targeting drugs. This would not be part of standard clinical practice but rather as an opportunity for trialists to consider when designing early phase pharmaceutical trials. ^{18}F-FES PET has been successfully utilized to determine target (ER) engagement by fulvestrant[47] and multiple novel ER-targeted therapeutics,[63–66] helping to determine the optimal

Table 1
Recruiting and/or active clinical trials of ^{18}F-FES PET

Predicting breast cancer treatment response	
NCT05068726	Clinical Utility of ^{18}F-FES PET/CT in Metastatic Breast Cancer Patients With ER-Positive and HER2-Negative Primary Lesions After Progression on First Line Hormonal Therapy
NCT04692103	Serial ^{18}F-FES PET Imaging to Evaluate Endocrine-targeted Therapy
NCT02409316	^{18}F-FES PET/CT Imaging to Evaluate in Vivo ER in Endocrine Refractory Metastatic Breast Cancer
NCT02398773	^{18}F-FES PET as a Predictive Measure for Endocrine Therapy in Patients With Newly Diagnosed Metastatic Breast Cancer
NCT02806050	Early Identification of Patients Who Benefit From Palbociclib in Addition to Letrozole
NCT03442504	Evaluation Study of the Prediction of the Response to Second-line Hormone Therapy by ^{18}F-FES PET in Patients With Metastatic Breast Cancer
NCT02409316	^{18}F-FES PET/CT Imaging to Evaluate in Vivo ER in Endocrine Refractory Metastatic Breast Cancer
NCT04727632	^{18}F-FES PET/CT Companion Imaging Study to the FORESEE: Functional Precision Oncology for Metastatic Breast Cancer Feasibility Trial
NCT05392985	Detection and Analysis of Metastatic Breast Cancer With Heterogeneous ER Expression
Breast cancer staging/restaging	
NCT04883814	^{18}F-FES PET/CT Compared to Standard-of-Care Imaging In Patients With Breast Cancer
NCT04252859	^{18}F-FES Positron Emission Tomography (PET)/CT Imaging of Invasive Lobular Carcinoma
NCT03726931	^{18}F-FES PET: Toward a New Standard to Stage Locally Advanced and Recurrent, Estrogen Receptor Positive (ER+) Breast Cancer? Pilot Study to Compare ^{18}F-FES-PET and ^{18}F-FDG-PET
Determining ER status	
NCT01916122	^{18}F-FES PET/CT for Imaging Estrogen Receptor Status
NCT01957332	Imaging Patients for Cancer Drug Selection – Metastatic Breast Cancer (IMPACT-MBC)
Reproducibility	
NCT05088785	Dynamic and Test-retest Whole Body ^{18}F-FES PET Imaging in Patients With Metastatic ER + Breast Cancer
Endometriosis	
NCT04347135	Pilot Study Evaluating Endometriosis With ^{18}F-FES PET/MRI
NCT04382911	Evaluation of Endometriosis With ^{18}F-FES PET/MRI
Ductal Carcinoma In Situ	
NCT03703492	Hybrid Molecular Imaging of ER in Breast Cancer Patients with DCIS
^{18}F-FES as a Pharmacodynamic Biomarker	
NCT03284957	Phase 1/2 Study of Amcenestrant (SAR439859) Single Agent and in Combination With Other Ant-cancer Therapies in Postmenopausal Women With Estrogen Receptor Positive Advanced Breast Cancer (AMEERA-1)
NCT04942054	A Phase 1 Study to Determine Safety, Tolerability, Pharmacokinetics, Pharmacodynamics and Preliminary Efficacy of SCO-120 in Hormone Receptor Positive, HER2 Negative Advanced Breast Cancer Patients
NCT04174352	A Pilot Study of ^{18}F-FES Imaging to Optimize Tamoxifen Dose for Metastatic Breast Cancer Patients With ESR1 Mutations

Data from ClinicalTrials.gov. Available at: https://clinicaltrials.gov/. Accessed Mar 20 2023.

dosage of drug needed for effective usage. In this scenario, molecular imaging with radioactive tracers is utilized to assist in the early development of nonradioactive treatments, a paradigm that could be utilized in tumors beyond breast cancer.

There is substantial ongoing research into potential future applications of ER-targeted imaging. One such potential application is for detection and quantification of disease in patients with tumors that are not adequately imaged by currently standard imaging methods, such as invasive lobular breast carcinoma (ILC). Approximately 15% of breast malignancies demonstrate ILC histology. It is underappreciated that ILC represents a distinct disease process from the more common invasive ductal carcinoma (IDC), with unique molecular, pathologic, clinical, and radiologic features.[67–73] ILC lacks the *CDH1* gene, which encodes for E-cadherin, a cell adhesion molecule.[67] Without E-cadherin, ILC does not grow in tight clusters of cells, but rather as noncohesive single files of cells, a pattern that can be recognized on histologic specimens.[74] This results in lower numbers of cells per volume of tissue and makes ILC more difficult to detect than IDC on mammography, ultrasound, MR, and ^{18}F-FDG PET.[68–72] Thus, there is a need for better methods of imaging ILC. Novel molecular approaches such as amino acid imaging have been attempted with some promise.[75–77] As nearly all ILC are ER-positive,[67,78] several have suggested ER-targeted imaging for patients with ILC. One review of prospective trials performed at Memorial Sloan Kettering Cancer Center demonstrated ^{18}F-FES PET was more sensitive for detecting ILC metastases than ^{18}F-FDG in a small number of patients.[79] Multiple ongoing prospective clinical trials are evaluating the potential clinical impact of ^{18}F-FES PET on patients with ER-positive breast cancer, including ILC (NCT04883814, NCT04252859, NCT03726931).

Several limitations should be considered when utilizing ^{18}F-FES PET. Some medications used for the treatment of breast cancer directly bind to the ER, including selective ER modulators (SERMs), such as tamoxifen, and selective ER degraders (SERDs), such as fulvestrant. Because these agents can block binding of ^{18}F-FES to the ER, the FDA label suggests patients should be withdrawn from these agents for 8 weeks (SERMs) to 28 weeks (SERDs) for optimal ^{18}F-FES PET performance.[80] This will limit the application of ^{18}F-FES PET in patients currently using these medications. The FDA label for ^{18}F-FES states that appropriate therapy with these agents should not be delayed in order to undergo ^{18}F-FES PET.[80] In addition, the high physiologic hepatic uptake and excretion in the liver limits the evaluation of ER-positive disease in the liver and gastrointestinal tract. As ^{18}F-FES detects the ER, tumors that do not express ER or do not express ER functional for ligand binding will not be detected on ^{18}F-FES. Thus, it should be realized that a negative ^{18}F-FES does not always exclude malignancy.

Table 1 summarizes ongoing trials for current and potential future clinical applications of ^{18}F-FES PET. In addition, there is growing interest in the development of more sensitive ER-targeting PET tracers.[81,82]

PROGESTERONE RECEPTOR-TARGETED IMAGING

PR, similar to ER, is routinely evaluated in breast cancer tissue samples by IHC.[83] Because PR is directly regulated by downstream ER effects,[84] it has been suggested that the presence of functional PR may identify tumors with functional ER and thus predict whether endocrine therapy will be effective.[85] PET tracers for PR have been developed,[85–87] of which the most notable is 21-[^{18}F]fluorofuranylnorprogesterone [^{18}F-FFNP].[85] ^{18}F-FFNP demonstrates increased avidity in tumor xenografts after estrogen exposure[88] and demonstrates substantially greater avidity for PR-positive tumors than PR-negative tumors in patients with breast cancer.[89] A recent phase 2 clinical trial notably reported that increased avidity of breast cancer tumors for ^{18}F-FFNP after a 1-day estradiol challenge could predict subsequent response to endocrine therapy with 100% sensitivity and specificity in 43 patients.[85] Although PR-targeted imaging is far earlier in its clinical validation than ER-targeted imaging, this study raises the promise of PR-targeted imaging as a valuable clinical biomarker in the future.

SUMMARY

ER-targeted imaging with ^{18}F-FES is FDA approved "for the detection of ER-positive lesions as an adjunct to biopsy in patients with recurrent or metastatic breast cancer." This broad label allows for multiple clinical applications of ^{18}F-FES PET in patients with ER-positive breast cancer. ^{18}F-FES PET has demonstrated value in resolving inconclusive findings on other imaging modalities and assessing ER status in lesions difficult to biopsy. Perhaps most impactful, ^{18}F-FES PET identifies patients unlikely to respond to endocrine therapies, despite ER-positivity by IHC. Thus, ^{18}F-FES PET can help select optimal patients for endocrine therapies and prevent patients from undergoing ineffective lines of endocrine-based therapy, as well as their associated side effects and costs. Because there are few benign lesions that express sufficient ER to demonstrate ^{18}F-FES-avidity on PET, a positive ^{18}F-FES PET has high specificity for ER-positive malignancy. ER-targeted PET brings the power of molecular imaging to the care of patients with breast cancer.

PR-targeted imaging is still early in clinical development. Currently, the most promising PR-targeted PET tracer is ^{18}F-FFNP, which in a phase 2 clinical trial demonstrated a remarkable 100% accuracy in predicting subsequent response to endocrine therapy.

ER-targeted and PR-targeted PET brings the power of molecular imaging to the care of patients with breast cancer. Molecular imaging for patients with breast cancer is an area of active research, which will likely result in further FDA-approved agents as the field develops.

CLINICS CARE POINTS

- ^{18}F-FES is a PET radiotracer that detects ER that is available to bind estogen ligand. Clinical applications of 18F-FES include: determining whether a pateint with ER-positive metastatic breast cancer should receive endocrine therapies, non-invasively determining the ER status of a lesion that is difficult to biopsy, and determining the status of lesions that are equivocal on other imaging modalites.

DISCLOSURE

G.A. Ulaner discloses grants, consulting fees, honoraria, and/or speaker fees from Lantheus, GE Heathcare, Curium, POINT, RayzeBio, Briacell, and ImaginAb. A.M. Fowler receives book chapter royalty from Elsevier, Inc and has served on an advisory board for GE Healthcare. The Department of Radiology at the University of Wisconsin School of Medicine and Public Health receives research support from GE Healthcare.

REFERENCES

1. Hennrich U, Benešová M. [(68)Ga]Ga-DOTA-TOC: the first FDA-approved (68)Ga-radiopharmaceutical for PET imaging. Pharmaceuticals (Basel) 2020; 13(3). https://doi.org/10.3390/ph13030038.
2. Strosberg J, El-Haddad G, Wolin E, et al. Phase 3 trial of (177)Lu-Dotatate for Midgut neuroendocrine tumors. N Engl J Med 2017;376(2):125–35.
3. FDA Approves (18)F-DCFPyL PET agent in prostate cancer. J Nucl Med 2021;62(8):11n.
4. Hennrich U, Eder M. [(68)Ga]Ga-PSMA-11: the first FDA-approved (68)Ga-radiopharmaceutical for PET imaging of prostate cancer. Pharmaceuticals (Basel) 2021;14(8). https://doi.org/10.3390/ph14080713.
5. Sartor O, de Bono J, Chi KN, et al. Lutetium-177-PSMA-617 for metastatic Castration-resistant prostate cancer. N Engl J Med 2021;385(12):1091–103.
6. Katzenellenbogen JA. The quest for improving the management of breast cancer by functional imaging: the discovery and development of 16α-[(18)F]fluoroestradiol (FES), a PET radiotracer for the estrogen receptor, a historical review. Nucl Med Biol 2021;92:24–37.
7. Henry KE, Ulaner GA, Lewis JS. Human epidermal growth factor receptor 2-targeted PET/single-photon emission computed tomography imaging of breast cancer: noninvasive measurement of a biomarker integral to tumor treatment and prognosis. Pet Clin 2017;12(3):269–88.
8. Fowler AM, Clark AS, Katzenellenbogen JA, Linden HM, Dehdashti F. Imaging diagnostic and therapeutic targets: steroid receptors in breast cancer. J Nucl Med 2016;57(Suppl 1):75S–80S.
9. Ducharme M, Mansur A, Sligh L, et al. Human Epidermal Growth Factor Receptor 2/Human Epidermal Growth Factor Receptor 3 PET Imaging: Challenges and Opportunities. Breast Cancer Res 2023;18(4) [Epub ahead of print].
10. Hwang KT, Kim J, Jung J, et al. Impact of breast cancer subtypes on prognosis of women with operable invasive breast cancer: a population-based study using SEER Database. Clin Cancer Res 2019;25(6):1970–9.
11. Harris L, Fritsche H, Mennel R, et al. American Society of Clinical Oncology 2007 update of recommendations for the use of tumor markers in breast cancer. J Clin Oncol 2007;25(33):5287–312.
12. (EBCTCG) EBCTCG. Effects of chemotherapy and hormonal therapy for early breast cancer on recurrence and 15-year survival: an overview of the randomised trials. Lancet 2005;365(9472):1687–717.
13. Ulaner GA, Riedl CC, Dickler MN, Jhaveri K, Pandit-Taskar N, Weber W. Molecular imaging of biomarkers in breast cancer. J Nucl Med 2016;57(Suppl 1): 53S–9S.
14. Davies C, Godwin J, Gray R, et al. Relevance of breast cancer hormone receptors and other factors to the efficacy of adjuvant tamoxifen: patient-level meta-analysis of randomised trials. Lancet 2011; 378(9793):771–84.
15. Kurland BF, Wiggins JR, Coche A, et al. Whole-body Characterization of estrogen receptor status in metastatic breast cancer with 16α-18F-Fluoro-17β-Estradiol positron emission tomography: meta-analysis and recommendations for integration into clinical applications. Oncologist 2020;25(10):835–44.
16. van Geel JJL, Boers J, Elias SG, et al. Clinical validity of 16α-[(18)F]Fluoro-17β-Estradiol positron emission

tomography/computed tomography to assess estrogen receptor status in newly diagnosed metastatic breast cancer. J Clin Oncol 2022. https://doi.org/10.1200/jco.22.00400. Jco2200400.

17. Ulaner GA, Mankoff DA, Clark AS, et al. Summary: appropriate use criteria for estrogen receptor-targeted PET imaging with 16α-(18)F-Fluoro-17β-Fluoroestradiol. J Nucl Med 2023;64(3):351–4.

18. Tsuchida T, Okazawa H, Mori T, et al. In vivo imaging of estrogen receptor concentration in the endometrium and myometrium using FES PET–influence of menstrual cycle and endogenous estrogen level. Nucl Med Biol 2007;34(2):205–10.

19. Moresco RM, Scheithauer BW, Lucignani G, et al. Oestrogen receptors in meningiomas: a correlative PET and immunohistochemical study. Nucl Med Commun 1997;18(7):606–15.

20. Has Simsek D, Kuyumcu S, Ozkan ZG, et al. Demonstration of in vivo estrogen receptor status with 16α- [(18)F]fluoro-17β-oestradiol (FES) PET/CT in a rare case of benign metastasizing leiomyoma. Eur J Nucl Med Mol Imaging 2021;48(12):4101–2.

21. Morel A, Maucherat B, Chiavassa S, Kraeber-Bodéré F, Rousseau C. Long-term trace of radiation pneumonitis with 18F-fluoroestradiol. Clin Nucl Med 2020;45(9):e403–5.

22. Venema CM, Apollonio G, Hospers GA, et al. Recommendations and technical Aspects of 16α-[18F] Fluoro-17β-Estradiol PET to image the estrogen receptor in vivo: the groningen experience. Clin Nucl Med 2016;41(11):844–51.

23. Ulaner GA. 16α-18F-fluoro-17β-Fluoroestradiol (FES): clinical applications for patients with breast cancer. Semin Nucl Med 2022. https://doi.org/10.1053/j.semnuclmed.2022.03.002. S0001-2998(22)00021-00026.

24. NCCN Clinical Practice Guidelines in Oncology. Breast Cancer. Version 3.2022. Available at: www.nccn.org Published 2022. Accessed January 31, 2023.

25. Fuster D, Duch J, Paredes P, et al. Preoperative staging of large primary breast cancer with [18F]fluorodeoxyglucose positron emission tomography/computed tomography compared with conventional imaging procedures. J Clin Oncol 2008;26(29):4746–51.

26. Groheux D, Giacchetti S, Espie M, et al. The yield of 18F-FDG PET/CT in patients with clinical stage IIA, IIB, or IIIA breast cancer: a prospective study. J Nucl Med 2011;52(10):1526–34.

27. Groheux D, Hindie E, Delord M, et al. Prognostic impact of (18)FDG-PET-CT findings in clinical stage III and IIB breast cancer. J Natl Cancer Inst 2012;104(24):1879–87.

28. Ulaner GA, Castillo R, Goldman DA, et al. 18)F-FDG-PET/CT for systemic staging of newly diagnosed triple-negative breast cancer. Eur J Nucl Med Mol Imaging 2016;43(11):1937–44.

29. Ulaner GA, Castillo R, Wills J, Gonen M, Goldman DA. 18F-FDG-PET/CT for systemic staging of patients with newly diagnosed ER-positive and HER2-positive breast cancer. Eur J Nucl Med Mol Imaging 2017;44(9):1420–7.

30. Wahl RL, Jacene H, Kasamon Y, Lodge MA. From RECIST to PERCIST: evolving Considerations for PET response criteria in solid tumors. J Nucl Med 2009;50(Suppl 1):122S–50S.

31. Ulaner GA, Saura C, Piha-Paul SA, et al. Impact of FDG PET imaging for expanding patient eligibility and measuring treatment response in a genome-Driven Basket trial of the pan-HER kinase inhibitor, Neratinib. Clin Cancer Res 2019;3(5):666–71.

32. Acheampong T, Kehm RD, Terry MB, Argov EL, Tehranifar P. Incidence trends of breast cancer molecular subtypes by Age and race/ethnicity in the US from 2010 to 2016. JAMA Netw Open 2020;3(8):e2013226.

33. Eggersmann TK, Degenhardt T, Gluz O, Wuerstlein R, Harbeck N. CDK4/6 inhibitors expand the therapeutic options in breast cancer: palbociclib, ribociclib and Abemaciclib. BioDrugs 2019;33(2):125–35.

34. Bui TBV, Burgering BMT, Goga A, Rugo HS, van 't Veer LJ. Biomarkers for cyclin-dependent kinase 4/6 inhibitors in the treatment of hormone receptor-positive/human epidermal growth factor receptor 2-negative advanced/metastatic breast cancer: translation to clinical practice. JCO Precis Oncol 2022;6:e2100473.

35. Goel S, Bergholz JS, Zhao JJ. Targeting CDK4 and CDK6 in cancer. Nat Rev Cancer 2022;22(6):356–72.

36. Linden HM, Stekhova SA, Link JM, et al. Quantitative fluoroestradiol positron emission tomography imaging predicts response to endocrine treatment in breast cancer. J Clin Oncol 2006;24(18):2793–9.

37. Hoefnagel LD, van de Vijver MJ, van Slooten HJ, et al. Receptor conversion in distant breast cancer metastases. Breast Cancer Res 2010;12(5):R75.

38. Kumar M, Salem K, Tevaarwerk AJ, Strigel RM, Fowler AM. Recent Advances in imaging steroid hormone receptors in breast cancer. J Nucl Med 2020;61(2):172–6.

39. Linden HM, Peterson LM, Fowler AM. Clinical potential of estrogen and progesterone receptor imaging. Pet Clin 2018;13(3):415–22.

40. Salem K, Kumar M, Powers GL, et al. 18)F-16α-17β-Fluoroestradiol binding specificity in estrogen receptor-positive breast cancer. Radiology 2018;286(3):856–64.

41. Mortimer JE, Dehdashti F, Siegel BA, Katzenellenbogen JA, Fracasso P, Welch MJ. Positron emission tomography with 2-[18F]Fluoro-2-deoxy-D-glucose and 16alpha-[18F]fluoro-17beta-estradiol in breast cancer: correlation with estrogen receptor status and response to systemic therapy. Clin Cancer Res 1996;2(6):933–9.

42. Dehdashti F, Flanagan FL, Mortimer JE, Katzenellenbogen JA, Welch MJ, Siegel BA. Positron emission tomographic assessment of "metabolic flare" to predict response of metastatic breast cancer to antiestrogen therapy. Eur J Nucl Med 1999;26(1): 51–6.

43. Mortimer JE, Dehdashti F, Siegel BA, Trinkaus K, Katzenellenbogen JA, Welch MJ. Metabolic flare: indicator of hormone responsiveness in advanced breast cancer. J Clin Oncol 2001;19(11):2797–803.

44. Dehdashti F, Mortimer JE, Trinkaus K, et al. PET-based estradiol challenge as a predictive biomarker of response to endocrine therapy in women with estrogen-receptor-positive breast cancer. Breast Cancer Res Treat 2009;113(3):509–17.

45. Linden HM, Kurland BF, Peterson LM, et al. Fluoroestradiol positron emission tomography reveals differences in pharmacodynamics of aromatase inhibitors, tamoxifen, and fulvestrant in patients with metastatic breast cancer. Clin Cancer Res 2011; 17(14):4799–805.

46. Peterson LM, Kurland BF, Schubert EK, et al. A phase 2 study of 16alpha-[18F]-fluoro-17beta-estradiol positron emission tomography (FES-PET) as a marker of hormone sensitivity in metastatic breast cancer (MBC). Mol Imaging Biol 2014;16(3):431–40.

47. van Kruchten M, de Vries EG, Glaudemans AW, et al. Measuring residual estrogen receptor availability during fulvestrant therapy in patients with metastatic breast cancer. Cancer Discov 2015; 5(1):72–81.

48. van Kruchten M, Glaudemans A, de Vries EFJ, Schroder CP, de Vries EGE, Hospers GAP. Positron emission tomography of tumour [(18)F]fluoroestradiol uptake in patients with acquired hormone-resistant metastatic breast cancer prior to oestradiol therapy. Eur J Nucl Med Mol Imaging 2015;42(11): 1674–81.

49. Park JH, Kang MJ, Ahn JH, et al. Phase II trial of neoadjuvant letrozole and lapatinib in Asian postmenopausal women with estrogen receptor (ER) and human epidermal growth factor receptor 2 (HER2)-positive breast cancer [Neo-ALL-IN]: highlighting the TILs, ER expressional change after neoadjuvant treatment, and FES-PET as potential significant biomarkers. Cancer Chemother Pharmacol 2016;78(4):685–95.

50. Kurland BF, Peterson LM, Lee JH, et al. Estrogen receptor binding (18F-FES PET) and glycolytic Activity (18F-FDG PET) predict progression-free survival on endocrine therapy in patients with ER+ breast cancer. Clin Cancer Res 2017;23(2):407–15.

51. Chae SY, Kim SB, Ahn SH, et al. A randomized feasibility study of (18)F-fluoroestradiol PET to predict pathologic response to neoadjuvant therapy in estrogen receptor-rich postmenopausal breast cancer. J Nucl Med 2017;58(4):563–8.

52. Boers J, Venema CM, de Vries EFJ, et al. Molecular imaging to identify patients with metastatic breast cancer who benefit from endocrine treatment combined with cyclin-dependent kinase inhibition. Eur J Cancer 2020;126:11–20.

53. He M, Liu C, Shi Q, et al. The predictive value of early changes in (18) F-fluoroestradiol positron emission tomography/computed tomography during fulvestrant 500 mg therapy in patients with estrogen receptor-positive metastatic breast cancer. Oncologist 2020;25(11):927–36.

54. Liu C, Xu X, Yuan H, et al. Dual tracers of 16α-[18F]fluoro-17β-Estradiol and [18F]fluorodeoxyglucose for prediction of progression-free survival after fulvestrant therapy in patients with HR+/HER2-metastatic breast cancer. Front Oncol 2020;10: 580277.

55. Peterson LM, Kurland BF, Yan F, et al. (18)F-fluoroestradiol PET imaging in a phase II trial of vorinostat to restore endocrine sensitivity in ER+/HER2-metastatic breast cancer. J Nucl Med 2021;62(2): 184–90.

56. Su Y, Zhang Y, Hua X, et al. High-dose tamoxifen in high-hormone-receptor-expressing advanced breast cancer patients: a phase II pilot study. Ther Adv Med Oncol 2021;13. 1758835921993436.

57. Liu C, Hu S, Xu X, et al. Evaluation of tumour heterogeneity by (18)F-fluoroestradiol PET as a predictive measure in breast cancer patients receiving palbociclib combined with endocrine treatment. Breast Cancer Res 2022;24(1):57.

58. Mariotto AB, Etzioni R, Hurlbert M, Penberthy L, Mayer M. Estimation of the number of women living with metastatic breast cancer in the United States. Cancer Epidemiol Biomarkers Prev 2017;26(6): 809–15.

59. van Kruchten M, Glaudemans AW, de Vries EF, et al. PET imaging of estrogen receptors as a diagnostic tool for breast cancer patients presenting with a clinical dilemma. J Nucl Med 2012;53(2):182–90.

60. Sun Y, Yang Z, Zhang Y, et al. The preliminary study of 16α-[18F]fluoroestradiol PET/CT in assisting the individualized treatment decisions of breast cancer patients. PLoS One 2015;10(1):e0116341.

61. Yang Z, Xie Y, Liu C, et al. The clinical value of (18)F-fluoroestradiol in assisting individualized treatment decision in dual primary malignancies. Quant Imaging Med Surg 2021;11(9):3956–65.

62. Boers J, Loudini N, Brunsch CL, et al. Value of (18)F-FES PET in solving clinical dilemmas in breast cancer patients: a retrospective study. J Nucl Med 2021;62(9):1214–20.

63. Wang Y, Ayres KL, Goldman DA, et al. 18F-Fluoroestradiol PET/CT measurement of estrogen receptor suppression during a phase I trial of the novel estrogen receptor-targeted therapeutic GDC-0810: using an imaging biomarker to guide drug dosage in

subsequent trials. Clin Cancer Res 2017;23(12): 3053–60.

64. Lin FI, Gonzalez EM, Kummar S, et al. Utility of (18) F-fluoroestradiol ((18)F-FES) PET/CT imaging as a pharmacodynamic marker in patients with refractory estrogen receptor-positive solid tumors receiving Z-endoxifen therapy. Eur J Nucl Med Mol Imaging 2017;44(3):500–8.

65. Jager A, de Vries EGE, der Houven van Oordt CWM, et al. A phase 1b study evaluating the effect of elacestrant treatment on estrogen receptor availability and estradiol binding to the estrogen receptor in metastatic breast cancer lesions using (18)F-FES PET/CT imaging. Breast Cancer Res 2020;22(1):97.

66. Iqbal R, Yaqub M, Oprea-Lager DE, et al. Biodistribution of (18)F-FES in patients with metastatic ER+ breast cancer undergoing treatment with rintodestrant (G1T48), a novel selective ER degrader. J Nucl Med 2022;63(5):694–9.

67. Ciriello G, Gatza ML, Beck AH, et al. Comprehensive molecular portraits of invasive lobular breast cancer. Cell 2015;163(2):506–19.

68. Berg WA, Gutierrez L, NessAiver MS, et al. Diagnostic accuracy of mammography, clinical examination, US, and MR imaging in preoperative assessment of breast cancer. Radiology 2004; 233(3):830–49.

69. Bos R, van Der Hoeven JJ, van Der Wall E, et al. Biologic correlates of (18)fluorodeoxyglucose uptake in human breast cancer measured by positron emission tomography. J Clin Oncol 2002;20(2): 379–87.

70. Ueda S, Tsuda H, Asakawa H, et al. Clinicopathological and prognostic relevance of uptake level using 18F-fluorodeoxyglucose positron emission tomography/computed tomography fusion imaging (18F-FDG PET/CT) in primary breast cancer. Jpn J Clin Oncol 2008;38(4):250–8.

71. Dashevsky BZ, Goldman DA, Parsons M, et al. Appearance of untreated bone metastases from breast cancer on FDG PET/CT: importance of histologic subtype. Eur J Nucl Med Mol Imaging 2015; 42(11):1666–73.

72. Hogan MP, Goldman DA, Dashevsky B, et al. Comparison of 18F-FDG PET/CT for systemic staging of newly diagnosed invasive lobular carcinoma versus invasive ductal carcinoma. J Nucl Med 2015;56(11): 1674–80.

73. Agostinetto E, Nader-Marta G, Paesmans M, et al. ROSALINE: a phase II, neoadjuvant study targeting ROS1 in combination with endocrine therapy in invasive lobular carcinoma of the breast. Future Oncol 2022;18(22):2383–92.

74. Van Baelen K, Geukens T, Maetens M, et al. Current and future diagnostic and treatment strategies for patients with invasive lobular breast cancer. Ann Oncol 2022. https://doi.org/10.1016/j.annonc.2022. 05.006.

75. Ulaner GA, Goldman DA, Gonen M, et al. Initial results of a prospective clinical trial of 18F-fluciclovine PET/CT in newly diagnosed invasive ductal and invasive lobular breast cancers. J Nucl Med 2016; 57(9):1350–6.

76. Tade FI, Cohen MA, Styblo TM, et al. Anti-3-18F-FACBC (18F-fluciclovine) PET/CT of breast cancer: an exploratory study. J Nucl Med 2016;57(9): 1357–63.

77. Ulaner GA, Goldman DA, Corben A, et al. Prospective clinical trial of 18F-fluciclovine PET/CT for determining the response to neoadjuvant therapy in invasive ductal and invasive lobular breast cancers. J Nucl Med 2017;58(7):1037–42.

78. Perou CM, Sorlie T, Eisen MB, et al. Molecular portraits of human breast tumours. Nature 2000; 406(6797):747–52.

79. Ulaner GA, Jhaveri K, Chandarlapaty S, et al. Head-to-Head evaluation of (18)F-FES and (18)F-FDG PET/CT in metastatic invasive lobular breast cancer. J Nucl Med 2021;62(3):326–31.

80. Available at: https://www.accessdata.fda.gov/drugs atfda_docs/nda/2020/212155Orig1s000lbl.pdf. Accessed January 31, 2023.

81. Paquette M, Lavallée É, Phoenix S, et al. Improved estrogen receptor assessment by PET using the novel radiotracer (18)F-4FMFES in estrogen receptor-positive breast cancer patients: an ongoing phase II clinical trial. J Nucl Med 2018;59(2): 197–203.

82. Paquette M, Espinosa-Bentancourt E, Lavallée É, et al. 18)F-4FMFES and (18)F-FDG PET/CT in estrogen receptor-positive endometrial carcinomas: preliminary report. J Nucl Med 2022;63(5):702–7.

83. Hammond ME, Hayes DF, Dowsett M, et al. American Society of Clinical Oncology/College of American Pathologists guideline recommendations for immunohistochemical testing of estrogen and progesterone receptors in breast cancer. J Clin Oncol 2010;28(16):2784–95. doi:JCO.2009.25.6529 [pii].

84. Horwitz KB, Koseki Y, McGuire WL. Estrogen control of progesterone receptor in human breast cancer: role of estradiol and antiestrogen. Endocrinology 1978;103(5):1742–51.

85. Dehdashti F, Wu N, Ma CX, Naughton MJ, Katzenellenbogen JA, Siegel BA. Association of PET-based estradiol-challenge test for breast cancer progesterone receptors with response to endocrine therapy. Nat Commun 2021;12(1):733.

86. Dehdashti F, McGuire AH, Van Brocklin HF, et al. Assessment of 21-[18F]fluoro-16 alpha-ethyl-19-norprogesterone as a positron-emitting radiopharmaceutical for the detection of progestin receptors in human breast carcinomas. J Nucl Med 1991; 32(8):1532–7.

87. Chan SR, Fowler AM, Allen JA, et al. Longitudinal noninvasive imaging of progesterone receptor as a predictive biomarker of tumor responsiveness to estrogen deprivation therapy. Clin Cancer Res 2015;21(5):1063–70.

88. Salem K, Kumar M, Yan Y, et al. Sensitivity and isoform specificity of (18)F-fluorofuranylnorprogesterone for measuring progesterone receptor protein response to estradiol challenge in breast cancer. J Nucl Med 2018;60(2):220–6.

89. Dehdashti F, Laforest R, Gao F, et al. Assessment of progesterone receptors in breast carcinoma by PET with 21-18F-fluoro-16α,17α-[(R)-(1'-α-furylmethylidene)dioxy]-19-norpregn-4-ene-3,20-dione. J Nucl Med 2012;53(3):363–70.

Human Epidermal Growth Factor Receptor 2/Human Epidermal Growth Factor Receptor 3 PET Imaging
Challenges and Opportunities

Maxwell Ducharme, BS[a], Ameer Mansur, BS[a,b], Luke Sligh, BS[a],
Gary A. Ulaner, MD, PhD[c,d], Suzanne E. Lapi, PhD[a,e,**],
Anna G. Sorace, PhD[a,b,*]

KEYWORDS

- Trastuzumab • Pertuzumab • Molecular imaging • Breast cancer • Peptide • Nanobody • Antibody

KEY POINTS

- HER2/HER3 imaging has shown value in clinical trials.
- HER2/HER3 PET can overcome challenges of receptor discordance intratumorally and between primary and metastatic lesions.
- Novel advancements in peptide and nanobody imaging provide opportunities for rapid images and faster radiotracer clearance.
- Paired HER2/HER3 theranostic on on the horizon with great promise.

HUMAN EPIDERMAL GROWTH FACTOR RECEPTOR 2/HUMAN EPIDERMAL GROWTH FACTOR RECEPTOR 3-POSITIVE BREAST CANCER INTRODUCTION

Breast cancer is the most diagnosed cancer in women, and extensive characterization of its biomarkers has allowed for advances in diagnosis, treatments, and imaging that have improved patient care. Early-stage, or localized, breast cancer is considered curable with standard treatments that include local therapy, such as surgical and radiation therapy, or systemic treatments, such as chemo, hormonal, or targeted therapies, that have provided a 5-year relative survival rate of 90% ("Cancer Facts & Figures 2022," 2022). Meanwhile, advanced or metastatic breast cancer is considered uncurable, with much lower survival rates and a clinical objective of alleviating symptoms of cancer burden and prolonging patient survival.[1] Immunohistochemical, genomic, and proliferation markers, assessed through pathologic analysis, are the bases of initial staging and treatment personalization.[2] Immunohistochemistry and fluorescence in situ hybridization allow for rapid quantization of these markers. However, the required biopsies are invasive and can contribute to inherent errors in tissue sampling and are incapable of identifying discordance in biomarker expression, intratumorally and between various sites of disease.[3] Thus, the need for noninvasive tools of biomarker assessment for patient

[a] Department of Radiology, University of Alabama at Birmingham, Birmingham, AL, USA; [b] Department of Biomedical Engineering, University of Alabama at Birmingham, Birmingham, AL, USA; [c] Molecular Imaging and Therapy, Hoag Family Cancer Institute, Irvine, CA, USA; [d] Department of Radiology and Translational Genomics, University of Southern California, Los Angeles, CA, USA; [e] Department of Chemistry, University of Alabama at Birmingham, Birmingham, AL, USA
* Corresponding author.
** Corresponding author.
E-mail addresses: lapi@uab.edu (S.E.L.); asorace@uabmc.edu (A.G.S.)

PET Clin 18 (2023) 543–555
https://doi.org/10.1016/j.cpet.2023.04.009
1556-8598/23/© 2023 Elsevier Inc. All rights reserved.

stratification and early response evaluation is well established.[4–6]

In human epidermal growth factor receptor 2 (HER2) positive breast cancer, an amplification of the HER2 gene and, therefore, overexpression of the HER2 receptor allows for targeted treatments that demonstrate side effects less severe than those typically associated with systemic therapy.[7] HER2-targeted treatments include monoclonal antibodies, such as trastuzumab and pertuzumab; antibody-drug conjugates, such as trastuzumab-emtansine (T-DM1); and HER2 kinase inhibitors including lapatinib, neratinib, and tucatinib.[8–10] Trastuzumab has been well established in the literature and clinical setting where its combination with standard chemotherapies has reduced recurrence rates by 40% and the risk of death by 34%.[9] Specifically, trastuzumab binding prevents activation of the HER2 intracellular tyrosine kinase domain, leading to cell-cycle arrest and eventual apoptosis in HER2-positive cells.[11] Despite advancements, most of the patients who receive trastuzumab-based regimens acquire resistance, which has spurred investigations of possible mechanisms of resistance.[11,12] Furthermore, the heterodimerization of HER2-HER3 has been identified as a potent stimulator of the PI3K/Akt, a downstream pathway associated with cell growth and survival. In addition, HER3 overexpression has been linked to poor prognosis observed in breast, head and neck, melanoma, gastric, and ovarian cancers[13–19] and has become a clear imaging and therapeutic target.[12,20] Because of its supportive role in HER signaling, the expression of HER3 may be altered in response to HER2, HER3, or PI3K inhibitors that diminish treatment efficacy.[9] Intra- and intertumoral heterogeneity of hormone and HER expression exacerbates these issues. Moreover, clinical trials have shown the prognostic impact of receptor status discordance in breast cancer.[21]

PET imaging can overcome challenges of receptor discordance intratumorally and between primary and metastatic lesions by providing a dynamic noninvasive assessment of receptor expression that offers several benefits over traditional pathological sampling. First, the assessment is done over the entire tumor volume rather than a small biopsy section tackling intratumoral discordance in receptor expression. Next, whole-body imaging provides benefits of assessing receptor expression in metastatic sites that may be impractical to biopsy and that have been shown to vary across lesions within the same patient.[20] Further, positron-emitting radiolabeled antibodies can target receptors used to identify and monitor expression changes throughout the course of therapy and could potentially be radiolabeled with therapeutic radioisotopes for the development of theragnostic strategies where the same compound is used for imaging or therapy. Numerous PET radiopharmaceuticals have been developed to evaluate HER2 and HER3 expression, which include [64Cu]-trastuzumab, [89Zr]-DFO-trastuzumab, [89Zr]-DFO-pertuzumab, [89Zr]-Anti-HER3 (GSK2849330), [89Zr]-lumretuzumab, and [177Lu]-DOTA-trastuzumab[20,22] as shown in **Fig. 1**. This review seeks to inform on challenges and opportunities in HER2 and HER3 PET imaging in both clinical and preclinical settings.

CLINICAL TRIALS: PET IMAGING OF HUMAN EPIDERMAL GROWTH FACTOR RECEPTOR 2/ HUMAN EPIDERMAL GROWTH FACTOR RECEPTOR 3

Human Epidermal Growth Factor Receptor 2

Although trastuzumab remains one of the first-line treatments for HER2-positive breast cancer, a variety of clinical trials exploring its use in PET imaging to determine patient HER2 status on both primary tumors and metastatic lesions have been (and are currently) ongoing. The first-in-human investigation of [89Zr]-trastuzumab was completed by Dijkers and colleagues to determine the optimal dosage and time of administration to image HER2 in 14 patients.[23] Although all patients received 38 ± 2 MBq ($\sim$1.5 mg) of [89Zr]-trastuzumab, patients who were currently undergoing trastuzumab therapy showed that coinjection of 10 mg unlabeled trastuzumab resulted in optimal pharmacokinetics for imaging, whereas trastuzumab-naïve patients required a 50 mg of unlabeled trastuzumab, demonstrating the ability to modulate the delivery of [89Zr]-trastuzumab with a variation in total mass of the injected antibody. Further, an injected radioactive dose of $\sim$37 MBq (1 mCi) of [89Zr]-trastuzumab proved to be sufficient for imaging up to 5 days postinjection. Although the study was not intended for direct comparison with HER2 staging or sensitivity/specificity, uptake of [89Zr]-trastuzumab was considered to agree with lesions identified from other imaging modalities. It was determined that future studies to evaluate the sensitivity and specificity of HER2 PET imaging with [89Zr]-trastuzumab would need to be completed to determine its accuracy with HER2 status from biopsies.

Adapting standards from Dijkers and colleagues, other clinical trials to determine dosimetry, sensitivity, and optimal imaging parameters of [89Zr]-trastuzumab were conducted. The ZEPHIR trial used [89Zr]-trastuzumab and [18F]-FDG to look at both HER2-negative and HER2-positive patients'

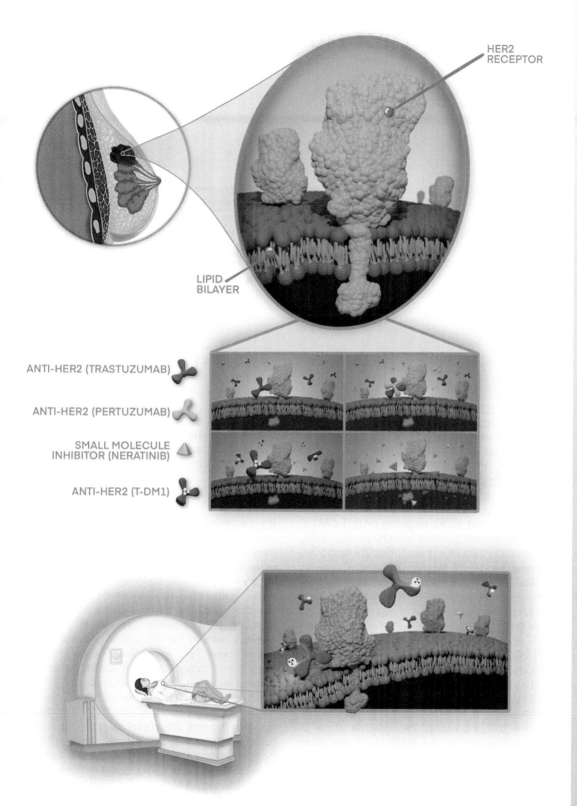

Fig. 1. Nuclear PET imaging and HER2 targets that demonstrate how high sensitivity of receptor targeting can provide key 3-dimensional information to improve detection, monitoring, and therapeutic guidance.

[^{89}Zr]-trastuzumab PET imaging

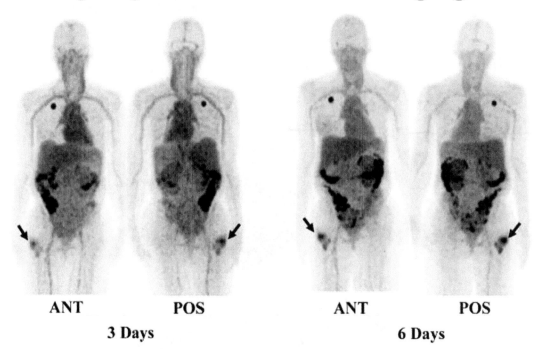

ANT   POS   ANT   POS

3 Days   **6 Days**

Fig. 2. HER2 clinical representative image. [^{89}Zr]trastuzumab anterior and posterior reprojection PET images of a patient with HER2-positive metastatic breast cancer (right femoral metastatic lesion, as indicated by the *arrow*) on day 3 and day 6 following administration of tracer. This research was originally published in Molecular Imaging and Biology. (*From* Laforest R, Lapi SE, Oyama R, et al. [89Zr]Trastuzumab: Evaluation of Radiation Dosimetry, Safety, and Optimal Imaging Parameters in Women with HER2-Positive Breast Cancer. Mol Imaging Biol. 2016;18(6):952-959.)

responses to the HER2 targeting drug T-DM1.[24] Out of 39 patients classified as HER2 positive using ^{89}Zr-trastuzumab, 28 showed objective response, whereas 14 out of 16 HER2-negative patients showed stable or progressive disease via computed tomography (CT); this resulted in a positive predictive value (PPV) and negative predictive value (NPV) of 72% and 88%, respectively. Moreover, when combined with clinical results from [^{18}F]-FDG, a PPV/NPV of 100% was obtained, demonstrating that [^{89}Zr]-trastuzumab can be used as a tool for predicting and evaluating treatment response in HER2-positive patients. Important dosimetry in work by Laforest and colleagues showed that increasing the injected dose of [^{89}Zr]-trastuzumab to 62 ± 2 MBq, with predosing with either 10 or 50 mg of unlabeled trastuzumab appropriately, resulted in the liver being the dose-limiting organ at an average dose of 1.54 mSv/MBq, with a whole-body effective dose of 0.47 mSv/MBq, as seen in **Fig. 2**.[22] However, with the increased injected dose, greater delineation of tumors was visible at 6 days postinjection, and

the percentage of known HER2-positive lesions with visible [^{89}Zr]-trastuzumab uptake was increased from 50% of subjects in the Dijkers study up to 83% in the higher dose study.[22,23]

Other clinical trials have focused on the use of [^{89}Zr]-trastuzumab to differentiate known HER2-positive and -negative lesions, to visualize possible HER2-positive metastasis in HER2-negative primary tumors, and to evaluate if HER2 status could be determined when standard workup was inconclusive.[25–27] Dehdashti and colleagues reported [^{89}Zr]-trastuzumab PET/CT was positive in 30/34 (88.2%) of HER2-positive patients and negative in 15/16 (93.7%) of HER2-negative patients. When excluding hepatic lesions, tumor SUVmax was significantly higher in HER2-positive patients compared with HER2-negative patients (P = .003), and a cutoff SUVmax of 3.2 demonstrated PPV, NPV, sensitivity, and specificity of 83.3%, 50.0%, 75.8%, and 61.5%, respectively, between HER2-positive and -negative lesions.[22] A different clinical trial showed that 55.6% (5 of 9) patients with confirmed

HER2-negative primary breast cancer had suggestive foci of [^{89}Zr]-trastuzumab enhancement on PET/CT. Resulting biopsies confirm that 2 of these patients had HER2-positive metastasis.[26] Bensch and colleagues further showed 15 of 20 patients with varying HER2 status from either multiple primary cancers, inaccessible metastasis, or equivocal HER2 status had [^{89}Zr]-trastuzumab PET imaging support the treatment decision.[27]

Other trials using [^{89}Zr]-trastuzumab PET have been conducted in HER2-positive esophagogastric cancer.[28,29] O'Donoghue and colleagues used [^{89}Zr]-trastuzumab to image HER2-positive lesions in 10 patients with esophagogastric cancer, and 8/10 of those patients had accumulation of the radiotracer 5 to 8 days postinjection. They also reported a whole-body effective dose of 0.48 mSv/MBq, which was similar to previously reported values.[22,28] The same group was also involved in phase II clinical trial using [^{89}Zr]-trastuzumab as a tool for both predictive responses to therapy and monitoring of afatinib with trastuzumab treatment. Successful images were acquired for at least one lesion in all patients, and it was concluded that lesions with heterogeneous uptake might indicate poor response to afatinib, whereas homogeneous uptake may be a marker of afatinib sensitivity.

Although [^{89}Zr] has been the preferred radionuclide for most of the trastuzumab PET imaging clinical trials, [^{64}Cu]-trastuzumab has also been investigated for similar uses. The overall idea of using [^{64}Cu]-trastuzumab has mostly centered on achieving adequate tumor-tissue contrast within 48 hours and in turn, decreasing the dose to the patient. The first-in-human study with [^{64}Cu]-trastuzumab completed by Tamura and colleagues showed the highest uptake in the tumors at 48 hours postinjection paving the way for future clinical trials.[30] It also reported that the whole-body effective dose with an average injection of 126 MBq was estimated at 0.036 ± 0.009 mSv/MBq, which was significantly lower than the reported dose from [^{89}Zr]-trastuzumab.[22,28,30] The same group also reported brain metastasis could be visualized with [^{64}Cu]-trastuzumab for all brain lesions greater than 1 cm in HER2-positive patients with primary breast cancer.[31] Although they were not able to obtain HER2 confirmation for most of the metastasis sites, one patient's lesions were resected and stained positive for HER2 using immunohistochemistry (IHC) in the same location as seen by autoradiography.[31] The second study completed by Mortimer and colleagues showed that there was significantly higher median SUV$_{max}$ in HER2-positive tumors compared with HER2-negative tumors at both 1

and 2 days postinjection ($P < .005$ for both days), indicating [^{64}Cu]-trastuzumab may have a role in optimizing treatments for patients.[32]

A few other clinical trials have explored different radiotracers as well. Two clinical trials conducted by Ulaner and colleagues based on preclinical work by Marquez and colleagues have explored the use of [^{89}Zr]-pertuzumab for PET imaging of HER2-positive breast cancer.[33–35] Their first study demonstrated that [^{89}Zr]-pertuzumab had similar dosimetry (ED of 0.54 ± 0.07) and optimal imaging times (5–8 days postinjection) as [^{89}Zr]-trastuzumab while identifying potential HER2 lesions that were subsequently proved to be HER2 positive after biopsy.[33] The second clinical trial focused on imaging potential HER2-positive metastasis from HER2-negative patients with breast cancer. Out of 24 patients, 6 had foci that were identified as potentially HER2 positive with 48 mg of unlabeled pertuzumab followed by ~2 mg of 74 MBq of [^{89}Zr]-pertuzumab, and 3/6 patients were confirmed HER2 positive after tissue sampling. Patients with previously unsuspected HER2-positive metastases that were discovered by [^{89}Zr]-pertuzumab PET/CT subsequently underwent HER2-targeted therapy with therapeutic response, demonstrating that this imaging approach could be used to identify patients eligible for HER2-targeted therapy that otherwise would not be considered for it. The ability to identify additional patients who may benefit from HER2-targeted therapies becomes even more critical given the recent demonstration by Modi and colleagues that even patients with "low" HER2 expression may benefit from newer HER2-targeted therapies.[36] Methods to further improve [^{89}Zr]-pertuzumab, including site-specific antibody radiolabeling, are in clinical trials (NCT04692831).[37]

Clinical trials have also looked at alternatives to antibodies for HER2 PET imaging. Beylergil and colleagues evaluated the F(ab')$_2$ of trastuzumab labeled with ^{68}Ga.[38] It was reported that with an injected dose of 236 MBq in 5 mg of mass the [^{68}Ga]-DOTA-F(ab')$_2$-trastuzumab was well tolerated with an effective dose of 0.0025 mSv/MBq and an average biological half-life of 3.6 ± 0.9 hours. Four HER2-positive patients (50%) showed uptake of the radiotracer after 3 hours in at least one target lesion.[38] Clinical studies with a ^{68}Ga-radiolabeled affibody, [^{68}Ga]-ABY-025, have also demonstrated clinical promise. A dosimetry study of [^{68}Ga]-ABY-025 showed highest dose was to the liver and kidneys with an average whole-body effective dose of 0.029 ± 0.003 mSv/MBq, whereas a trial by Sörensen and colleagues reported that the same affibody had 5 times greater uptake in HER2-positive lesions compared with HER2-negative lesions (P = .005) 4 hours postinjection.[39,40] Lastly, a phase I clinical trial involving a HER2-specific nanobody was evaluated by Keyaerts and colleagues.[41] This small naturally derived antibody fragment from camelid heavy chain–only antibodies showed uptake in 13 of 15 primary tumors while also showing at least 1 metastasis site in all patients 1.5 hours postinjection. The dose to the patients were highest in the kidney/bladder, whereas the whole-body effective dose was 0.043 ± 0.005 mSv/MBq.

Human Epidermal Growth Factor Receptor 3

HER3 has been less explored as a molecular imaging target than HER2. Notable examples in clinical trials have mainly focused on intact antibodies labeled with long-lived positron emitters such as [89]Zr and [64]Cu.

The first HER3 imaging clinical trial was reported in 2016 with [^{64}Cu]DOTA-patritumab.[42] This phase I first-in-human trial aimed to investigate safety, dosimetry, and apparent receptor occupancy with administration of unlabeled patritumab. Patients were imaged at 3, 24, and 48 hours after injection with the highest tumor to blood ratios obtained after 48 hours. PET imaging in the dosimetry cohort demonstrated the critical dose organ to be the liver (0.46 ± 0.086 mGy/MBq), as expected due to the route of excretion. In the receptor occupancy cohort, the tumor-to-blood ratio decreased after administration of stable patritumab at 9.0 mg/kg;

however, no correlation was observed in the tumor to muscle SUV$_{ratio}$ in this cohort.

PET imaging with [[89]Zr]GSK2849330, fully human monoclonal antibody, was explored in patients with solid tumors to assess HER3 target engagement, as shown in **Fig. 3**.[43] This study includes imaging before and after increasing doses of unlabeled GSK2849330 to assess target engagement with the drug. Imaging at several time points revealed imaging 5 days after injection yielded the best tumor contrast. A comparison of imaging preadministration and postadministration of unlabeled GSK2849330 at 24 to 30 mg/kg showed a decrease in uptake, which correlated with the administered dose, with saturation observed at the highest levels. Modeling data of target engagement from this study were able to yield a 50% inhibitory mass dose (ID50) of 2 mg/kg.

A similar prior study with [[89]Zr]-lumretuzumab, a glycoengineered humanized monoclonal antibody, was also carried out in a larger pool of patients with HER3-expressing tumors.[44] This trial included 20 patients who were imaged either with a coinjection of escalating doses of unlabeled lumretuzumab or before and after higher doses, 400 to 1600 mg, of the drug. PET imaging revealed the SUV$_{mean}$ was highest with a coinjection of 100 mg of lumretuzumab and that tumor visualization was best at 7 days postinjection. Of 216 total lesions that were greater than 1 cm, 68% were

[89]Zr-GSK2849330 PET/CT of pelvic metastasis

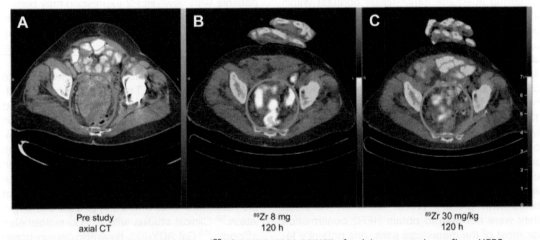

Pre study axial CT   [89]Zr 8 mg 120 h   [89]Zr 30 mg/kg 120 h

Fig. 3. HER3 clinical representative image. [[89]Zr]-GSK2849330 PET/CT of pelvic metastasis confirms HER3 expression, with coorespondign CT (A). Dose-dependent inhibition of tumor uptake of [[89]Zr]-GSK2849330 by unlabeled mAb confirmed target engagement of mAb to the HER3 receptor (B). A Patlak analysis to model irreversible tumor accumulation observed a marked reduction in radiotracer accumulation rate at the highest dose of 30 mg/kg (shown in C), suggesting saturation of the target. mAb, monoclonal antibody. (This research was originally published in JNM. Menke-van der Houven van Oordt CW, McGeoch A, Bergstrom M, et al. Immuno-PET Imaging to Assess Target Engagement: Experience from 89Zr-Anti-HER3 mAb (GSK2849330) in Patients with Solid Tumors. J Nucl Med. 2019;60(7):902-909. © SNMMI.)

visible on the PET images [^{89}Zr]-lumretuzumab. PET imaging before and after therapeutic amounts of lumretuzumab showed decreasing tumor uptake in a dose-dependent fashion. However, saturation of the tumor receptor sites was not observed in this study.

Challenges with Human Epidermal Growth Factor Receptor 2/Human Epidermal Growth Factor Receptor 3 Imaging

Standardization of HER2/HER3 imaging for clinical applications is not without challenges, as there are normal tissues with a range of HER2 expression, such as kidney and bladder, muscle, and components of the respiratory system.[45] Further, normal excretion and processing of peptides and antibody-based probes results in high uptake in certain organs (some of which have tumors that would need to be imaged).[46] As HER2-positive primary tumors have a high rate of metastasis to the liver, and antibody-based probes have high hepatic uptake, this poses a potential challenge for routine use of radiolabeled HER2/HER3 antibodies for receptor imaging of metastasis. However, there are clinically relevant and Food and Drug Administration (FDA)-approved antibody-imaging strategies and antibody-drug conjugate strategies that focused on HER2 as the targeting moiety of interest that have demonstrated effective targeting. A key component in future clinical applicability is also the design of appropriate image analysis approaches to quantify overexpression of HER2/HER3 that allow for quantitative analysis of receptor expression heterogeneity, which is one of the key advantages of imaging over traditional biopsies.

PRECLINICAL MOLECULAR IMAGING OF HUMAN EPIDERMAL GROWTH FACTOR RECEPTOR 2/HUMAN EPIDERMAL GROWTH FACTOR RECEPTOR 3 ON THE HORIZON

As promising clinical trials for HER2/HER3 PET imaging continue, new preclinical antibodies, antibody fragments, and peptides are constantly being evaluated and developed. Although HER2 clinical trials involving trastuzumab and pertuzumab are the most mature, development of antibody fragments for HER2 PET imaging illustrate potential with opportunities to leverage the strengths of targeted imaging while minimizing some of the weaknesses of antibodies (ie, long circulation time). Similar to the clinical trial evaluating F(ab')$_2$ of trastuzumab, [^{64}Cu]-NOTA-pertuzumab F(ab')$_2$ has shown high binding and affinity for HER2 in vivo.[38,47] Lam and colleagues reported a K_d of 2.6 ± 0.3 nM after synthesis and conjugation. [^{64}Cu]-NOTA-pertuzumab F(ab')$_2$ had the highest

%ID/g at a dose of 50 μg (1–3 MBq) in SKOV-3 xenografts, and visible images could be acquired at 24 hours postinjection. Confirmation of specificity for HER2 was confirmed by blocking with unlabeled pertuzumab with a 3.7-fold decreased uptake of [^{64}Cu]-NOTA-pertuzumab F(ab')$_2$. Further, the estimated whole-body effective dose to humans calculated using OLINDA was 0.015 mSv/MBq, which is lower than previous clinical studies with [^{89}Zr]-pertuzumab.[33,47] Alternatively, because HER2 forms heterodimers with other HER family members, the development of a bispecific radioimmunoconjugate is under development by Kwon and colleagues for HER2 and epidermal growth factor receptor (EGFR) (HER1).[48] The bispecific [^{64}Cu]-NOTA-Fab-PEG$_{24}$-EGF had significantly higher uptake in modified MDA-MB-231/h2N (EGFR^{moderate}/HER2^{moderate}) tumor xenografts at 48 hours postinjection (4.9 ± 0.4 %ID/g) compared with the radiolabeled compounds targeting individual receptors ($P < .05$).

Development of HER3 targeting radiotracers also shows great promise in preclinical research. Warnders and colleagues combined 3 different nanobodies to make a biparatopic construct ([^{89}Zr]-MSB0010853) that has 2 different nanobodies targeting HER3, with one-third to bind to albumin to extend its biological half-life.[49] [^{89}Zr]-MSB0010853 showed strong binding and specificity to HER3 in vitro to H441 cells. Both protein dose and time-dependent biodistribution studies with [^{89}Zr]-MSB0010853 demonstrated that a 25 μg injection and imaging 24 hours postinjection had the highest SUV$_{mean}$ in xenograft tumors (0.6 ± 0.2); however, tumors were visible up to 96 hours despite minimal internalization in vitro. There was also a significant difference in HER3-positive H441 xenografts compared with HER3-negative Calu-1 xenografts 24 hours postinjection (6.2 ± 1.1 vs 2.3 ± 0.3 %ID/g; $P = .04$). The affibody Z$_{08698}$ has been evaluated extensively, originally structured as ^{68}Ga-(HE)$_3$-Z$_{08698}$-NOTA and later modified with a variety of alternative chelators and linkers.[50] Compared with [^{68}Ga]-(HE)$_3$-Z$_{08698}$-NOTA, switching the chelator to NODAGA while keeping the (HE)$_3$ linker improved some in vitro and in vivo characteristics. [^{68}Ga]-(HE)$_3$-Z$_{08698}$-NODAGA had less release of ^{68}Ga in both PBS and human serum than its NOTA predecessor. Binding to HER3-positive BxPC3 was confirmed for both affibodies, and a significant decrease in binding ($P < .05$) was obtained when blocked with excess unlabeled affibody. In vivo biodistribution studies also showed differences between the 2 affibodies. ^{68}Ga-(HE)$_3$-Z$_{08698}$-NODAGA had a significantly higher tumor-to-blood ratio than [^{68}Ga]-(HE)$_3$-Z$_{08698}$-NOTA ($P < .05$) despite a nonsignificant difference in tumor binding. The kidneys had greater than 100% %ID/g for both affibodies, prompting the need for future development to lower renal retention. Most importantly, both affibodies showed clear PET images of HER3-positive tumors 3 hours postinjection; therefore, [68 Ga]-(HE)$_3$-Z$_{08698}$-NODAGA was the optimal affibody, as it had higher tumor-to-blood and tumor-to-liver ratio.[50]

As biological half-lives for antibodies are typically days and antibody fragments have variable biological half-lives depending on the fragment used, the development of HER2-/HER3-targeting peptides have the potential for rapid images with faster radiotracer clearance. There have been a handful of HER2-targeting peptides that have been investigated for imaging HER2 using PET.[51,52] Kumar and colleagues developed 3 different peptides using the KCCYSL peptide motif combined with ^{64}Cu to evaluate imaging characteristics.[51] [64Cu]-DO3A-GSG-KCCYSL, [64Cu]-TE2A-GSG-KCCYSL, and [64Cu]-NO2A-GSG-KCCYSL all showed high affinity to HER2 with IC50 values between 31 and 45 nM with in vitro stability in serum up to 2 hours. The study determined that 2 hours after injection was the optimal time to visualize tumor uptake in mice bearing MDA-MB-435 xenografts. Out of the compounds studied, [64Cu]-NO2A-GSG-KCCYSL had both the highest tumor uptake (0.61 ± 0.06 % ID/g) and the highest tumor-to-blood ratio (7.62).[51] Ardakani and colleagues evaluated a different peptide sequence, [68 Ga]-DOTA-(Ser)$_3$-LTVSPWY, for PET imaging.[52] After confirming in vitro binding affinity and specificity, tumor images in SKOV-3 xenografts were visualized

1 hour postinjection with an uptake of 0.56 ± 0.26 %ID/g. In vivo specificity was also confirmed by blocking with nonlabeled peptide significantly decreasing radiopeptide uptake (P < .05). Further, preclinical evaluation of a HER2-specific nanobody, 5F7, was labeled with [18F], allowing slightly longer imaging windows, while retaining high specificity to HER2, as shown in **Fig. 4**[53] One of the most promising HER3-targeting peptides was evaluated by Larimer and colleagues after discovery in a 7-mer bacteriophage library.[54] [68 Ga]-NOTA-HER3P1 showed an affinity of ~270 nM for HER3 in vitro. [68 Ga]-NOTA-HER3P1 had successful image acquisition 1 hour postinjection with an uptake of 0.50 ± 0.18 %ID/g with higher tumor-to-blood ratios between 1.60 and 3.32 in high HER3 tumors versus low HER3 tumors (0.69–0.94).[54]

FUTURE DIRECTIONS

As HER2/HER3 imaging biomarkers are being developed for nuclear imaging, there is a push for multiparametric and/or multimodality imaging to combine anatomical and functional imaging metrics that relate to underlying biology with molecular expression profiles. For example, this could be combining information from FDG-PET with HER2/3-PET imaging for initial disease characterization or combining molecular expression with therapeutic response imaging metrics (such as quantitative MR imaging that has demonstrated to have strong predictive capabilities in breast cancer). The development of this field has potential to drive forward noninvasive tumor characterization that can be a

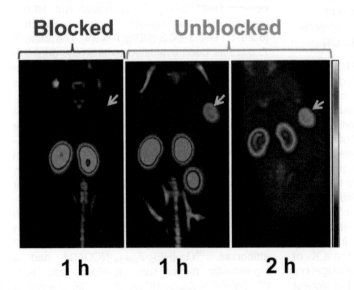

Blocked   **Unblocked**

1 h   **1 h**   **2 h**

Fig. 4. Preclinical representative image. Small animal PET/CT images at 24 and 48 hours postinjection [18F]-RL-I-5F7 in mice with subcutaneous BT-474 human breast cancer xenografts (indicated by *green arrows*), comparing specificity of the imaging probe with trastuzumab-blocked imaging and unblocked imaging. The imaging reveals high uptake in tumor, with no uptake in other organs other than kidneys and bladder. In addition, blocking reduced tumor uptake by greater than 90%, demonstrating high specificity to HER2. (This research was originally published in JNM. Vaidyanathan G, McDougald D, Choi J, et al. Preclinical Evaluation of 18F-Labeled Anti-HER2 Nanobody Conjugates for Imaging HER2 Receptor Expression by Immuno-PET. J Nucl Med. 2016;57(6):967-973. © SNMMI.)

game changer for patients with tumors that overexpress HER2/HER3.

Although only 20% of patients with breast cancer demonstrate an overexpression of HER2, which has been the primary driver for development of this technology, roughly 50% of primary breast tumors show a low-level expression of HER2 (HER2-low), which is defined by a score of 1+ on immunohistochemistry and negative results on in situ hybridization.[55] In 2022, "low HER2" became a definable subtype of cancer and has redefined treatment options for these patients, which includes approximately 60% of metastatic patients.[36] Effective treatment and long-term survival outcomes have been improved with antibody drug conjugates, such as trastuzumab deruxtecan; therefore, it is assumed that trastuzumab appropriately targets this patient population. The DESTINY-Breast04 trial aimed to categorize the HER2 low breast cancer patient population with IHC and in situ hybridization, allowing this subtype to be defined. Therapeutic results from these trials have potential to improve the treatment outcome for a large population of patients historically categorized as having HER2-negative breast cancer and enhance the need for improved and effective imaging strategies to define the inter- and intraheterogeneity of HER2 expression in metastatic HER2-positive breast cancers.[36] Further, there is an opportunity to use imaging to accurately score HER2-low, as traditional methodology has been questioned and deemed to not be accurate, leading to potential mismanagement of patients, leading back to new potential options for imaging-driven therapies.[56]

Imaging to characterize primary and secondary tumors to assess therapeutic strategies can be categorized into multiple approaches: (1) HER2/HER3 to guide initial systemic targeted therapy and response kinetics to direct timing or decision-making for traditional therapeutic interventions, (2) matched imaging/therapy radiopharmaceutical (theranostic) approaches that aim to image to direct therapy. Matched theranostic radiopharmaceuticals for imaging and therapy such as [^{89}Zr]-trastuzumab, followed by [^{177}Lu]-trastuzumab, have been demonstrated to be safely administered to patients with HER2-overexpressing metastatic brain lesions.[57] Further, dosimetry analysis has demonstrated this radiotherapeutic targeted to HER2 to be relatively tolerable; this follows upon the success of similar FDA-approved strategies, such as imaging/therapy pairs in prostate cancer

Table 1
HER2/HER3 PET imaging probes

	Probe	Status/Phase	Type	ClinicalTrials.gov Identifier
HER2	[^{64}Cu]-trastuzumab	Clinical	Antibody	NCT00605397 NCT01093612 NCT02226276 NCT01939275
	[^{89}Zr]-DFO-trastuzumab	Clinical	Antibody	NCT03321045 NCT02065609 NCT01420146
	[^{89}Zr]- pertuzumab	Clinical	Antibody	NCT04692831
	[^{68}Ga]-ABY-025	Clinical	Affibody	NCT02095210 NCT01858116
	[^{68}Ga]-DOTA-F(ab')2 -trastuzumab	Clinical	Fab antibody	NCT00613847
	HER2 nanobody (Ablynx) [^{18}F]GE-226	Clinical	Nanobody	Not available NCT03827317
	[^{68}Ga]-(HE)$_3$-Z$_{08698}$-NODAGA	Preclinical		
	[^{68}Ga]-DOTA-(Ser)$_3$-LTVSPWY	Preclinical		
	[^{64}Cu]-DO3A-GSG-KCCYSL [^{64}Cu]-TE2A-GSG-KCCYSL [^{64}Cu]-NO2A-GSG-KCCYSL	Preclinical	Peptide	
	[^{68}Ga]-NOTA-HER3P1	Preclinical	Peptide	
	[^{68}Ga]-DOTA-(Ser)3-LTVSPWY	Preclinical	Peptide	
	[^{18}F]-RL-I	Preclinical	Nanobody	
HER3	^{89}Zr-Anti-HER3 (GSK2849330)	Clinical	Antibody	NCT01966445 NCT02345174
	89Zr-lumretuzumab	Clinical	Antibody	NCT01482377

targeting prostate-specific membrane antigen and neuroendocrine tumors targeting SSTR2 expression. In addition, inherently paired isotopes [^{64}Cu] and [^{67}Cu] may allow for expansion of this field. For example, [^{67}Cu]-labeled pertuzumab coadministered with trastuzumab has demonstrated ability to enhance tumor response to therapy by combining radiation therapy with directed targeted therapy.[58] In addition, as there is known discordance and heterogeneity of HER2 expression across primary and metastatic tumors and this is known to affect therapeutic response to a wide range of drug response (chemotherapy, targeted therapy, radiotherapeutics, antibody drug conjugates), imaging has become critical to push the field of therapy toward patient personalization and optimization.

Although HER2 is mostly commonly overexpressed in breast cancers, there is a growing body of literature that is exploring subtypes of other solid tumors that have overexpression of HER2, including head and neck cancers, biliary tract, colorectal,[59] non–small lung and bladder cancers (~10% head and neck tumors, ~3%–5% colorectal).[60,61] Furthermore, HER2-positive breast cancer often metastasizes to the visceral organs, such as liver and brain, making evaluation of metastatic disease with full-length antibodies potentially challenging.[62] Although delivery to the brain with antibody therapies has been in question, it is important to note that several studies have demonstrated uptake of HER2-labeled antibodies in brain lesions.[33] However, with greater than 5% of discordance between metastatic disease and primary, it is of utmost importance to appropriately guide therapeutic options.[63]

SUMMARY

PET imaging can play a pivotal role in noninvasively evaluating HER2 and HER3 expression, creating opportunities for more precise targeted therapy. The research conducted including (but not limited to) radiotracers, [^{64}Cu]-trastuzumab, [^{89}Zr]-trastuzumab, [^{89}Zr]-pertuzumab, [^{89}Zr]-Anti-HER3 (GSK2849330), and [^{89}Zr]-lumretuzumab, has allowed for development and innovation of optimized treatment in clinical and preclinical environments with theranostic approaches such as [^{177}Lu]-DOTA-trastuzumab on the horizon. An overview of current ongoing efforts is shown in **Table 1**. Through these studies, challenges were identified and addressed to improve HER2/HER3 imaging. Future PET studies and new directions for this technology hold great potential and play a critical role in furthering the field.

CLINICS CARE POINTS

- HER2/HER3 receptor status can be dynamic and tracers that allow for faster imaging times with radpid clearance would enable improved clinical guidance for treatment decision making.
- HER2/HER3 imaging may play a role in other cancer types other than breast cancer.

DISCLOSURE

G.A. Ulaner: Consultant/speaker/advisory board memeber for GE Healthcare, Lantheus, POINT, and Nuclidium. The other authors have nothing to disclose.

FUNDING

DOE DESC0021279, 1R01CA279143, 1R01CA24 0589.

REFERENCES

1. Harbeck N, Gnant M. Breast cancer. Lancet 2017;389: 1134–50. https://doi.org/10.1016/s0140-6736(16) 31891-82.
2. Loibl S, Poortmans P, Morrow M, et al. Breast cancer. Lancet 2021;397:1750–69. https://doi.org/10.1016/s0140-6736(20)32381-33.
3. Henry KE, Ulaner GA, Lewis JS. Human epidermal growth factor receptor 2-targeted PET/single-photon emission computed tomography imaging of breast cancer: noninvasive measurement of a biomarker integral to tumor treatment and prognosis. Pet Clin 2017;12:269–88. https://doi.org/10.1016/j.cpet.2017.02.0014.
4. Boers J, de Vries EFJ, Glaudemans A, et al. Application of PET tracers in molecular imaging for breast cancer. Curr Oncol Rep 2020;22:85. https://doi.org/10.1007/s11912-020-00940-95.
5. Paydary K, Seraj SV, Zadeh MZ, et al. The evolving role of FDG-PET/CT in the diagnosis, staging, and treatment of breast cancer. Mol Imaging Biol 2019; 21:1–10. https://doi.org/10.1007/s11307-018-1181-36.
6. Sorace AG, Elkassem AA, Galgano AJ, et al. Imaging for response assessment in cancer clinical trials. Semin Nucl Med 2020;50:488–504. https://doi.org/10.1053/j.semnuclmed.2020.05.0017.
7. Teven CM, Schmid DB, Sisco M, et al. Systemic therapy for early-stage breast cancer: what the plastic surgeon should know. Eplasty 2017;17:e7.

8. Perez EA, Cortés J, Gonzalez-Angulo AM, et al. HER2 testing: current status and future directions. Cancer Treat Rev 2014;40:276–84. https://doi.org/10.1016/j.ctrv.2013.09.0019.

9. Pernas S, Barroso-Sousa R, Tolaney SM. Optimal treatment of early stage HER2-positive breast cancer. Cancer 2018;124:4455–66. https://doi.org/10.1002/cncr.3165710.

10. Schlam I, Swain SM. HER2-positive breast cancer and tyrosine kinase inhibitors: the time is now. NPJ Breast Cancer 2021;7:56. https://doi.org/10.1038/s41523-021-00265-111.

11. Nahta R, Esteva FJ. Herceptin: mechanisms of action and resistance. Cancer Lett 2006;232:123–38. https://doi.org/10.1016/j.canlet.2005.01.04112.

12. Vu T, Claret FX. Trastuzumab: updated mechanisms of action and resistance in breast cancer. Front Oncol 2012;2:62. https://doi.org/10.3389/fonc.2012.0006213.

13. Ahmed A. Prevalence of Her3 in gastric cancer and its association with molecular prognostic markers: a Saudi cohort based study. Libyan J Med 2019;14:1574532. https://doi.org/10.1080/19932820.2019.157453214.

14. Hayashi M, Inokuchi MI, Takagi Y, et al. High expression of HER3 is associated with a decreased survival in gastric cancer. Clin Cancer Res 2008;14:7843–9. https://doi.org/10.1158/1078-0432.Ccr-08-106415.

15. Hüser L, Kokkaleniou M-M, Granados K, et al. HER3-receptor-mediated STAT3 activation plays a central role in adaptive resistance toward vemurafenib in melanoma. Cancers 2020;12. https://doi.org/10.3390/cancers1212376116.

16. Kumai T, Ohkuri T, Nagato T, et al. Targeting HER-3 to elicit antitumor helper T cells against head and neck squamous cell carcinoma. Sci Rep 2015;5:16280. https://doi.org/10.1038/srep1628017.

17. Lyu H, Han A, Polsdofer E, et al. Understanding the biology of HER3 receptor as a therapeutic target in human cancer. Acta Pharm Sin B 2018;8:503–10. https://doi.org/10.1016/j.apsb.2018.05.01018.

18. Mizuno T, Kojima Y, Yonemori K, et al. Neoadjuvant chemotherapy promotes the expression of HER3 in patients with ovarian cancer. Oncol Lett 2020;20:336. https://doi.org/10.3892/ol.2020.1220019.

19. Reschke M, Mihic-Probst D, van der Horst EH, et al. HER3 is a determinant for poor prognosis in melanoma. Clin Cancer Res 2008;14:5188–97. https://doi.org/10.1158/1078-0432.Ccr-08-018620.

20. Henry KE, Ulaner GA, Lewis JS. Clinical potential of human epidermal growth factor receptor 2 and human epidermal growth factor receptor 3 imaging in breast cancer. Pet Clin 2018;13:423–35. https://doi.org/10.1016/j.cpet.2018.02.01021.

21. Yang Z, Li N, Li X, et al. The prognostic impact of hormonal receptor and HER-2 expression discordance in metastatic breast cancer patients. OncoTargets Ther 2020;13:853–63. https://doi.org/10.2147/ott.S23149322.

22. Laforest R, Lapi SE, Oyama R, et al. [(89)Zr]Trastuzumab: evaluation of radiation dosimetry, safety, and optimal imaging parameters in women with HER2-positive breast cancer. Mol Imaging Biol 2016;18:952–9. https://doi.org/10.1007/s11307-016-0951-z23.

23. Dijkers EC, Munnink OTH, Kosterink JG, et al. Biodistribution of 89Zr-trastuzumab and PET imaging of HER2-positive lesions in patients with metastatic breast cancer. Clin Pharmacol Ther 2010;87:586–92. https://doi.org/10.1038/clpt.2010.1224.

24. Gebhart G, Lamberts LE, Wimana Z, et al. Molecular imaging as a tool to investigate heterogeneity of advanced HER2-positive breast cancer and to predict patient outcome under trastuzumab emtansine (T-DM1): the ZEPHIR trial. Ann Oncol 2016;27:619–24. https://doi.org/10.1093/annonc/mdv57725.

25. Dehdashti F, Wu N, Bose R, et al. Evaluation of [(89)Zr]trastuzumab-PET/CT in differentiating HER2-positive from HER2-negative breast cancer. Breast Cancer Res Treat 2018;169:523–30. https://doi.org/10.1007/s10549-018-4696-z26.

26. Ulaner GA, Hyman DM, Ross DS, et al. Detection of HER2-positive metastases in patients with HER2-negative primary breast cancer using 89Zr-Trastuzumab PET/CT. J Nucl Med 2016;57:1523–8. https://doi.org/10.2967/jnumed.115.17203127.

27. Bensch F, Brouwers AH, Hooge MN, et al. 89)Zr-trastuzumab PET supports clinical decision making in breast cancer patients, when HER2 status cannot be determined by standard work up. Eur J Nucl Med Mol Imaging 2018;45:2300–6. https://doi.org/10.1007/s00259-018-4099-828.

28. O'Donoghue JA, Lewis JS, Pandit-Taskar N, et al. Pharmacokinetics, biodistribution, and radiation dosimetry for (89)Zr-Trastuzumab in patients with esophagogastric cancer. J Nucl Med 2018;59:161–6. https://doi.org/10.2967/jnumed.117.19455529.

29. Sanchez-Vega F, Hechtman JF, Castel P, et al. EGFR and MET amplifications determine response to HER2 inhibition in ERBB2-amplified esophagogastric cancer. Cancer Discov 2019;9:199–209. https://doi.org/10.1158/2159-8290.Cd-18-059830.

30. Tamura K, Kurihara H, Yonemori K, et al. 64Cu-DOTA-trastuzumab PET imaging in patients with HER2-positive breast cancer. J Nucl Med 2013;54:1869–75. https://doi.org/10.2967/jnumed.112.1186 1231.

31. Kurihara H, Hamada A, Yoshida M, et al. 64)Cu-DOTA-trastuzumab PET imaging and HER2 specificity of brain metastases in HER2-positive breast cancer patients. EJNMMI Res 2015;5:8. https://doi.org/10.1186/s13550-015-0082-632.

32. Mortimer JE, Bading JR, Park JM, et al. Tumor uptake of (64)Cu-DOTA-trastuzumab in patients with

metastatic breast cancer. J Nucl Med 2018;59: 38–43. https://doi.org/10.2967/jnumed.117.1938 8833.

33. Ulaner GA, Lyashchenko SK, Riedl C, et al. First-in-human human epidermal growth factor receptor 2-targeted imaging using (89)Zr-Pertuzumab PET/CT: dosimetry and clinical application in patients with breast cancer. J Nucl Med 2018;59:900–6. https://doi.org/10.2967/jnumed.117.20201034.

34. Ulaner GA, Carrasquillo JA, Riedl CC, et al. Identification of HER2-positive metastases in patients with HER2-negative primary breast cancer by using HER2-targeted (89)Zr-Pertuzumab PET/CT. Radiology 2020;296:370–8. https://doi.org/10.1148/radiol.202019282835.

35. Marquez BV, Ikotun OF, Zheleznyak A, et al. Evaluation of (89)Zr-pertuzumab in breast cancer xenografts. Mol Pharm 2014;11:3988–95. https://doi.org/10.1021/mp500323d36.

36. Modi S, Jacot W, Yamashita T, et al. Trastuzumab deruxtecan in previously treated HER2-low advanced breast cancer. N Engl J Med 2022;387:9–20. https://doi.org/10.1056/NEJMoa220369037.

37. Vivier D, Fung K, Rodriguez C, et al. The influence of glycans-specific bioconjugation on the FcγRI binding and in vivo performance of (89)Zr-DFO-Pertuzumab. Theranostics 2020;10:1746–57. https://doi.org/10.7150/thno.3908938.

38. Beylergil V, Morris PG, Smith-Jones PM, et al. Pilot study of 68Ga-DOTA-F(ab')2-trastuzumab in patients with breast cancer. Nucl Med Commun 2013; 34:1157–65. https://doi.org/10.1097/MNM.0b013 e328365d99b39.

39. Sandström M, Lindskog KM, Velikyan I, et al. Biodistribution and radiation dosimetry of the anti-HER2 affibody molecule 68Ga-ABY-025 in breast cancer patients. J Nucl Med 2016;57:867–71. https://doi.org/10.2967/jnumed.115.16934240.

40. Sörensen J, Velikyan I, Sandberg D, et al. Measuring HER2-receptor expression in metastatic breast cancer using [68Ga]ABY-025 affibody PET/CT. Theranostics 2016;6:262–71. https://doi.org/10.7150/thno.1350241.

41. Keyaerts M, Xavier C, Heemskerk J, et al. Phase I study of 68Ga-HER2-Nanobody for PET/CT assessment of HER2 expression in breast carcinoma. J Nucl Med 2016;57:27–33. https://doi.org/10.2967/jnumed.115.16202442.

42. Lockhart AC, Liu Y, Dehdashti F, et al. Phase 1 evaluation of [(64)Cu]DOTA-Patritumab to assess dosimetry, apparent receptor occupancy, and safety in subjects with advanced solid tumors. Mol Imaging Biol 2016;18:446–53. https://doi.org/10.1007/s11307-015-0912-y43.

43. Menke-van der Houven van Oordt CW, McGeoch A, Bergstrom M, et al. Immuno-PET imaging to assess target engagement: experience from (89)Zr-Anti-HER3 mAb (GSK2849330) in patients with solid tumors. J Nucl Med 2019;60:902–9. https://doi.org/10.2967/jnumed.118.21472644.

44. Bensch F, Lamberts LE, Smeenk MM, et al. 89)Zr-Lumretuzumab PET imaging before and during HER3 antibody lumretuzumab treatment in patients with solid tumors. Clin Cancer Res 2017;23: 6128–37. https://doi.org/10.1158/1078-0432.Ccr-17-031145.

45. Uhlén M, Fagerberg L, Hallstrom BM, et al. Proteomics. Tissue-based map of the human proteome. Science 2015;347:1260419. https://doi.org/10.1126/science.126041946.

46. Boyle CC, Paine AJ, Mather SJ. The mechanism of hepatic uptake of a radiolabelled monoclonal antibody. Int J Cancer 1992;50:912–7. https://doi.org/10.1002/ijc.291050061647.

47. Lam K, Chan C, Reilly RM. Development and preclinical studies of (64)Cu-NOTA-pertuzumab F(ab')(2) for imaging changes in tumor HER2 expression associated with response to trastuzumab by PET/CT. MAbs 2017;9:154–64. https://doi.org/10.1080/19420862.2016.125538948.

48. Kwon LY, Scollard DA, Reilly RM. 64Cu-labeled Trastuzumab Fab-PEG24-EGF radioimmunoconjugates bispecific for HER2 and EGFR: pharmacokinetics, biodistribution, and tumor imaging by PET in comparison to monospecific agents. Mol Pharm 2017;14: 492–501. https://doi.org/10.1021/acs.molpharmaceut.6b0096349.

49. Warnders FJ, Terwisscha van Scheltinga AGT, Knuehl C, et al. Human epidermal growth factor receptor 3-specific tumor uptake and biodistribution of (89)Zr-MSB0010853 visualized by real-time and noninvasive PET imaging. J Nucl Med 2017;58:1210–5. https://doi.org/10.2967/jnumed.116.18158650.

50. Dahlsson Leitao C, et al. Molecular design of HER3-targeting affibody molecules: influence of chelator and presence of HEHEHE-tag on biodistribution of (68)Ga-Labeled tracers. Int J Mol Sci 2019;20. https://doi.org/10.3390/ijms2005108051.

51. Kumar SR, et al. In vitro and in vivo evaluation of Cu-radiolabeled KCCYSL peptides for targeting epidermal growth factor receptor-2 in breast carcinomas. Cancer Biother Radiopharm 2010;25: 693–703. https://doi.org/10.1089/cbr.2010.082052.

52. Biabani Ardakani J, Akhlaghi M, Nikkholgh B, et al. Targeting and imaging of HER2 overexpression tumor with a new peptide-based (68)Ga-PET radiotracer. Bioorg Chem 2021;106:104474. https://doi.org/10.1016/j.bioorg.2020.10447453.

53. Vaidyanathan G, McDougald D, Choi J, et al. Preclinical evaluation of 18F-Labeled anti-HER2 nanobody conjugates for imaging HER2 receptor expression by immuno-PET. J Nucl Med 2016;57: 967–73. https://doi.org/10.2967/jnumed.115.1713 0654.

54. Larimer BM, Phelan N, Wehrenberg-Klee E, et al. Phage display selection, in vitro characterization, and correlative PET Imaging of a novel HER3 peptide. Mol Imaging Biol 2018;20:300–8. https://doi.org/10.1007/s11307-017-1106-655.

55. Gampenrieder SP, Rinnerthaler G, Tinchon C, et al. Landscape of HER2-low metastatic breast cancer (MBC): results from the Austrian AGMT_MBC-Registry. Breast Cancer Res 2021;23:112. https://doi.org/10.1186/s13058-021-01492-x56.

56. Fernandez AI, Liu M, Bellizzi A, et al. Examination of low ERBB2 protein expression in breast cancer tissue. JAMA Oncol 2022;8:607–10. https://doi.org/10.1001/jamaoncol.2021.723958.

57. Bhusari P, Vatsa R, Singh G, et al. Development of Lu-177-trastuzumab for radioimmunotherapy of HER2 expressing breast cancer and its feasibility assessment in breast cancer patients. Int J Cancer 2017;140:938–47. https://doi.org/10.1002/ijc.3050059.

58. Hao G, Mastren T, Silvers W, et al. Copper-67 radioimmunotheranostics for simultaneous immunotherapy and immuno-SPECT. Sci Rep 2021;11:3622. https://doi.org/10.1038/s41598-021-82812-160.

59. Oh D-Y, Bang Y-J. HER2-targeted therapies — a role beyond breast cancer. Nat Rev Clin Oncol 2020;17:33–48. https://doi.org/10.1038/s41571-019-0268-361.

60. Djaballah SA, Daniel F, Milani A, et al. HER2 in colorectal cancer: the long and winding road from negative predictive factor to positive actionable target. American Society of Clinical Oncology Educational Book; 2022. p. 219–32. https://doi.org/10.1200/edbk_35135462.

61. Birkeland AC, Yanik M, Tillman BN, et al. Identification of targetable ERBB2 aberrations in head and neck squamous cell carcinoma. JAMA Otolaryngol Head Neck Surg 2016;142:559–67. https://doi.org/10.1001/jamaoto.2016.033563.

62. Lyu X, Luo B. Prognostic factors and survival prediction in HER2-positive breast cancer with bone metastases: a retrospective cohort study. Cancer Med 2021;10:8114–26. https://doi.org/10.1002/cam4.432664.

63. Houssami N, Macaskill P, Balleine RL, et al. HER2 discordance between primary breast cancer and its paired metastasis: tumor biology or test artefact? Insights through meta-analysis. Breast Cancer Res Treat 2011;129:659–74. https://doi.org/10.1007/s10549-011-1632-x.

Other Novel PET Radiotracers for Breast Cancer

Sophia R. O'Brien, MD[a],*, Rebecca Ward, MD[a], Grace G. Wu, BA[a],
Sina Bagheri, MD[a], Mahsa Kiani, MD[a], Ashrit Challa[a],
Gary A. Ulaner, MD, PhD[b,c], Austin R. Pantel, MD, MSTR[a],
Elizabeth S. McDonald, MD, PhD, FSBI[a],*

KEYWORDS

• PET/CT • Breast cancer • Fluciclovine • PARP • FAPI • FLT • FMISO • ImmunoPET

KEY POINTS

• There are many novel PET radiotracers which may one day play a role in the diagnosis, staging, management, and even treatment of breast cancer.
• [18F]fluciclovine, currently Food and Drug Association-approved for use in patients with prostate cancer, may have greater uptake in invasive lobular carcinoma of the breast than that seen on [18F]fluorodeoxyglucose PET/CT.
• Multiple poly-adenosine disphosphate (ADP)-ribose polymerase (PARP) radiotracers have been investigated in patients with breast cancer and may one day allow identification of patients who could benefit from PARP inhibitor therapy.
• Fibroblast activation protein inhibitor (FAPI) radiotracers have demonstrated potential use as theranostics in patients with breast cancer, with creation of both diagnostic imaging agents and treatment radiopharmaceuticals.
• [18F]fluoro-3′-deoxy-3′-L-fluorothymidine (FLT) and [18F]fluoromisonidazole (FMISO) may have prognostic implications in patients with breast cancer and potentially guide management.

INTRODUCTION

Many novel PET radiotracers have demonstrated potential use in breast cancer. Although not currently approved for clinical use in the breast cancer population, these innovative imaging agents may one day have a role in the diagnosis, staging, management, and even treatment of breast cancer.

18F-FLUCICLOVINE PET IMAGING

Anti-1-amino-3-[18F]flurocyclobutane-1-carboxylic acid ([18F]fluciclovine) is a synthetic amino acid analog PET tracer.[1,2] It was approved by the US Food and Drug Association for imaging of patients with prostate cancer in 2016. [18F]fluciclovine is transported into cells by amino acid transporters, which are upregulated in a number of malignancies besides prostate cancer.[3] For instance, [18F]fluciclovine uptake is substantially increased in breast cancer cells compared to normal breast parenchyma.[2] In general, the higher the breast cancer tumor grade, the higher the [18F]fluciclovine uptake.[4] As such, [18F]fluciclovine has been investigated as an imaging agent for primary and metastatic breast

[a] Department of Radiology, Hospital of the University of Pennsylvania, 1 Donner, 3400 Spruce Street, Philadelphia, PA 19104, USA; [b] Molecular Imaging and Therapy, Hoag Family Cancer Institute, Irvine, CA 92618, USA; [c] Radiology and Translational Genomics, University of Southern California, Los Angeles, CA 90033, USA
* Corresponding authors.
E-mail addresses: Sophia.Obrien@pennmedicine.upenn.edu (S.R.O.); elizabeth.mcdonald@pennmedicine.upenn.edu (E.S.M.)
Twitter: @SophiaObrien (S.R.O.); @Sina_Bagherii (S.B.)

PET Clin 18 (2023) 557–566
https://doi.org/10.1016/j.cpet.2023.05.001

malignancies. Multiple groups have demonstrated that [18F]fluciclovine may have greater uptake in invasive lobular carcinoma of the breast (ILC) than [18F]fluorodeoxyglucose (FDG)-uptake.[2,4] This is an important finding, as FDG PET is less useful for the evaluation of ILC than for invasive ductal carcinomas of the breast (IDC), and thus other radiotracers may be needed for optimal evaluation of ILC.[5–8] Neoadjuvant therapy response in breast cancers may also be quantified by [18F]fluciclovine PET.[9]

PET IMAGING WITH POLY (ADP-RIBOSE) POLYMERASE RADIOTRACERS

Poly (ADP-ribose) polymerases (PARPs) are a class of proteins involved in DNA damage repair, cell proliferation, and cell death. Effective in vivo whole-body imaging and quantification of PARP expression has been investigated in multiple cancers, including breast cancers which are known to be highly heterogeneous.[10] PARP-1 is the major therapeutic target for PARP inhibitors (PARPi). A biomarker capable of identifying patients based on tumor expression of PARP-1 could inform care in a variety of solid tumor types. Multiple radiolabeled PARPi have been developed for this purpose, based on either olaparib-like structures[11-18] or rucaparib-like structures (Mach et al.[19–21]). Excellent reviews on the subject have been published[22,23]. Some radiolabeled PARPi are being studied as radionuclide therapy agents[13,24–26]. This section focuses on [18F]fluorthanatrace ([18F]FTT) since it is the only PARP-radiotracer that has been investigated in clinical trials in patients with breast cancer.

Pre-clinical studies have demonstrated the binding characteristics of a PARP-1 radiotracer, [18F]FTT, and analog with longer isotope half-life, [125I]KX-1, and their specificity for active PARP-1[19,21,27]. The set of data includes work in a set of ovarian cancer cell constructs with a mix of BRCA competency and PARP-1 expression, which showed that PARP-1 expression is predictive in cell lines, even when BRCA1 is intact[28]. In ovarian cancer, in vitro studies have shown that the level of PARP-1 expression is predictive of responsiveness to PARPi and PARP-1 expression is required for PARPi efficacy[19,28]. Pilot human studies[29] have demonstrated the potential of FTT for PARPi response prediction in the clinical setting. We have demonstrated that PARP-1 expression (as measured by [18F]FTT) is highly variable in breast cancer and not predicted by tumor subtype or BRCA status.[30] This was followed by a pilot human study demonstrating in vivo measurement of drug-target engagement in the setting of PARP inhibitor administration.[31] In that study, in vivo quantification of [18F]FTT uptake was correlated with data derived from ex vivo competition experiments in corresponding tumor samples (**Fig. 1**A and B; **Fig. 2**). There are many possibilities for future tracer development in conjunction with PARPi treatments including combination therapy and theranostics.

FIBROBLAST ACTIVATION PROTEIN INHIBITOR PET IMAGING

Cancer-associated fibroblasts (CAFs) are a subpopulation of tumor stromal cells that are found in over 90% of epithelial tumors. Unlike normal cells, CAFs highly express fibroblast activation protein (FAP), a membrane serine protease that is thought to play various roles in cancer progression. Owing to its specific expression and biological function in tumor environments, FAP is a promising target for imaging and therapy in a variety of malignancies, including breast cancer.[32]

In 2018, researchers at the University of Heidelberg developed novel quinoline-based, DOTA-chelator-labeled FAP-specific inhibitors (FAPI): FAPI-02 and FAPI-04.[33,34] Loktev and colleagues synthesized and demonstrated promising in vitro and in vivo results with FAPI-02, namely, rapid internalization into FAP-positive cancer cells and FAP-positive tumor xenografts. When PET/computed tomography (CT) was performed on a subject with metastatic breast cancer, robust accumulation of ^{68}Ga-FAPI-02 was observed in breast cancer at 10 minutes and 1 hour, with rapid bloodstream clearance and low uptake into normal tissue.[33] Lindner and colleagues subsequently developed FAPI-04 and observed comparably rapid tracer accumulation into tumors, fast physiological clearance, and high image contrast.

FAP has been shown to be abundantly expressed in multiple breast cancer subtypes.[35] In a 2019 retrospective study involving over 80 patients and 28 tumor types, Kratochwil and colleagues[36] found that breast cancer was among the tumor types that displayed the highest average SUV_{max} (> 12) on ^{68}Ga-FAPI-04 PET/CT imaging. In 2021, two comparative studies by Komek and colleagues[37] and Elboga and colleagues[38] found ^{68}Ga-FAPI-04 PET/CT imaging to have improved tumor-to-background ratios (TBRs), and superior sensitivity of lesion detection as compared to FDG PET in patients with breast cancer.

FAPI uptake has been shown to vary based on pathologic grade and molecular subtype of breast neoplasms. In 2021, Dendl and colleagues examined ^{68}Ga-FAPI tracer activity in a cohort of women with gynecological malignancies,

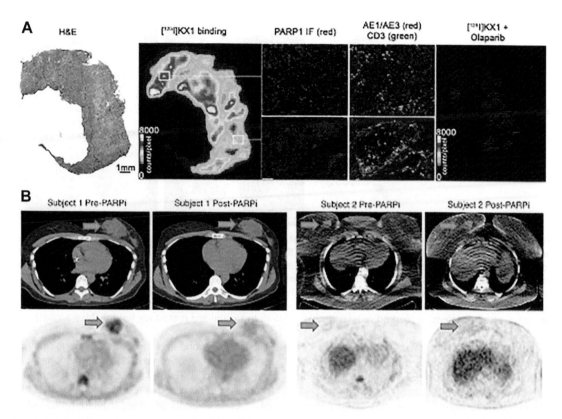

Fig. 1. The baseline expression of PARP-1 in breast cancer was suppressed after PARPi treatment. (*A*) A breast cancer tumor section shows a decrease in PARP radiotracer uptake with the use of olaparib. Quantitative analysis of radioligand binding was conducted through autoradiography and was followed by staining with hematoxylin and eosin (H&E). Cryosections were used for chromogenic PARP-1 immunofluorescence (*red*) with DAPI counterstaining (*blue*). AE1/AE3 staining was performed to identify epithelial tumor cells (*red*), and CD3 staining was used to identify tumor-infiltrating T cells (*green*). Autoradiography reveals the heterogeneous expression of PARP-1 at the microscopic level with a correlation between the intensity of [125I]KX1 uptake and PARP-1 expression as measured by immunofluorescence. The addition of 20 μM olaparib to a sequential section of [125I]KX1 results in a reduction of tracer to background levels. The scale bar on the H&E-stained slide of the whole specimen is 1 mm. (*B*) [18F]FTT PET/CT images were taken before and approximately 1 week after PARPi treatment for two women with advanced triple-negative breast cancer. Subject 1 had a left breast mass (*blue arrows* column 1 and 2) with moderate [18F]FTT uptake pre-therapy (SUVmax breast 4.7 g/mL) which was blocked after treatment (SUVmax breast 2.4 g/mL) and resulted in a response to PARPi. Subject 2 had a left breast mass (*blue arrows* column 3 and 4) with minimal pretreatment uptake (SUVmax breast 2.3 g/mL) and similar post-therapy uptake (SUVmax breast 2.4 g/mL) and experienced progression on PARPi. ER/PR, estrogen receptor/progesterone receptor; SUV, standardized uptake value. (*From* McDonald ES, Pantel AR, Shah PD, et al. In vivo visualization of PARP inhibitor pharmacodynamics. JCI Insight. 2021;6(8):e146592. Published 2021 Apr 22.)

including breast cancer. ^{68}Ga-FAPI PET/CT demonstrated high tracer uptake and excellent TBRs compared with ^{18}F-FDG PET/CT and also demonstrated higher uptake in histologically high-grade compared with low-grade breast cancers.[39] On ^{68}Ga-FAPI-04 PET/CT, Elboga and colleagues reported higher mean SUV$_{max}$ values in patients with human epidermal growth factor 2 (HER2) expression. Given that high FAP expression has been associated with aggressive tumor subtypes,[40] some investigators posit that FAPI may play a role in prognostic assessment of breast cancer.[41]

FAPI tracers have been studied for a possible role in breast cancer staging. In 2022, Backhaus and colleagues assessed the potential value of FAPI PET/MR imaging in supporting clinical staging alongside conventional US, mammogram, and CT imaging. They observed strong ^{68}Ga-FAPI-46 uptake in index lesions and marked tracer accumulation in all biopsy-proven lymph node metastases.[42] In addition, several case reports between 2020 and 2022 demonstrated higher ^{68}Ga-FAPI uptake in, and superior detection of, various metastatic lesions compared with [18F]FDG, including retroperitoneal lymph node and

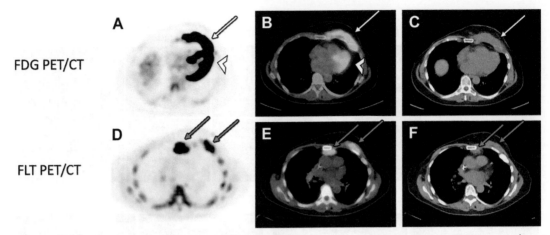

Fig. 2. A 74-year-old woman with ER/PR + HER2 negative breast cancer with biopsy-proven metastases to bones and left axillary nodes. FDG PET/CT (*A*) axial FDG PET, (*B*) fused FDG PET/CT, and (*C*) CT demonstrate an infiltrative soft tissue mass involving the left pectoralis musculature with osseous invasion representing the patient's hypermetabolic metastatic breast cancer (*white arrows*). Note is made of physiologic myocardial uptake on FDG-PET (*white arrowheads*). FLT PET/CT *D*) axial FLT PET, (*E*) fused FLT PET/CT, and (*F*) CT demonstrate marked uptake of FLT in the left chest wall invasive soft tissue mass, seen extending behind the sternum at this slightly higher anatomic slice, representing marked cellular proliferation in the visualized metastatic lesions (*blue arrows*).

rectal metastases[43] and bone metastases.[44,45] Currently, there are five ongoing clinical trials examining FAPI-based PET imaging in patients with breast cancer.[46–50]

False-positive breast uptake has been seen in FAPI PET imaging following hormonal stimulation from estradiol injection, ovulation, and lactation, with higher mean SUV_{max} uptake values in premenopausal versus postmenopausal normal breast tissue.[39,51–53] In addition, increased ^{68}Ga-FAPI-04 uptake has been seen in benign intramammary lymphoid tissue.[54] Further studies are needed to fully characterize and identify possible ways to mitigate false-positive FAPI-tracer uptake in the breasts and elsewhere.

FAPI tracers have also been used in case reports as both diagnostic and therapeutic tracers in patients with breast cancer. The use of ^{90}Y-FAPI-04 to treat a patient with metastatic breast cancer revealed persistent tumor accumulation 24 hours post injection, supporting potential therapeutic application of FAPI-based radiopharmaceuticals.[34] In 2018, Lindner and colleagues[34] treated a patient with confirmed FAP-positive metastatic breast cancer on ^{68}Ga-FAPI-04 PET/CT with 2.9GBq of ^{90}Y-FAPI-04 and reported significant reduction of required pain medication and no adverse events. Ballal and colleagues administered 3.2 GBq of [^{177}Lu]Lu-DOTA.SA.FAPi therapy to a late-stage patient with breast cancer (FAP-positive on [^{68}Ga] Ga-DOTA.SA.FAPi imaging) with new symptomatic brain metastasis. Following therapy, the patient's headaches decreased in intensity, with no observed treatment-related adverse events; however, although radiotracer accumulation was noted

in primary lesions and metastases, image findings proving stability or regression of the lesions were not reported.[55] Baum and colleagues achieved promising in-human therapeutic results with a trial of ^{177}Lu-FAP-2286 peptide-targeted radionuclide therapy in patients with confirmed FAPI-positive disease seen on ^{68}Ga-FAP-2286 or ^{68}Ga-FAPI-04 PET. They demonstrated a favorable safety profile as well as high uptake and long retention in primary and metastatic lesions.[56] However, Rathke and colleagues[57] cautioned that tracer uptake may not be associated with clinical response, reporting disease progression and mortality 11 months post-^{90}Y-FAPI-04 treatment in a ^{68}Ga-FAPI-04 uptake-positive metastatic breast cancer patient who displayed high tumor tracer accumulation. Variable adverse events, such as leukocytopenia,[56] thyroiditis,[58] and moderate stress-induced ischemia,[59] have also been observed with FAPI-based therapy.

In summary, FAPI radiotracers are promising tools for breast cancer diagnosis and therapy; however, the current literature consists largely of small retrospective studies and case reports. Larger prospective studies are needed to investigate potential clinical use of FAPI.

[^{18}F]Fluoro-3'-DEOXY-3'-L-FLUOROTHYMIDINE PET IMAGING

[^{18}F]fluoro-3'-deoxy-3'-L-fluorothymidine ([^{18}F]FLT) images cellular proliferation, a sine qua non of malignancy. This radiotracer has exhibited some success in several diseases and settings, including serving as a biomarker in breast cancer trials paired with targeted therapy.

Radiolabeled thymidine has been investigated as a marker of cellular proliferation as thymidine is the only pyrimidine or purine base that is unique to DNA (cytosine is common to both DNA and RNA; uracil is found in RNA but not DNA). Both 11C-thymidine and F-18-labeled compounds have been studied, with the former impractical for routine clinical translation secondary to short half-life and rapid metabolism necessitating complex analysis.[60–62] With respect to the biological and chemical properties of [^{18}F]FLT, the fluorinated thymidine, [^{18}F]FLT, is phosphorylated by thymidine kinase 1 (TK$_1$) into [^{18}F]FLT-monophosphate through the thymidine salvage pathway. This phosphorylated compound may undergo additional phosphorylations but is not further incorporated into DNA, distinguishing the fluorinated compound from native thymidine and 11C-thymidine. There may be subsequent dephosphorylation but at a rate much slower than initial TK1 phosphorylation. It follows that the retention of [^{18}F]FLT in the cell is a function of TK1 activity, the rate-limiting step of this process.[63] TK$_1$ does not exhibit enzymatic activity in quiescent cells but reaches a maximum in the late G1 and S phases of the cell cycle in proliferating cells.[64,65] Given TK1 activity correlates with cellular proliferation, [^{18}F]FLT offers a noninvasive approach to query cellular proliferation that has potential for clinical translation.

Physiologic uptake of [^{18}F]FLT is seen in bone marrow and liver, limiting the detection of disease in these organs. [^{18}F]FLT is excreted through the kidneys with resultant tracer seen in the urinary tract and bladder, similarly hampering evaluation of these organs. No physiologic uptake is seen in the brain, myocardium, or skeletal muscles, in contrast to FDG-PET.[65] Overall, though, the utilization of [^{18}F]FLT for detection of tumors is quite limited compared with FDG, especially outside of the brain.[62] Similar to FDG, [^{18}F]FLT may demonstrate uptake in inflammation, as demonstrated in head and neck tumors with increased uptake seen in nonmetastatic lymph nodes due to reactive B-lymphocyte proliferation.[66]

Given the biologic target of [^{18}F]FLT, this radiotracer has been most extensively studied as a biomarker to monitor response to targeted therapies. In breast cancer, this has been most extensively studied in the ACRIN 6688 trial, a prospective multicenter phase II study designed to test if [^{18}F]FLT could predict pathologic complete response to neoadjuvant chemotherapy (NAC) in patients with primary breast cancer. Subjects were imaged with [^{18}F]FLT PET at three times: at baseline, after one cycle of NAC, and at the completion of NAC. A percent difference between the baseline PET and PET after the first cycle of NAC was marginally significant between subjects that obtained a pathologic complete response (pCR) and those that did not; the difference between baseline and the PET after completion of NAC reached significance. In both cases, a greater decrease in [^{18}F]FLT SUVmax was seen in the pCR group. Of course, the measure of early therapeutic response after one cycle of NAC has greater clinical relevance, suggesting the potential to modify treatments based on likelihood of response. This study also demonstrated a correlation between post-NAC [^{18}F]FLT SUVmax and Ki-67 on surgical samples. More studies are necessary to corroborate these results, in particular with more uniform NAC regimes, to extend FLT clinical practice for this use.[67]

Although [^{18}F]FLT-PET has demonstrated success in preclinical studies, its role in clinical practice is yet to be determined. Future studies are needed to determine the role of [^{18}F]FLT-PET in guiding breast cancer management.

[^{18}F]Fluoromisonidazole PET IMAGING

Cellular hypoxia has been associated with a majority of neoplasms, leading to dysfunctional vascularization, increased cellular mobility, and metastasis.[68] As radiation therapy and some chemotherapeutic medications require oxygen to generate free radicals that kill cancer cells, hypoxic malignant cells are largely resistant to radiotherapy and chemotherapy.[69] In addition, it has been shown that hypoxic triple-negative breast cancer cells are more likely to metastasize, less sensitive to chemotherapy, and more likely to recur.[70] Therefore, identification of hypoxic activity in tumor cells could potentially guide management decisions. Although methods exist for identifying hypoxic activity in tumor cells, such as the Eppendorf polarographic needle electrode, these methods are invasive and limited to tumors that are accessible percutaneously.[71,72]

In 1984, [^{18}F]fluoromisonidazole ([^{18}F]FMISO) was developed as a PET tracer for noninvasive detection of hypoxia in cancer cells.[70,73] [^{18}F]FMISO has demonstrated success in identifying tumor hypoxia in various cancer types, such as breast, lung, brain, and head and neck.[74–77] As a radiolabeled 2-nitroimidazole, [^{18}F]FMISO binds selectively to macromolecules within hypoxic cells. Because [^{18}F]FMISO is hydrophilic, it readily diffuses across cell membranes and shows passive distribution in normal tissues. In normoxic cells (non-hypoxic cells), the [^{18}F]FMISO electron is removed by oxygen molecules acting as a strong oxidant, allowing for passive diffusion of [^{18}F]FMISO from the cell.[68] In hypoxic cells, [^{18}F]

FMISO captures electrons in the mitochondrial electron transfer system and irreversibly binds to high-weight molecules, becoming trapped in the cell. Since FMISO metabolites are trapped solely in hypoxic cells, increased [^{18}F]FMISO uptake is seen in neoplasm hypoxia.[75,78] Concentration in non-hypoxic tissues is always lower than plasma, with the exception of the intestines, kidney, bladder, and liver.

The detection of cellular hypoxia by [^{18}F]FMISO PET could potentially guide clinical management. Cheng and colleagues[79] found a correlation between baseline [^{18}F]FMISO uptake and poor clinical outcomes after 3 or more months of primary endocrine therapy with letrozole, suggesting hypoxia as a poor prognostic factor in the endocrine receptor-positive breast cancer population. Another study group interested in early imaging changes in patients treated with neoadjuvant bevacizumab in stage II/III breast cancers found that [^{18}F]FMISO uptake was significantly higher in stage III and triple-negative breast cancers than in stage II breast cancers. [^{18}F]FMISO PET SUV_{max} was correlated with vascular endothelial growth factor receptor expression. [^{18}F]FMISO SUV_{max} at baseline was also significantly correlated with Ki-67 values and ^{18}FFLT SUV_{max} at baseline, indicating it may also be a prognostic marker. Average [^{18}F]FMISO uptake across groups did not differ after bevacizumab therapy; however, [^{18}F]FMISO uptake differed significantly between tumors which demonstrated no significant decreased cellularity on postsurgery pathology ("G1 tumors") versus those which demonstrated 30% to 90% reduction in tumor cells on postsurgery pathology ("G3 tumors"). After bevacizumab therapy, G1 tumors demonstrated an increase in hypoxia on [^{18}F]FMISO imaging, whereas G3 tumors demonstrated a decrease in hypoxia. Overall, these findings suggest that [^{18}F]FMISO should be used in conjunction with other modalities, pathology, and clinical factors to accurately identify patients who may respond to neoadjuvant therapy with bevacizumab.[80]

As with other radiotracers, there are limitations to PET imaging with [^{18}F]FMISO. For instance, the lack of active transport of the tracer and slow reaction mechanisms require long examination protocols to quantify regions of tumor hypoxia.[81] In addition, in regions of severe hypoxia, the degree of hypoxia is underestimated by [^{18}F]FMISO uptake, likely secondary to nonlinear uptake of tracer at greater levels of hypoxia.[78] Therefore, although [^{18}F]FMISO PET is a promising noninvasive modality for hypoxia detection, these aforementioned limitations must be taken into consideration when used in a research setting and possibly in the clinic in the future.

ImmunoPET IMAGING

ImmunoPET uses PET-radionuclides attached to monoclonal antibodies for targeted molecular imaging of cancer cells and tumor microenvironments.[82] Multiple immunoPET tracers have been investigated in breast cancer. Programmed death ligand 1 (PD-L1) is an immune checkpoint inhibitor expressed in some triple-negative breast cancers. A radiolabeled anti-PD-L1 antibody, [^{89}Zr]-atezolizumab, has been used to image patients with breast cancer and has potential to guide selection of patients with breast cancer for inclusion in immune-checkpoint inhibitor clinical trials.[83–85] HER2-overexpression in breast cancer is associated with poorer outcomes, which are somewhat mitigated by HER2-directed therapies; however, heterogeneous HER2 expression within a single tumor, across metastatic sites, and over time may hinder patient response to HER2-targeted therapy.[86,87] ImmunoPET radiotracers based on monoclonal antibodies for the HER receptor, including [^{89}Zr]-pertuzumab and [^{89}Zr]-trastuzumab, have been evaluated in preclinical and phase 1 clinical studies as a way to noninvasively image HER2-expression at all sites of metastatic breast cancer, allowing for assessment of disease heterogeneity and potentially guiding management.[88,89] Radiolabeled antibodies to other prognostic biomarkers in breast cancer have also been developed and there are many ongoing studies of these tracers.[90,91] ImmunoPET is an exciting and dynamic field of study with the potential to become a major component of precision medicine for patients with breast cancer in the future.

SUMMARY

There are many innovative and emerging PET radiotracers which may one day play a role in the diagnosis, staging, management, and even treatment of breast cancer.

CLINICS CARE POINTS

- Invasive lobular carcinoma, notoriously occult on many imaging modalities and often demonstrating minimal FDG uptake, may have greater 18F-fluciclovine uptake than FDG uptake, potentially allowing for better disease staging and restaging.

- PARP radiotracers noninvasively measure the expression of PARP-1, the major target of PARP inhibitor drugs.

- FAPI has been used as a theranostic in a small number of patients but pre-treatment FAPI uptake did not always correlate with treatment response. Larger, prospective studies are needed.

- [^{18}F]FLT images cellular proliferation and may one day be used to assess response to ongoing neo-adjuvant chemotherapy, but more studies are needed.

- High baseline [^{18}F]FMISO uptake, indicating cellular hypoxia, has been correlated with poor clinical outcomes of primary endocrine therapy, indicating a potential use in treatment decisions.

- ImmunoPET tracers have been used in preclinical and phase 1 clinical studies to noninvasively assess HER2-expression across all sites of metastatic breast cancer, which may one day be leveraged for management decisions.

DISCLOSURE

The authors have nothing to disclose.

REFERENCES

1. Ulaner GA, Schuster DM. Amino acid metabolism as a target for breast cancer imaging. Pet Clin 2018; 13(3):437–44.

2. Tade FI, Cohen MA, Styblo TM, et al. Anti-3-[^{18}F] FACBC [^{18}F]Fluciclovine) PET/CT of breast cancer: an exploratory study. J Nucl Med 2016;57(9):1357–63.

3. Savir-Baruch B, Schuster DM. Prostate cancer imaging with [^{18}F]fluciclovine. Pet Clin 2022;17(4):607–20.

4. Ulaner GA, Goldman DA, Gonen M, et al. Initial results of a prospective clinical trial of [^{18}F]Fluciclovine PET/CT in newly diagnosed invasive ductal and invasive lobular breast cancers. J Nucl Med 2016; 57(9):1350–6.

5. Avril N, Rose CA, Schelling M, et al. Breast imaging with positron emission tomography and fluorine-18 fluorodeoxyglucose: use and limitations. J Clin Oncol 2000;18(20):3495–502.

6. Bos R, van Der Hoeven JJ, van Der Wall E, et al. Biologic correlates of (18)fluorodeoxyglucose uptake in human breast cancer measured by positron emission tomography. J Clin Oncol 2002;20(2):379–87.

7. Dashevsky BZ, Goldman DA, Parsons M, et al. Appearance of untreated bone metastases from breast cancer on FDG PET/CT: importance of histologic subtype. Eur J Nucl Med Mol Imaging 2015; 42(11):1666–73.

8. Hogan MP, Goldman DA, Dashevsky B, et al. Comparison of [^{18}F]FDG PET/CT for systemic staging of newly diagnosed invasive lobular carcinoma versus invasive ductal carcinoma. J Nucl Med 2015;56(11):1674–80.

9. Ulaner GA, Goldman DA, Corben A, et al. Prospective clinical trial of [^{18}F]Fluciclovine PET/CT for determining the response to neoadjuvant therapy in invasive ductal and invasive lobular breast cancers. J Nucl Med 2017;58(7):1037–42.

10. McDonald ES, Clark A, Tchou J, et al. Clinical diagnosis and management of breast cancer. J Nuc Med 2016;57: 9S–16S.

11. Kossatz S, Weber WA, Reiner T. Optical imaging of PARP1 in response to radiation in oral squamous cell carcinoma. PLoS One 2016;11(1):e0147752.

12. Carney B, Carlucci G, Salinas B, et al. Non-invasive PET imaging of PARP1 expression in glioblastoma models. Mol Imaging Biol 2016;18(3):386–92.

13. Jannetti SA, Carlucci G, Carney B, et al. PARP-1-targeted radiotherapy in mouse models of glioblastoma. J Nucl Med 2018;59(8):1225–33.

14. Carlucci G, Carney B, Brand C, et al. Dual-modality optical/PET imaging of PARP1 in glioblastoma. Mol Imaging Biol 2015;17(6):848–55.

15. Reiner T, Keliher EJ, Earley S, et al. Synthesis and in vivo imaging of a [^{18}F]labeled PARP1 inhibitor using a chemically orthogonal scavenger-assisted high-performance method. Angew Chem Int Ed Engl 2011;50(8):1922–5.

16. Zmuda F, Malviya G, Blair A, et al. Synthesis and evaluation of a radioiodinated tracer with specificity for Poly(ADP-ribose) Polymerase-1 (PARP-1) in Vivo. J Med Chem 2015;58(21):8683–93.

17. Huang T, Hu P, Banizs AB, et al. Initial evaluation of Cu-64 labeled PARPi-DOTA PET imaging in mice with mesothelioma. Bioorg Med Chem Lett 2017; 27(15):3472–6.

18. Wilson TC, Xavier MA, Knight J, et al. PET imaging of PARP expression using [^{18}F]Olaparib. J Nucl Med 2019;60(4):504–10.

19. Makvandi M, Xu K, Lieberman BP, et al. A radiotracer strategy to quantify PARP-1 expression in vivo provides a biomarker that can enable patient selection for PARP inhibitor therapy. Cancer Res 2016;76(15):4516–24.

20. Michel LS, Dyroff S, Brooks FJ, et al. PET of Poly (ADP-Ribose) polymerase activity in cancer: preclinical assessment and first in-human studies. Radiology 2017;282(2):453–63.

21. Zhou D, Chu W, Xu J, et al. Synthesis, [(1)(8)F] radiolabeling, and evaluation of poly (ADP-ribose) polymerase-1 (PARP-1) inhibitors for in vivo imaging of PARP-1 using positron emission tomography. Bioorg Med Chem 2014;22(5):1700–7.

22. Puentes LN, Makvandi M, Mach RH. Molecular imaging: PARP-1 and Beyond. J Nucl Med 2021; 62(6):765–70.

23. Carney B, Kossatz S, Reiner T. Molecular imaging of PARP. J Nucl Med 2017;58(7):1025–30.

24. Makvandi M, Samanta M, Martorano P, et al. Preclinical investigation of astatine-211-parthanatine for high-risk neuroblastoma. Commun Biol 2022; 5(1):1260.

25. Riad A, Gitto SB, Lee H, et al. PARP theranostic auger emitters are cytotoxic in BRCA mutant ovarian cancer and viable tumors from ovarian cancer patients enable ex-vivo screening of tumor response. Molecules 2020;25(24). https://doi.org/10.3390/molecules25246029.

26. Wilson TC, Jannetti SA, Guru N, et al. Improved radiosynthesis of (123)I-MAPi, an auger theranostic agent. Int J Radiat Biol 2023;99(1):70–6.

27. Edmonds CE, Makvandi M, Lieberman BP, et al. [(18)F]FluorThanatrace uptake as a marker of PARP1 expression and activity in breast cancer. Am J Nucl Med Mol Imaging 2016;6(1): 94–101.

28. Makvandi M, Pantel A, Schwartz L, et al. A PET imaging agent for evaluating PARP-1 expression in ovarian cancer. J Clin Invest 2018;128(5): 2116–26.

29. Pantel AR, Gitto SB, Makvandi M, et al. [18F]FluorThanatrace ([18F]FTT) PET Imaging of PARP-inhibitor drug-target engagement as a biomarker of response in ovarian cancer, a pilot study. Clin Cancer Res 2022. https://doi.org/10.1158/1078-0432. CCR-22-1602.

30. McDonald ES, Doot RK, Pantel AR, et al. Positron emission tomography imaging of poly–(adenosine diphosphate–ribose) polymerase 1 expression in breast cancer: a nonrandomized clinical trial. JAMA Oncol 2020;6(6):921–3.

31. McDonald ES, Pantel AR, Shah PD, et al. In vivo visualization of PARP inhibitor pharmacodynamics. JCI Insight 2021;6(8).

32. Fitzgerald AA, Weiner LM. The role of fibroblast activation protein in health and malignancy. Cancer Metastasis Rev 2020;39(3):783–803.

33. Loktev A, Lindner T, Mier W, et al. A tumor-imaging method targeting cancer-associated fibroblasts. J Nucl Med 2018;59(9):1423–9.

34. Lindner T, Loktev A, Altmann A, et al. Development of quinoline-based theranostic ligands for the targeting of fibroblast activation protein. J Nucl Med 2018; 59(9):1415–22.

35. Tchou J, Zhang PJ, Bi Y, et al. Fibroblast activation protein expression by stromal cells and tumor-associated macrophages in human breast cancer. Hum Pathol 2013;44(11):2549–57.

36. Kratochwil C, Flechsig P, Lindner T, et al. 68Ga-FAPI PET/CT: tracer uptake in 28 different kinds of cancer. J Nucl Med 2019;60(6):801–5.

37. Kömek H, Can C, Güzel Y, et al. 68)Ga-FAPI-04 PET/CT, a new step in breast cancer imaging: a comparative pilot study with the (18)F-FDG PET/CT. Ann Nucl Med 2021;35(6):744–52.

38. Elboga U, Sahin E, Kus T, et al. Superiority of (68) Ga-FAPI PET/CT scan in detecting additional lesions compared to [18F]FDG PET/CT scan in breast cancer. Ann Nucl Med 2021;35(12): 1321–31.

39. Dendl K, Koerber SA, Finck R, et al. 68Ga-FAPI-PET/CT in patients with various gynecological malignancies. Eur J Nucl Med Mol Imaging 2021;48(12): 4089–100.

40. Costa A, Kieffer Y, Scholer-Dahirel A, et al. Fibroblast heterogeneity and immunosuppressive environment in human breast cancer. Cancer Cell 2018;33(3): 463–479 e10.

41. Vallejo-Armenta P, Ferro-Flores G, Santos-Cuevas C, et al. [(99m)Tc]Tc-iFAP/SPECT tumor stroma imaging: acquisition and analysis of clinical images in six different cancer entities. Pharmaceuticals 2022; 15(6). https://doi.org/10.3390/ph15060729.

42. Backhaus P, Burg MC, Roll W, et al. Simultaneous FAPI PET/MRI targeting the fibroblast-activation protein for breast cancer. Radiology 2022;302(1): 39–47.

43. Xu W, Meng T, Shang Q, et al. Uncommon metastases from occult breast cancer revealed by [18F]FDG and 68 Ga-FAPI PET/CT. Clin Nucl Med 2022;47(8): 751–3.

44. Pang Y, Zhao L, Chen H. 68Ga-FAPI Outperforms [18F]FDG PET/CT in identifying bone metastasis and peritoneal carcinomatosis in a patient with metastatic breast cancer. Clin Nucl Med 2020;45(11): 913–5.

45. Shang Q, Hao B, Xu W, et al. (68)Ga-FAPI PET/CT detected non-FDG-avid bone metastases in breast cancer. Eur J Nucl Med Mol Imaging 2022;49(6): 2096–7.

46. Characterizing Breast Cancer With 68Ga-FAPI PET/CT. Available at: https://ClinicalTrials.gov/show/NCT05574907. Accessed February 16, 2023.

47. Characterizing Breast Cancer With Al[18F]NOTA-FAPI-04 PET/CT. Available at: https://ClinicalTrials.gov/show/NCT05574920. Accessed February 16, 2023.

48. Comparison of 68Ga GaFAPI-46 PET/CT and [18F] FDG PET/CT Findings in Breast Carcinoma. Available at: https://ClinicalTrials.gov/show/NCT05339113. Accessed February 16, 2023.

49. Experimental PET Imaging Scans Before Cancer Surgery to Study the Amount of PET Tracer Accumulated in Normal and Cancer Tissues. Available at: https://ClinicalTrials.gov/show/NCT04147494. Accessed February 16, 2023.

50. Novruzov F, Mehdi E, Orucova N, et al. Head to head comparison of 68Ga-FAPI-46 PET/ CT and [18F]FDG PET/CT in breast carcinoma staging: a clinical trial update from Azerbaijan. J Nucl Med 2022; 63(supplement 2):2372.

51. Sonni I, Lee-Felker S, Memarzadeh S, et al. 68Ga-FAPi-46 diffuse bilateral breast uptake in a patient

with cervical cancer after hormonal stimulation. Eur J Nucl Med Mol Imaging 2021;48(3):924–6.

52. Wang LJ, Zhang Y, Wu HB. Intense diffuse uptake of 68Ga-FAPI-04 in the breasts found by PET/CT in a patient with advanced nasopharyngeal carcinoma. Clin Nucl Med 2021;46(5):e293–5.

53. Dendl K, Koerber SA, Adeberg S, et al. Physiological FAP-activation in a postpartum woman observed in oncological FAPI-PET/CT. Eur J Nucl Med Mol Imaging 2021;48(6):2059–61.

54. Gündoğan C, Güzel Y, Can C, et al. False-positive 68Ga-fibroblast activation protein-specific inhibitor uptake of benign lymphoid tissue in a patient with breast cancer. Clin Nucl Med 2021;46(8): e433–5.

55. Ballal S, Yadav MP, Kramer V, et al. A theranostic approach of [(68)Ga]Ga-DOTA.SA.FAPi PET/CT-guided [(177)Lu]Lu-DOTA.SA.FAPi radionuclide therapy in an end-stage breast cancer patient: new frontier in targeted radionuclide therapy. Eur J Nucl Med Mol Imaging 2021;48(3):942–4.

56. Baum RP, Schuchardt C, Singh A, et al. Feasibility, biodistribution, and preliminary dosimetry in peptide-targeted radionuclide therapy of diverse adenocarcinomas using (177)Lu-FAP-2286: first-in-humans results. J Nucl Med 2022; 63(3):415–23.

57. Rathke H, Fuxius S, Giesel FL, et al. Two tumors, one target: preliminary experience with 90Y-FAPI therapy in a patient with metastasized breast and colorectal cancer. Clin Nucl Med 2021;46(10): 842–4.

58. Can C, Gundogan C, Guzel Y, et al. 68Ga-FAPI uptake of thyroiditis in a patient with breast cancer. Clin Nucl Med 2021;46(8):683–5.

59. Chandra P, Nath S, Krishnamoorthy J, et al. Incidental detection of ischemic myocardium on (68) Ga-FAPI PET/CT. Nucl Med Mol Imaging 2021; 55(4):194–8.

60. Pantel AR, Viswanath V, Muzi M, et al. Principles of tracer kinetic analysis in oncology, part II: examples and future directions. J Nucl Med 2022;63(4): 514–21.

61. Pantel AR, Viswanath V, Muzi M, et al. Principles of tracer kinetic analysis in oncology, part I: principles and overview of methodology. J Nucl Med 2022; 63(3):342–52.

62. Bading JR, Shields AF. Imaging of cell proliferation: status and prospects. J Nucl Med 2008;49(Suppl 2): 64s–80s.

63. Muzi M, Mankoff DA, Grierson JR, et al. Kinetic modeling of 3'-deoxy-3'-fluorothymidine in somatic tumors: mathematical studies. J Nucl Med 2005; 46(2):371–80.

64. Sergeeva O, Zhang Y, Kenyon J, et al. Liver background uptake of [18F]FLT in PET imaging. Am J Nucl Med Mol Imaging 2020;10(5):212–25.

65. Been LB, Suurmeijer AJ, Cobben DC, et al. [18F]FLT-PET in oncology: current status and opportunities. Eur J Nucl Med Mol Imaging 2004;31(12):1659–72.

66. Troost EG, Vogel WV, Merkx MA, et al. 18FFLT PET does not discriminate between reactive and metastatic lymph nodes in primary head and neck cancer patients. J Nucl Med 2007;48(5): 726–35.

67. Kostakoglu L, Duan F, Idowu MO, et al. A phase II study of 3'-Deoxy-3'-18Ffluorothymidine PET in the assessment of early response of breast cancer to neoadjuvant chemotherapy: results from ACRIN 6688. J Nucl Med 2015;56(11):1681–9.

68. Muz B, de la Puente P, Azab F, et al. The role of hypoxia in cancer progression, angiogenesis, metastasis, and resistance to therapy. Hypoxia 2015;3: 83–92.

69. Rockwell S, Dobrucki IT, Kim EY, et al. Hypoxia and radiation therapy: past history, ongoing research, and future promise. Curr Mol Med 2009;9(4):442–58.

70. Godet I, Mamo M, Thurnheer A, et al. Post-hypoxic cells promote metastatic recurrence after chemotherapy treatment in TNBC. Cancers 2021;13(21). https://doi.org/10.3390/cancers13215509.

71. Asano A, Ueda S, Kuji I, et al. Intracellular hypoxia measured by [18F]-fluoromisonidazole positron emission tomography has prognostic impact in patients with estrogen receptor-positive breast cancer. Breast Cancer Res 2018;20(1):78.

72. Scigliano S, Pinel S, Poussier S, et al. Measurement of hypoxia using invasive oxygen-sensitive electrode, pimonidazole binding and [18F]FDG uptake in anaemic or erythropoietin-treated mice bearing human glioma xenografts. Int J Oncol 2008;32(1): 69–77.

73. Dubois L, Landuyt W, Haustermans K, et al. Evaluation of hypoxia in an experimental rat tumour model by [18F]fluoromisonidazole PET and immunohistochemistry. Br J Cancer 2004;91(11): 1947–54.

74. Thureau S, Piton N, Gouel P, et al. First comparison between [18F]-FMISO and [18F]-Faza for Preoperative pet imaging of hypoxia in lung cancer. Cancers 2021;13(16).

75. Bruehlmeier M, Roelcke U, Schubiger PA, et al. Assessment of hypoxia and perfusion in human brain tumors using PET with 18Ffluoromisonidazole and 15O-H2O. J Nucl Med 2004;45(11):1851–9.

76. Eschmann SM, Paulsen F, Reimold M, et al. Prognostic impact of hypoxia imaging with 18Fmisonidazole PET in non-small cell lung cancer and head and neck cancer before radiotherapy. J Nucl Med 2005;46(2):253–60.

77. Pantel AR, Mankoff DA. Molecular imaging to guide systemic cancer therapy: illustrative examples of PET imaging cancer biomarkers. Cancer Lett 2017; 387:25–31.

78. The MICAD Research Team. [^{18}F]Fluoromisonidazole. In: Molecular Imaging and Contrast Agent Database (MICAD). National Center for Biotechnology Information (US); 2004. Available at: http://www.ncbi.nlm.nih.gov/books/NBK23099/. Accessed December 12, 2022.

79. Cheng J, Lei L, Xu J, et al. ^{18}Ffluoromisonidazole PET/CT: a potential tool for predicting primary endocrine therapy resistance in breast cancer. J Nucl Med 2013;54(3):333–40.

80. López-Vega JM, Álvarez I, Antón A, et al. Early imaging and molecular changes with neoadjuvant bevacizumab in stage II/III breast cancer. Cancers 2021; 13(14). https://doi.org/10.3390/cancers13143511.

81. Couturier O, Luxen A, Chatal JF, et al. Fluorinated tracers for imaging cancer with positron emission tomography. Eur J Nucl Med Mol Imaging 2004;31(8):1182–206.

82. Manafi-Farid R, Ataeinia B, Ranjbar S, et al. Immuno-PET: antibody-based PET imaging in solid tumors. Front Med 2022;9:916693.

83. Li M, Ehlerding EB, Jiang D, et al. In vivo characterization of PD-L1 expression in breast cancer by immuno-PET with (89)Zr-labeled avelumab. Am J Transl Res 2020;12(5):1862–72.

84. Jagoda EM, Vasalatiy O, Basuli F, et al. Immuno-PET imaging of the programmed cell death-1 ligand (PD-L1) using a zirconium-89 labeled therapeutic antibody, avelumab. Mol Imaging 2019;18. https://doi.org/10.1177/1536012119829986. 1536012119829986.

85. Bensch F, van der Veen EL, Lub-de Hooge MN, et al. 89)Zr-atezolizumab imaging as a non-invasive approach to assess clinical response to PD-L1 blockade in cancer. Nat Med 2018;24(12):1852–8.

86. Mendes D, Alves C, Afonso N, et al. The benefit of HER2-targeted therapies on overall survival of patients with metastatic HER2-positive breast cancer–a systematic review. Breast Cancer Res 2015;17:140.

87. Massicano AVF, Marquez-Nostra BV, Lapi SE. Targeting HER2 in nuclear medicine for imaging and therapy. Mol Imaging 2018;17. https://doi.org/10.1177/1536012117745386. 1536012117745386.

88. Ulaner GA, Lyashchenko SK, Riedl C, et al. First-in-human human epidermal growth factor receptor 2-targeted imaging using (89)Zr-Pertuzumab PET/CT: dosimetry and clinical application in patients with breast cancer. J Nucl Med 2018;59(6):900–6.

89. Dehdashti F, Wu N, Bose R, et al. Evaluation of [(89)Zr]trastuzumab-PET/CT in differentiating HER2-positive from HER2-negative breast cancer. Breast Cancer Res Treat 2018;169(3):523–30.

90. Pichon B, Rousseau C, Blanc-Lapierre A, et al. Targeting stereotactic body radiotherapy on metabolic PET- and immuno-PET-positive vertebral metastases. Biomedicines 2020;8(12). https://doi.org/10.3390/biomedicines8120548.

91. Rousseau C, Ruellan AL, Bernardeau K, et al. Syndecan-1 antigen, a promising new target for triple-negative breast cancer immuno-PET and radioimmunotherapy. A preclinical study on MDA-MB-468 xenograft tumors. EJNMMI Res 2011;1(1):20.

AI-Enhanced PET and MR Imaging for Patients with Breast Cancer

Valeria Romeo, MD, PhD[a],*, Linda Moy, MD[b], Katja Pinker, MD, PhD[c]

KEYWORDS

• PET/MR imaging • Breast cancer • Artificial intelligence • Radiomics

KEY POINTS

• PET/MR imaging can be empowered by radiomics and artificial intelligence (AI) to meet the new needs of clinical and surgical oncology in breast cancer management.
• Preoperative and noninvasive assessment of tumor molecular profile, lymph node spread, recurrence risk, and early response to primary systemic therapy are the main goals of AI-enhanced diagnostic imaging.
• Standardization of AI methods and models' validation are the essential prerequisites for their clinical implementation.

INTRODUCTION

Breast cancer is the most frequent solid tumor affecting women worldwide.[1] Notably, although the 5-year-survival rate for patients diagnosed with stage I breast cancer approaches 100%, patients with later stage breast cancer often have a poor prognosis.[2] Hence, much effort has been expended to develop advanced strategies not only for treatment but also for early diagnosis. Some of the exciting developments in the field of breast cancer in the recent decades stem from the increased understanding of tumor biology and the emergence of targeted treatment approaches. In addition, there have been many technological developments in diagnostic imaging allowing physiological data to be obtained beyond morphological data.[3]

Such developments in diagnostic imaging involve techniques such as PET and advanced MR imaging sequences including diffusion-weighted imaging (DWI), which interrogates the microstructure; perfusion-weighted imaging, which interrogates neoangiogenesis; and magnetic resonance spectroscopy, which interrogates cancer-related metabolites.[4] Although most of these techniques are still confined to the research realm, they are promising to assess different aspects of tumor biology and several quantitative parameters derived from these techniques have been linked with tumor aggressiveness and metastatic potential. In this context, simultaneous PET/MR imaging, the newest hybrid imaging modality, has shown great promise, especially for local/distant staging and treatment monitoring.[5–7] In addition, the ability of PET/MR imaging to obtain biologically related quantitative data can be further enhanced with artificial intelligence (AI),[8] using either traditional handcrafted radiomics coupled with machine learning (ML) or deep learning (DL). The underlying principle of AI applications in medical imaging is that imaging features can be extracted from medical images that encode both simple patterns and many higher order patterns not discernible with the naked eye and that can be useful for diagnosis, prognostication, and prediction.[8–12]

[a] Department of Advanced Biomedical Sciences, University of Naples Federico II, Via S. Pansini 5, Naples 80138, Italy; [b] Department of Radiology, New York University School of Medicine, 160 East 34th Street, New York, NY 10016, USA; [c] Department of Radiology, Breast Imaging Service, Memorial Sloan Kettering Cancer Center, 300 East 66th Street, New York, NY 10065, USA
* Corresponding author.
E-mail address: valeria.romeo@unina.it

PET Clin 18 (2023) 567–575
https://doi.org/10.1016/j.cpet.2023.05.002
1556-8598/23/© 2023 Elsevier Inc. All rights reserved.

In this article, we explain how the most advanced imaging modalities used in patients with breast cancer, PET and MR imaging, can be empowered by radiomics and AI to meet the new needs of clinical and surgical oncology in breast cancer management. In the first section, we present a summary of the current trends of breast cancer management and the questions to be answered. In the second section, we present a state-of-art review on radiomics and AI applications to PET and MR imaging, addressing the questions raised in the first section.

Clinical Needs for Breast Cancer

Tissue characterization and molecular profiling
Current knowledge shows us that breast cancer is a heterogeneous disease, related to the identification of breast cancer molecular profiles with different degrees of biological aggressiveness and molecular targets, leading to different patient outcomes and prognoses.[13,14] As such, each patient represents a specific case, requiring a personalized therapeutic approach, and the preoperative knowledge of the breast cancer molecular profile is essential to establish the most appropriate treatment. Such assessment is currently performed through the analysis of a histological sample of tumor tissue obtained by a core biopsy, a procedure not free from risk that, additionally, does not provide information on the whole lesion.[15] Depending on the breast cancer molecular profile, different therapeutic approaches can be offered, with primary systemic therapy (PST) being increasingly used. In addition, the shifting of breast cancer to a different molecular subtype can occur based on tumor clonal diversity and the development of treatment-resistant clones, such that the noninvasive assessment of tumor heterogeneity through a "virtual biopsy" would be extremely advantageous.

Preoperative assessment of axillary lymph node involvement
Although the available imaging modalities have reached a high accuracy for breast cancer diagnosis, due especially to the high sensitivity of dynamic contrast-enhanced (DCE) MR imaging, the preoperative assessment of axillary lymph node involvement remains an unsolved issue. Indeed, for the latter, there is a high variability in diagnostic performance between the available imaging modalities, with ultrasound still representing the most sensitive modality (87%), even if affected by a variable specificity (53%–97%).[16] At present, sentinel lymph node biopsy (SLNB) remains the gold standard for assessing axillary lymph node involvement.[17] This issue is critical because a reassessment of treatment strategy is required when axillary lymph node involvement unrecognized at imaging is found after SLNB, especially for patients who could have benefited from PST. On the other side, a more conservative axillary surgical approach is preferred in selected cases, in the context of deescalation treatment, to avoid side effects related to axillary node dissection, such as arm lymphedema.[18,19] According to current guidelines, axillary node dissection can be avoided not only in patients with negative lymph node after SLNB but also after PST in clinically node-positive patients presenting as cN0 after treatment and in patients with fewer than 3 positive axillary lymph nodes at SLNB who are receiving breast/axillary radiation.[18,20]

Primary Systemic Therapy

Recurrence risk assessment and early prediction of response
In locally advanced breast cancer, PST can make surgery feasible in nonoperable cases as well as allow a more conservative surgical approach. Furthermore, with PST, the in vivo assessment of response is still possible, allowing the possibility to change/stop treatment in nonresponder cases, with a tangible impact on patient outcome and prognosis.[21] As such, even considering the new trends on deescalation surgery,[22] PST is still increasingly recommended even in operable but selected cases.[23] Indeed, PST-related issues must be considered, such as systemic/cardiac toxicity, psychological implications, and the possible occurrence of tumor progression related to chemotherapy-induced changes of the breast cancer molecular profile.[24–26] Therefore, a careful assessment of PST clinical indications is mandatory. So far, PST is highly recommended in specific breast cancer subtypes such as human epidermal growth factor receptor 2 (HER2+) breast cancer, in combination with targeted drugs, and triple-negative breast cancer, for which no targeted approaches are currently available.[23] For luminal subtypes, hormone treatment is indicated in luminal A breast cancer, whereas the usefulness of PST in luminal B breast cancer is still debated. At present, patients with luminal B breast cancer are referred to PST in locally advanced, nonoperable cases (eg, with axillary lymph node involvement or T4 stages) or to multigene tests (eg, Oncotype DX, Mammaprint, PAM50) on tumor sample after surgical excision to assess the risk of tumor recurrence and therefore the cost/effectiveness of an adjuvant systemic treatment.[22,23] Similarly, since functional response to treatment seems to precede morphological changes, the

possibility for early prediction of the response to PST based on multiparametric/multimodal quantitative imaging obtained preoperatively or during early imaging assessment through AI-enhanced analysis could further stratify and select patients for whom the cost–benefit ratio is advantageous. A summary of clinical and surgical needs is illustrated in **Fig. 1**.

Clinical Needs Addressed from the "Artificial Intelligence Perspective"

Artificial intelligence basics concepts: machine and deep learning

The rationale behind AI is that, if properly instructed, computers can learn to analyze a multitude of data to make predictions and improve their performance with the experience. Two different approaches can be used for this purpose: traditional radiomics and ML, and DL.

Traditional radiomics and ML extracts quantitative imaging features that are used to identify a phenotypical fingerprint or "radiomics signature." The cancer is annotated by expert readers or automated software reflecting the distribution of pixels at different complexity levels. The radiomics pipeline for ML studies is usually made of different steps, including image preprocessing, segmentation, radiomics features extraction and selection, and running of the ML algorithms.[27]

DL uses a complex network inspired by the human brain architecture to devise its own features. Currently, in medical image analysis, DL algorithms use convolutional neural networks, which comprise multiple layers of processing designed to optimize millions of variables, the so-called weights and biases, to extract hierarchical patterns, to retain the most important information and use them for classification.[10,28] The majority of DL models utilize a supervised learning approach in which training is done using a multitude of labeled examples that can be on different levels (examination, breast, pixel). Although big datasets are not necessarily required by ML systems, they are essential for DL studies, which must learn features from the data. Consequently, high computational time and costs are required for running DL software, depending on the architecture and the size of the dataset. An advantage of DL over ML is that it can process a huge amount of data but is considered a "black box." Once a model is developed, an essential condition is that results obtained in a "training" population have to be validated preferentially in an external "test" set, that is, from a different institution. Simplified ML and DL pipelines are illustrated in **Fig. 2**.

Tissue characterization and molecular profiling

Although breast MR imaging has a high sensitivity for breast cancer detection, the possibility to use AI to noninvasively discriminate benign from malignant breast lesions, and in addition to determine the molecular profile of breast cancer, is attractive and has been recently explored using different imaging modalities. In highly suspicious breast lesions (eg, breast imaging reporting and data system [BI-RADS] 4 and 5), a combined MR imaging and PET approach could be of value to provide tumor diagnosis, profiling, and staging at the same time. Therefore, initial experience was recently published on the use of ML for breast cancer diagnosis and phenotyping using simultaneously acquired PET and MR imaging images.

In 2018, an unsupervised clustering based on PET and MR imaging radiomics features was performed by Huang and colleagues, extracting a

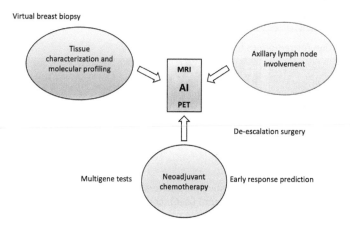

Fig. 1. Clinical areas of interest for AI applications in breast cancer, represented by tumor *characterization/molecular profiling*, which, along with the preoperative assessment of *axillary lymph node involvement* and multigene tests, helps in defining clinical indications for *neoadjuvant chemotherapy*. An accurate definition of axillary status, in terms of the number of involved lymph nodes, and neoadjuvant chemotherapy allow for a more conservative surgical approach, the so called "deescalation" treatment. One of the most promising and fascinating clinical applications of PET/MR imaging functional imaging coupled with AI is also the early prediction of the response to neoadjuvant chemotherapy, which would help in further selecting the ideal candidates among patients with breast cancer.

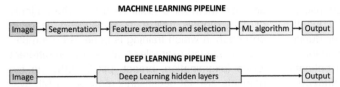

MACHINE LEARNING PIPELINE

Image → Segmentation → Feature extraction and selection → ML algorithm → Output

DEEP LEARNING PIPELINE

Image → Deep Learning hidden layers → Output

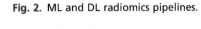

Fig. 2. ML and DL radiomics pipelines.

total of 84 radiomics features of 113 patients. Three groups were identified, significantly associated with tumor grade, stage, breast cancer subtypes, and disease recurrence status. This preliminary experience suggested that both MR imaging and PET could be able to decipher breast cancer biological behavior while providing imaging biomarkers predictive of tumor recurrence.[29] In a further investigation, an ML-based model for breast cancer diagnosis using a combination of radiomic features, quantitative MR imaging diffusion and perfusion parameters, and PET parameters was proposed. The integrated model combining mean transit time and mean apparent diffusion coefficient (ADCmean) with radiomic features extracted from PET and ADC images obtained an area under the curve (AUC) of 0.983.[30]

The same group also developed a method for breast cancer phenotyping to discriminate triple negative from other breast cancer subtypes. After the calculation of quantitative parameters and

radiomic features from PET and MR images (**Fig. 3**), different combinations of such data were explored. The best performing ML method used radiomic features extracted from ADC and PET images and obtained an AUC, sensitivity, and specificity of 0.887, 79.7%, and 86%, respectively.[31]

Similarly, Umutlu and colleagues developed different ML models for breast cancer characterization, in terms of molecular subtype (luminal A vs luminal B, luminal A vs others), ER/PgR status, HER2 expression, Ki67 levels, and tumor grade, using combination of MR imaging and/or PET features. As a result, the AUC of the developed models ranged from 0.771 (tumor grade prediction model, based on PET features) to 0.97 (Ki67 levels prediction model, based on MR imaging and PET features).[32]

Overall, the combined use of MR imaging and PET could provide morphological tumor information along with functional and histological data, thus representing a "one-stop-shop" tool for a

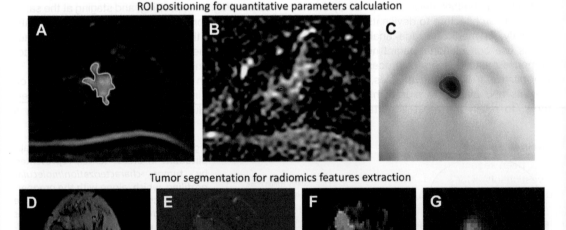

ROI positioning for quantitative parameters calculation

Tumor segmentation for radiomics features extraction

Fig. 3. Examples of 2D ROI placement for the extraction of quantitative parameters (mean transit time; plasma flow; volume distribution; ADC mean; and SUVmax, mean, and minimum) (*A–C*), and whole tumor segmentation for radiomics features (first, second, and higher order) extraction (*D–G*) from primary breast cancer tumor lesions on DCE (*A, E*), DWI (*B, F*), PET (*C, G*), and T2-weighted (*D*) images. (*From* Romeo V, Kapetas P, Clauser P, et al. A Simultaneous Multiparametric 18F-FDG PET/MRI Radiomics Model for the Diagnosis of Triple Negative Breast Cancer. *Cancers (Basel)*. 2022;14(16):3944. Published 2022 Aug 16.)

comprehensive breast cancer diagnosis and staging. Such an approach would have a significant implication for patients' management. Indeed, the performance of a "virtual biopsy" would dramatically reduce patients' discomfort as well as allow a comprehensive assessment of whole-lesion heterogeneity and the monitoring of tumor feature changes during PST, to assess for tumor resistance and progression.

Preoperative assessment of axillary lymph node involvement

At present, little evidence is available on the use of ML/DL applied to PET and MR imaging for the preoperative evaluation of axillary lymph node status. The rationale of current investigations is that axillary dissemination of breast cancer cells strongly depends on primary lesion heterogeneity, such that the majority of AI analyses are conducted to extract radiomic features from primary breast cancer lesions. In this task, preliminary investigations report a good performance of ML algorithms using radiomic feature extracted from breast cancer lesions on MR imaging and PET images in the prediction of axillary status (positive vs negative), with an AUC, sensitivity, and specificity of 0.810, 63.8%, and 82.2%, respectively.[32]

Besides preliminary studies exploring the potential of both MR imaging and PET for the assessment of axillary lymph node status, several investigations have been published during the past years to assess the individual contribution of these modalities. Regarding MR imaging, a recent systematic review and meta-analysis by Zhang and colleagues, including 13 studies on the use of ML applied to DCE MR imaging images for the prediction of axillary lymph node metastasis in 1618 patients, reported a pooled sensitivity, specificity, diagnostic odds ratio, and AUC of 0.82, 0.83, 21.56, and 0.89, respectively.[33] Studies on the use of ML applied to PET have also been recently conducted. In an interesting investigation, Chen and colleagues aimed to develop and validate an ML model applied to ^{18}F-fluorodeoxyglucose positron emission tomography/computed tomography (^{18}F-FDG PET/CT) for the prediction of clinically occult axillary lymph node metastasis (cN0) in 180 patients.[34] Different ML algorithms were used, with random forest resulting as the best performing one, showing a mean AUC of 0.817, and a mean accuracy of 81.2%.

The possibility to combine PET with additional clinical and imaging data has also been explored by Cheng and colleagues, who developed different ML model, including clinical (physical examination), histological (ER status), imaging

(ultrasound and PET) and radiomics data.[35] In the validation set, the combined model, made of 6 clinicopathologic factors and 5 radiomic features extracted from dedicated PET, yielded the highest diagnostic performance (AUC = 0.93, sensitivity = 92.11, specificity = 83.67, accuracy = 87.36). ML has also been recently used to combine clinically assessable features on MR imaging and PET and possibly compare/overcome the performance of expert radiologists.[36] A total of 303 PET/MR imaging examinations were collected from 3 different institutions. The authors found no difference between the performance of ML and radiologists in assessing the presence of axillary lymph node metastases, with a diagnostic accuracy of 91.2% and 89.3%, respectively. When using MR imaging alone, the accuracy was 87.5% for both ML and radiologists, showing no significant difference with that of PET/MR imaging. Among PET/MR imaging features, the most relevant were FDG uptake and lymph node size. With an adjusted threshold, a decision tree was built, which could help in reducing the number of invasive procedures, such as sentinel lymph node biopsy, in 68.2% of cases.

With all these premises, it seems that information provided by histology, clinical examination, conventional, and radiomic image features of different imaging modalities could allow an accurate, noninvasive, detection of axillary lymph node metastasis in breast cancer. On this basis, ML is promising as an effective tool for the elaboration of these complex data, supporting clinicians in their clinical practice as a potential clinical decision-making instrument. Because surgical treatment changes according to the number of affected axillary lymph nodes, a significant improvement could be to preoperatively predict the involvement of more than 2 axillary lymph nodes, in a way that patients could be directly addressed to axillary lymph node dissection.

Primary Systemic Therapy

Recurrence risk assessment

New genomic tests are currently available to assess the recurrence risk in patients with breast cancer and therefore to identify those who would benefit from systemic treatment, especially in hormone receptor-positive subtypes. Although these tests are currently performed on postoperative surgical specimens, the prediction of recurrence score from pretreatment imaging examinations would be advantageous, allowing high-risk patients to undergo the systemic treatment in a neoadjuvant setting, with all the related, previously discussed benefits. Among these tests, Oncotype

DX score is one of the most widely used. Indeed, several investigations have been carried out for its early prediction, using semantic MR imaging features and multivariate models.[37,38] ML techniques have been recently used for this purpose along with clinical variables and multiparametric radiomics, obtaining an AUC of 0.89 in discriminating between low and intermediate/high-risk groups.[39] In a recently published article, ML was applied to MR imaging alone for the noninvasive prediction of Oncotype DX score.[40] Despite the use of a limited sample size (248 patients from a publicly available dataset), encouraging findings are reported (accuracy in the test set = 63 and AUC of 0.66), suggesting a possible role of this modality for recurrence prediction. DL systems were also used for discriminating between patients at low and intermediate/high risk of breast cancer recurrence, with an overall accuracy of 84%.[41] Still, more evidence is needed to fully explore the potential of AI as a clinical decision-making tool for breast cancer recurrence risk assessment.

Early prediction of the response to primary systemic therapy

The possibility for early prediction of response to PST using cytotoxic chemotherapy in breast cancer has extensively been investigated. In this task, radiomics is one of the most promising tools because of its ability to describe imaging heterogeneity patterns invisible to human assessment, and before any morphological changes can be appreciated. Among the available imaging modalities, MR imaging and PET are the best candidates because both examinations capture functional, quantitative data related to tumor neoangiogenesis (DCE-MR imaging), cellularity (DWI), and metabolism (PET).

Specifically, neoadjuvant chemotherapy acts at the level of tumor cell density, due to its cytotoxic effect that increases the extravascular/extracellular space and that reduces tumor vascularization and permeability. In addition, the antiangiogenetic effect of neoadjuvant chemotherapy affects tumor metabolism, which also tends to decrease early in patients who respond to PST. As a result, several studies have assessed the usefulness of quantitative parameters reflecting such functional changes as well as radiomic features for the detection of early PST-related changes. Consequently, systematic reviews and meta-analyses are now available to summarize the current evidence on this matter.

In a recent article by O'Donnell and colleagues, different breast MR imaging radiomics methods were analyzed and compared using a network meta-analysis, including quantitative functional parameters, radiomic features, and different time points of MR imaging examinations (before, during, and after PST).[42] The authors demonstrated that radiomic features performed better than quantitative parameters, and during PST and post-PST were the best time points for the prediction of the response. Another systematic review and meta-analysis, which included 34 studies on MR imaging radiomics, showed a pooled AUC of 0.78 (95% CI: 0.74–0.81) for the prediction of pathological complete response to PST. However, the authors also found substantial heterogeneity in the included studies.[43]

The role of ^{18}F-FDG PET/CT for the prediction of response to PST has also been widely explored. In a recent systematic review, the promise of PET-derived radiomic features was reported, with possible improvements when clinical features were also included in the model.[44] In a retrospective study by Li and colleagues, 100 ^{18}F-FDG PET/CT examinations were collected and used for the extraction of 2210 PET-derived radiomics features.[45] The random forest ML classifier was used and obtained a prediction accuracy of 0.857 (AUC = 0.844) on the training set and 0.767 (AUC = 0.722) on the test set. When patient age was also included in the model, the accuracy of the predictive model increased to 0.857 (AUC = 0.958) and 0.8 (AUC = 0.73) in the training and test set, respectively.

More recently, studies combining clinical imaging data and/or radiomic features obtained from both PET and MR imaging images were conducted, using either ML or DL approaches. In a first experience, Choi and colleagues investigated the ability of DL applied to ^{18}F-FDG PET/CT and MR images for the prediction of pathological complete response after PST in 56 patients, comparing its performance with that of conventional quantitative data obtained from pretreatment and interim (after the first PST cycle) PET and DWI examinations (**Fig. 4**).[46] Among the quantitative data, early variation in the standard uptake value (SUV) showed the highest AUC of 0.805 (95% CI: 0.677–0.899). Of note, the accuracy of PET data improved after the application of DL (from 0.687 to 0.980) but this did not occur for DWI data. A first experience of ML applied to pretreatment simultaneous ^{18}F-FDG PET/MR imaging for the prediction of the response has been recently reported by Umutlu and colleagues. A total of 73 ^{18}F-FDG PET/MR imaging examinations were retrospectively collected and analyzed for the extraction of 101 radiomics features.[47] The support vector machine algorithm was used, with a 5-fold cross validation, obtaining the highest accuracy, sensitivity, and specificity

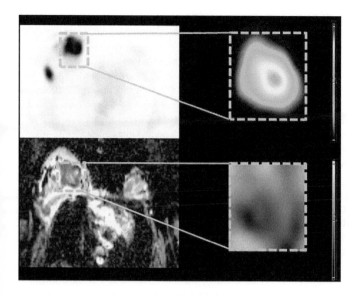

Fig. 4. Image cropping for DL technique. The cubic shaped region-of-interest was selected at the largest cross-sectional area of the lesion and resized to 64 × 64 pixels. FDG and ADC images were obtained from PET/CT and MR imaging scans, respectively. Baseline images were defined as PET0 and ADC0, respectively, and interim images were defined as PET1 and ADC1, respectively. (*From* Choi JH, Kim HA, Kim W, et al. Early prediction of neoadjuvant chemotherapy response for advanced breast cancer using PET/MRI image deep learning. *Sci Rep.* 2020;10(1):21149. Published 2020 Dec 3.)

(0.8, 81%, and 73.8%, respectively) when radiomic features from both ^{18}F-FDG PET and MR imaging were combined. In a subgroup analysis according to the different breast cancer molecular subtypes, the best performance (AUC = 0.94) was observed in HR+/HER2− group.

Based on the available evidence, the use of AI techniques could enable the early prediction of the response to PST even on pretreatment PET/MR imaging examinations, whereas interim examinations seem to be the most effective for a "clinical assessment," performed on the early variation of quantitative, mainly PET, parameters.

All that glitters is not gold: the dark shadows of artificial intelligence

Preliminary evidence suggests a possible expanding role of AI to provide radiologists and clinicians with information that is not readily available from conventional images, such as molecular expression, response to treatment, and prognosis. However, there are still no robust data to suggest its imminent use in clinical practice. Indeed, as several studies highlighted, there is a huge heterogeneity in the applied AI methods, to the extent that guidelines and recommendations have been released in a bid to standardize image acquisition, processing, and analysis.[27,48,49] The need to assess the generalizability and robustness of the developed algorithms through external validation has also been pointed out. Once these methodological issues will be solved, the discussion of medico-legal implications of the clinical use of AI software is necessary for clinical adaption of radiomic tools. Indeed, clinicians may be responsible for decisions they did not make or the AI system

may have a higher diagnostic accuracy than radiologists.[50]

SUMMARY

AI-empowered PET and MR imaging will play a central role in the assessment of patients with breast cancer. The ideal clinical scenario would be the "one-stop-shop" protocol to become a reality while providing a set of comprehensive information from diagnosis to clinical management. It should be considered that other breast imaging modalities, such as ultrasound and mammography, will remain the backbone of breast imaging, especially considering their lower costs compared with MR imaging and PET. However, in the oncologic setting, whole-body imaging modalities such as PET are preferred for their ability to detect distant metastasis, and MR imaging is the imaging modality with the highest sensitivity for the detection of breast cancer. Furthermore, both techniques represent an objective tool for tumor staging, treatment monitoring, and response assessment. Regarding functional and biological information that can be obtained through AI application, each modality seems most promising in a specific task. Indeed, while MR imaging has extensively been applied for breast cancer molecular subtyping and assessment of axillary lymph node involvement, PET shows high sensitivity in the early prediction of the response to PST, both using either pretreatment PET-derived features or the early variation of quantitative metabolic parameters at interim examinations. Additionally, several investigations demonstrated a significant improvement in the prediction task when clinical data are also added to the model. This combination of clinical and imaging data supports the idea that a comprehensive information package, including PET, MR imaging, and clinical information may further empower the performance of AI systems. However, a great deal remains to be done, in terms of standardization procedures and models validation. A major obstacle is also represented by the limited availability of hybrid PET/MR imaging scanners and their high related costs. Actions are being taken to overcome these issues, while providing recommendations and building public datasets. In conclusion, AI studies on PET/MR imaging systems in the breast cancer field are strongly encouraged, particularly in a multicenter setting, in an attempt to increase the robustness of the developed models and the standardization of MR imaging and PET imaging biomarkers.

CLINICS CARE POINTS

- Non-invasive tissue characterization, assessment of lymph nodes involvement and prediction of response to primary systemic therapy are the major clinical needs for breast cancer treatment.
- AI-empowered PET and MRI can significantly contribute to pre-operatively and non-invasively manage breast cancer patients.
- Huge efforts are still needed to fully address the role of AI applied to imaging techniques and traslate its use into clinical practice.

DISCLOSURE

The authors have nothing to disclose.

REFERENCES

1. Bray F, Ferlay J, Soerjomataram I, et al. Global cancer statistics 2018: GLOBOCAN estimates of incidence and mortality worldwide for 36 cancers in 185 countries. Cancer J. Clin 2018. https://doi.org/10.3322/caac.21492.
2. Kalli S, Semine A, Cohen S, et al, American Joint committee on cancer's staging system for breast cancer. What the Radiologist Needs to Know. Radiographics 2018;38:1921–33.
3. Padhani AR, Miles KA. Multiparametric imaging of tumor response to therapy. Radiology 2010. https://doi.org/10.1148/radiol.10091760.
4. García-Figueiras R, Baleato-González S, Padhani AR, et al. How clinical imaging can assess cancer biology. Insights Imaging 2019;10:28.
5. Bruckmann NM, Morawitz J, Fendler WP, et al. A role of PET/MR in breast cancer? Semin Nucl Med 2022; 52:611–8.
6. Romeo V, Helbich TH, Pinker K. Breast PETMRI hybrid imaging and targeted tracers. J. Magn. Reson. Imaging 2022. https://doi.org/10.1002/jmri.28431.
7. Fowler AM, Strigel RM. Clinical advances in PET–MRI for breast cancer. Lancet Oncol 2022;23:e32–43.
8. Gillies RJ, Kinahan PE, Hricak H. Radiomics: images are more than pictures. They Are Data, Radiology 2016;278:563–77.
9. Shah SM, Khan RA, Arif S, et al. Artificial intelligence for breast cancer analysis: trends and directions. Comput Biol Med 2022;142:105221.
10. Reig B, Heacock L, Geras KJ, et al. Machine learning in breast MRI. J. Magn. Reson. Imaging 2020;52:998–1018.
11. Lo Gullo R, Daimiel I, Morris EA, et al. Combining molecular and imaging metrics in cancer: radiogenomics. Insights Imaging 2020;11:1.
12. Kohli M, Prevedello LM, Filice RW, et al. Implementing machine learning in radiology practice and research. Am J Roentgenol 2017. https://doi.org/10.2214/AJR.16.17224.
13. Polyak K. Heterogeneity in breast cancer. J Clin Invest 2011;121:3786–8.
14. Cleator S, Ashworth A. Molecular profiling of breast cancer: clinical implications. Br J Cancer 2004;90:1120–4.
15. Helbich TH, Matzek W, Fuchsjger MH. Stereotactic and ultrasound-guided breast biopsy. Eur Radiol 2004;14:383–93.
16. Marino MA, Avendano D, Zapata P, et al. Lymph node imaging in patients with primary breast cancer: concurrent diagnostic tools. Oncol 2020. https://doi.org/10.1634/theoncologist.2019-0427.
17. Thompson JL, Wright GP. Contemporary approaches to the axilla in breast cancer. Am J Surg 2022. https://doi.org/10.1016/j.amjsurg.2022.11.036.
18. Noguchi M, Inokuchi M, Yokoi-Noguchi M, et al. Conservative axillary surgery is emerging in the surgical management of breast cancer. Breast Cancer 2023;30:14–22.
19. Angarita FA, Brumer R, Castelo M, et al. De-escalating the management of in situ and invasive breast cancer. Cancers 2022;14:4545.
20. Lyman GH, Temin S, Edge SB, et al. Sentinel lymph node biopsy for patients with early-stage breast cancer: American society of clinical oncology clinical practice guideline update. J Clin Oncol 2014;32:1365–83.
21. Romeo V, Accardo G, Perillo T, et al. Assessment and prediction of response to neoadjuvant chemotherapy in breast cancer: a comparison of imaging modalities and future perspectives. Cancers 2021;13:3521.
22. Varsanik MA, Shubeck SP. De-escalating breast cancer therapy. Surg. Clin. North Am 2023;103:83–92.

23. Spring LM, Bar Y, Isakoff SJ. The evolving role of neoadjuvant therapy for operable breast cancer. J Natl Compr Cancer Netw 2022;20:723–34.

24. De La Cruz LM, Harhay MO, Zhang P, et al. Impact of neoadjuvant chemotherapy on breast cancer subtype: does subtype change and, if so, how? Ann Surg Oncol 2018;25:3535–40.

25. Kittaneh M, Montero AJ, Glück S. Molecular profiling for breast cancer: a comprehensive review. Biomark Cancer 2013;5:BIC.S9455.

26. Goncalves R, Bose R. Using multigene tests to select treatment for early-stage breast cancer. J Natl Compr Cancer Netw 2013;11:174–82.

27. Stanzione A, Cuocolo R, Ugga L, et al. Oncologic imaging and radiomics: a walkthrough review of methodological challenges. Cancers 2022;14:4871.

28. Afshar P, Mohammadi A, Plataniotis KN, et al. From handcrafted to deep-learning-based cancer radiomics: challenges and opportunities. IEEE Signal Process Mag 2019;36:132–60.

29. Huang S, Franc BL, Harnish RJ, et al. Exploration of PET and MRI radiomic features for decoding breast cancer phenotypes and prognosis. Npj Breast Cancer 2018;4:24.

30. Romeo V, Clauser P, Rasul S, et al. AI-enhanced simultaneous multiparametric 18F-FDG PET/MRI for accurate breast cancer diagnosis. Eur. J. Nucl. Med. Mol. Imaging 2022;49:596–608.

31. Romeo V, Kapetas P, Clauser P, et al. A simultaneous multiparametric 18F-FDG PET/MRI radiomics model for the diagnosis of triple negative breast cancer. Cancers 2022;14:3944.

32. Umutlu L, Kirchner J, Bruckmann NM, et al. Multiparametric integrated 18F-FDG PET/MRI-Based radiomics for breast cancer phenotyping and tumor decoding. Cancers 2021;13:2928.

33. Zhang J, Li L, Zhe X, et al. The diagnostic performance of machine learning-based radiomics of DCE-MRI in predicting axillary lymph node metastasis in breast cancer: a meta-analysis. Front Oncol 2022;12:1–10.

34. Chen K, Yin G, Xu W. Predictive value of 18F-FDG PET/CT-Based radiomics model for occult axillary lymph node metastasis in clinically node-negative breast cancer. Diagnostics 2022;12:997.

35. Cheng J, Ren C, Liu G, et al. Development of high-resolution dedicated PET-based radiomics machine learning model to predict axillary lymph node status in early-stage breast cancer. Cancers 2022;14:950.

36. Morawitz J, Sigl B, Rubbert C, et al. Clinical decision support for axillary lymph node staging in newly diagnosed breast cancer patients based on 18 F-FDG PET/MRI and machine-learning. J Nucl Med 2022. https://doi.org/10.2967/jnumed.122.264138.

37. Saha A, Harowicz MR, Wang W, et al. A study of association of Oncotype DX recurrence score with DCE-MRI characteristics using multivariate machine learning models. J Cancer Res Clin Oncol 2018. https://doi.org/10.1007/s00432-018-2595-7.

38. Kim HJ, Choi WJ, Kim HH, et al. Association between Oncotype DX recurrence score and dynamic contrast-enhanced MRI features in patients with estrogen receptor-positive HER2-negative invasive breast cancer. Clin. Imaging 2021;75:131–7.

39. Jacobs MA, Umbricht CB, Parekh VS, et al. Integrated multiparametric radiomics and informatics system for characterizing breast tumor characteristics with the OncotypeDX gene assay. Cancers 2020;12:2772.

40. Romeo V, Cuocolo R, Sanduzzi L, et al. MRI radiomics and machine learning for the prediction of Oncotype dx recurrence score in invasive breast cancer. Cancers 2023;15:1840.

41. Ha R, Chang P, Mutasa S, et al. Convolutional neural network using a breast MRI tumor dataset can predict Oncotype dx recurrence score. J. Magn. Reson. Imaging 2019;49:518–24.

42. O'Donnell JPM, Gasior SA, Davey MG, et al. The accuracy of breast MRI radiomic methodologies in predicting pathological complete response to neoadjuvant chemotherapy: a systematic review and network meta-analysis. Eur J Radiol 2022;157:110561.

43. Pesapane F, Agazzi GM, Rotili A, et al. Prediction of the pathological response to neoadjuvant chemotherapy in breast cancer patients with MRI-radiomics: a systematic review and meta-analysis. Curr Probl Cancer 2022;46:100883.

44. Sollini M, Cozzi L, Ninatti G, et al. PET/CT radiomics in breast cancer: mind the step. Methods 2020. https://doi.org/10.1016/j.ymeth.2020.01.007.

45. Li P, Wang X, Xu C, et al. 18F-FDG PET/CT radiomic predictors of pathologic complete response (pCR) to neoadjuvant chemotherapy in breast cancer patients. Eur. J. Nucl. Med. Mol. Imaging 2020. https://doi.org/10.1007/s00259-020-04684-3.

46. Choi JH, Kim H-A, Kim W, et al. Early prediction of neoadjuvant chemotherapy response for advanced breast cancer using PET/MRI image deep learning. Sci Rep 2020;10:21149.

47. Umutlu L, Kirchner J, Bruckmann N-M, et al. Multiparametric 18F-FDG PET/MRI-Based radiomics for prediction of pathological complete response to neoadjuvant chemotherapy in breast cancer. Cancers 2022;14:1727.

48. Mongan J, Moy L, Kahn CE. Checklist for artificial intelligence in medical imaging (CLAIM): a guide for authors and reviewers. Radiol Artif Intell 2020;2: e200029.

49. Lambin P, Leijenaar RTH, Deist TM, et al. Radiomics: the bridge between medical imaging and personalized medicine. Nat Rev Clin Oncol 2017;14:749–62.

50. Carter SM, Rogers W, Than K, et al. The ethical , legal and social implications of using arti fi cial intelligence systems in breast cancer care. Breast 2020; 49:25–32.

Moving?

Make sure your subscription moves with you!

To notify us of your new address, find your **Clinics Account Number** (located on your mailing label above your name), and contact customer service at:

Email: journalscustomerservice-usa@elsevier.com

800-654-2452 (subscribers in the U.S. & Canada)
314-447-8871 (subscribers outside of the U.S. & Canada)

Fax number: 314-447-8029

Elsevier Health Sciences Division
Subscription Customer Service
3251 Riverport Lane
Maryland Heights, MO 63043

*To ensure uninterrupted delivery of your subscription, please notify us at least 4 weeks in advance of move.

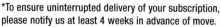

Printed and bound by CPI Group (UK) Ltd, Croydon, CR0 4YY

03/10/2024

01040363-0012